Clinical Imaging Physics

Clinical Imaging Physics

Current and Emerging Practice

Edited by

Ehsan Samei, PhD
Departments of Radiology,
Medical Physics, Physics,
Biomedical Engineering, and
Electrical and Computer Engineering
Duke University Medical Center
Durham, NC, USA

Douglas E. Pfeiffer, MS
Boulder Community Health
Boulder, CO, USA

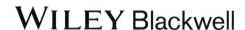

Registered Office(s)
John Wiley & Sons, Inc., 111 River Street, Hoboken, NJ 07030, USA
John Wiley & Sons Ltd, The Atrium, Southern Gate, Chichester, West Sussex, PO19 8SQ, UK

Editorial Office
9600 Garsington Road, Oxford, OX4 2DQ, UK

For details of our global editorial offices, customer services, and more information about Wiley products visit us at www.wiley.com.

Wiley also publishes its books in a variety of electronic formats and by print-on-demand. Some content that appears in standard print versions of this book may not be available in other formats.

Library of Congress Cataloging-in-Publication Data

Names: Samei, Ehsan, editor. | Pfeiffer, Douglas E., editor.
Title: Clinical imaging physics : current and emerging practice / edited by
    Ehsan Samei, Douglas E. Pfeiffer.
Description: Hoboken, NJ : Wiley-Blackwell, 2020. | Includes
    bibliographical references and index.
Identifiers: LCCN 2020001250 (print) | LCCN 2020001251 (ebook) |
    ISBN 9781118753453 (hardback) | ISBN 9781118753606 (adobe pdf) |
    ISBN 9781118753545 (epub)
Subjects: MESH: Diagnostic Imaging–methods | Biophysical Phenomena
Classification: LCC RC78.7.D53 (print) | LCC RC78.7.D53 (ebook) | NLM WN
    180 | DDC 616.07/54–dc23
LC record available at https://lccn.loc.gov/2020001250
LC ebook record available at https://lccn.loc.gov/2020001251

Cover Design: Wiley
Cover Image: © Ehsan Samei, 2020

Set in 9.5/12.5pt STIXTwoText by SPi Global, Pondicherry, India
Printed and bound in Singapore by Markono Print Media Pte Ltd

10 9 8 7 6 5 4 3 2 1

To my parents, Parvaneh Lotfi and Mohammad Ali Samei
Who gave much and loved much
And Whose legacy of loving beauty and caring selflessly continues to inspire.

Ehsan Samei

To my wife, Fionnuala Dundon
Whose victory against cancer made what we do very real.

Douglas E. Pfeiffer

Contents

List of Contributors

Eric Berns, PhD
Radiological Sciences
University of Colorado
Aurora, CO
USA

Paul Carson, PhD
Department of Radiology
University of Michigan
Ann Arbor, MI
USA

Michael Flynn, PhD
Diagnostic Radiology
Henry Ford Health System
Henry Ford Hospital
Detroit, MI
USA

David Gauntt, PhD
Department of Radiology
University of Alabama at Birmingham
Birmingham, AL
USA

Nicholas J. Hangiandreou, PhD
Department of Radiology
Mayo Clinic Rochester
Rochester, MN
USA

Andrew Karellas, PhD
Department of Medical Imaging
College of Medicine
University of Arizona
Tucson, AZ
USA

Zheng Feng Lu, PhD
Department of Radiology
University of Chicago
Chicago, IL
USA

Mahadevappa Mahesh, PhD
The Russell H. Morgan Department of
Radiology and Radiological Science
Johns Hopkins University
Baltimore, MD
USA

Steven Mann, PhD
Clinical Imaging Physics Group
Duke University
Durham, NC
USA

Melissa Martin, MS
Therapy Physics, Inc.
Signal Hill, CA
USA

Jeffrey Nelson, MHP
Clinical Imaging Physics Group
Duke University
Durham, NC
USA

Donald Peck, PhD
Department of Radiology
Michigan Technological University
Henry Ford Health System
Houghton, MI
USA

Douglas E. Pfeiffer, MS
Boulder Community Health
Boulder, CO
USA

David Pickens, PhD
Department of Radiology
Vanderbilt University
Nashville, TN
USA

Ronald Price, PhD
Department of Radiology
Vanderbilt University
Nashville, TN
USA

Ehsan Samei, PhD
Departments of Radiology,
Medical Physics, Physics,
Biomedical Engineering, and
Electrical and Computer Engineering
Duke University Medical Center
Durham, NC
USA

Beth A. Schueler, PhD
Department of Radiology
Mayo Clinic Rochester
Rochester, MN
USA

Keith J. Strauss, MS
Department of Radiology and Medical Imaging
Children's Hospital Medical Center
Cincinnati, OH
USA

Srinivasan Vedantham, PhD
Department of Medical Imaging
College of Medicine
University of Arizona
Tucson, AZ
USA

Jered Wells, PhD
Clinical Imaging Physics Group
Duke University
Durham, NC
USA

Joshua Wilson, PhD
Clinical Imaging Physics Group
Duke University
Durham, NC
USA

Introduction

Medical imaging is a cornerstone of healthcare. A technology that was initially grown from a physics experiment, medical imaging has been developed and advanced over decades by medical physicists who have played central roles in the development and the practice of the discipline. In a period of just over a century, medical physics has brought rapid growth and continuous innovation to the presence of imaging in medicine. While innovative technologies have offered enhanced opportunities for high-quality imaging care, optimized and evidence-based use of these advanced technologies cannot be assumed. Thus, clinically, physicists have also played key roles in ensuring compliance with the quality and safety standards that they themselves fostered. However, this clinical role has not kept up with the advancement of the technologies. In the midst of diverse imaging options, and in the current drive towards consistent, patient-centered, and safe practice of medical imaging, there is need for a renewed presence of medical physics in clinical practice in order to enable and ensure optimized, quantitative, and safe use of the imaging technologies. In doing so, medical physics can move beyond the current compliance and safety testing towards intentionally-targeted, evidence-based use of the technology to serve clinical care.

Clinical Imaging Physics: Current and Emerging Practice aims to serve as a reference for the application of medical physics in clinical medical imaging. The "clinical" aspect is the primary focus of the book. The book aims to not only provide a single reference for the existing practice of medical physics (what we call Medical Physics 1.0), but also to address the growing need to establish an updated approach to clinical medical imaging physics (so called Medical Physics 3.0) in light of new realities in healthcare practice (see Chapter 1). It is envisioned that the book will become a resource to redefine the expanding role of clinical medical physics in addressing topics such as physics support of new technologies, operational engagement of physics in clinical practice, and metrologies that are most closely reflective of the clinical utility of imaging methods.

The book covers all imaging modalities in use in clinical medicine today. For each modality, the book provides a "state of practice" (Medical Physics 1.0) description, a reflection of the medical physics service pertaining to the modality as it is practiced today. That is followed with an "emerging practice" (Medical Physics 3.0) with content on how clinical medical physics is evolving. The 1.0/3.0 segmentation can be thought of as a classical/new or present/developing treatment of the subject. In this fashion, the book summarizes both the current state of practice and also provides definitions on how the field is developing. The authors are luminaries in the field of clinical

Clinical Imaging Physics: Current and Emerging Practice, First Edition. Edited by Ehsan Samei and Douglas E. Pfeiffer.
© 2020 John Wiley & Sons, Inc. Published 2020 by John Wiley & Sons, Inc.

medical physics, as they help direct the development of the field of clinical imaging physics. It is hoped that the book will offer helpful and clarifying contributions in the current changing healthcare environment.

Ehsan Samei
Durham, NC, USA

Douglas E. Pfeiffer
Boulder, CO, USA

1

What Is Clinical Imaging Physics?*

Ehsan Samei

Departments of Radiology, Medical Physics, Physics, Biomedical Engineering, and Electrical and Computer Engineering, Duke University Medical Center, Durham, NC, USA

1.1 Introduction

Medical imaging started with physics. Since November 8, 1895 when the German Physicist and first physics Nobel laureate Wilhelm Roentgen discovered the mysterious "x" rays, physics has had a central role in the development and continuous advancement of nearly every medical imaging modality in use today. Thus, the research role of physicists in the research and development of medical imaging is well established. The use of the images in the care of the patient has also been largely undertaken by interpreting physicians (mostly radiologists) who undergo years of specialized training to be qualified for the task. But what about clinical physics? Is there an essential role for the presence and contribution of physicists in the *clinical practice* of medical imaging? The answer is an obvious yes, but how is this role defined? What are the essential ingredients for effective contribution of medical physics to the clinical imaging practice? In this chapter we outline the basic components and expectation of quality physics support of clinical practice across the current medical imaging modalities (Table 1.1).

1.2 Key Roles of the Clinical Physicist

1.2.1 Offering "Scientist in the Room"

In recent years we have seen a drive toward evidence-based medicine [2], ensuring that clinical practice is informed by science. Physics is a foundational scientific discipline. Physicists are trained and skilled in the language and methods of science. Their perspective can thus play an essential role toward evidence-based practice. Likewise, the current emphasis on comparative effectiveness and meaningful use puts extra scrutiny on the actual, as opposed to presumed, utility of technology and processes [3–6]. This highlights the need for a scientific approach toward practice, again with an obvious role for physics. In line with these moves, medicine is also seeing a slow shift toward quantification, using biometrics that personalize the care of the patient in numerical terms [7]. This provides for better evidence-based practice for both diagnostic and interventional care. Again,

---

* Some of the content of this chapter is based on a prior publication [1].

Clinical Imaging Physics: Current and Emerging Practice, First Edition. Edited by Ehsan Samei and Douglas E. Pfeiffer.
© 2020 John Wiley & Sons, Inc. Published 2020 by John Wiley & Sons, Inc.

Table 1.1   Key expectations and activities of modern clinical imaging physics practice.

Attribute	Practice
1) Offering "scientist in the room"	Providing scientific and quantitative perspective in the clinic toward evidence-based, quantitative, and personalized practice
2) Assurance of quality and safety	Assuring quality, safety, and precision of the imaging operation across complex sources of variability throughout the clinical practice
3) Regulatory compliance	Assuring adherence to practice for quality and safety regulatory requirements as well as guidelines of professional practice
4) Relevant technology assessment	Quantifying the performance of imaging technology through surrogates that can be related to clinical performance or outcome – evaluations performed in the context of acceptance testing and quality control
5) Use optimization	Prospectively optimizing the use of the imaging technology to ensure adherence to balanced performance in terms of dose and image quality
6) Performance monitoring	Retrospective auditing of the actual quality and safety of the imaging process through monitoring systems – quality control at the practice level; troubleshooting
7) Technology acquisition	Guidance on comparative effectiveness and wise selection of new imaging technologies and applications for the clinic
8) Technology commissioning	Effective commissioning of new imaging technologies and applications into the clinic to ensure optimum and consistent use and integration
9) Manufacturer cooperation	Serving as a liaison with the manufacturers of the imaging systems to facilitate communication and partnership in devising new applications
10) Translational practice	Engaging in quality improvement projects (clinical scholarship) and ensuring discoveries are extended to clinical implementation
11) Research consultancy	Providing enabling resources and advice to enhance the research activities involving medical imaging
12) Providing education	Providing targeted education for clinicians and operators on the technical aspects of the technology and its features

physics is a discipline grounded in mathematics and analytics with direct potential for the practice of quantitative imaging. Finally, the mantra of value-based medicine [8] highlights new priorities for safety, benefit, consistency, stewardship, and ethics. To practice value-based care, the value needs to be quantified, which again brings forth the need for numerical competencies that physics can provide. Physicists have an essential role in the clinical imaging practice to serve as the "scientists in the room."

1.2.2   Assurance of Quality and Safety

The overarching reason for the presence of medical physicists in the clinic is to assure the quality and safety of the practice. Medical imaging devices are diverse and complex. Their heterogeneity manifests itself in their diversity of type, make and model, and technical parameters. Combined with the diversity in patients, human operators, and stakeholders of varying (sometimes competing) interests, the practice left on its own creates variability in the quality of care. This variability is not insignificant and has a cost. A recent report from the National Academy of Medicine reports most people will experience at least one diagnostic error in their lifetime [9]. In fact 10% of patient deaths and 6–17% of hospital adverse events are due to diagnostic errors. Medical imaging being largely a diagnostic process contributes to these statistics. The presence of clinical physicists in the clinic directly tackles this challenge. By overseeing the setup and use of the equipment and imaging processes, physicists offer an essential scrutiny of the operation to enhance consistency and minimize the likelihood of mishaps.

1.2.3 Regulatory Compliance

Toward the assurance of quality and safety, regulatory compliance and adherence to professional guidelines and standards offer a "scaffolding," a safeguard against quality issues that have been documented previously. Apart from federal and state regulation, The Technical Joint Commission (TJC), Centers for Medicare and Medicaid Service (CMS), Environmental Protection Agency (EPA), American College of Radiology (ACR), American Association of Physicists in Medicine (AAPM), and others provide useful standards, the meeting of which require active engagement of clinical imaging physicists. However necessary, the regulation and compliance-weighted focus of the current clinical physics practice may not be enough; the newest clinical practice guidelines from the ACR and AAPM highlight this limitation [10, 11]. Physics is most relevant to the extent that it seeks to address clinical needs and limitations. Regulations, by necessity and their reactive tendencies, are always a step behind clinical opportunities, needs, and realities. Clinical physics practice should extend beyond compliance and should inform the development and refinement of regulations and accreditation programs.

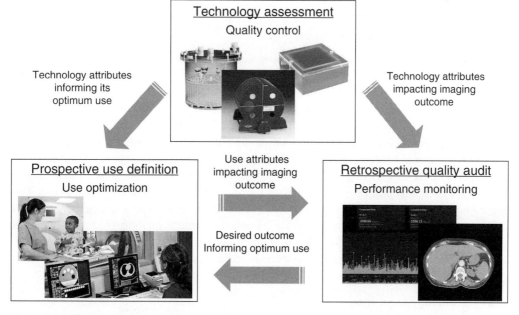

Figure 1.1 The three major components of clinical imaging physics practice according to the Medical Physics 3.0 paradigm. Attributes and assessment of technology (represented in the upper square) inform its optimum use (left square), and the two of them impact image outcome (right square). Outcome analysis conversely informs the optimum use of the technology.

1.2.4 Relevant Technology Assessment

The modern practice of clinical physics, as encouraged through the Medical Physics 3.0 paradigm [12], is based on three elements (Figure 1.1). One primary goal of clinical physics practice is technology assessment based on metrics that reflect the attributes of those technologies and relate to expected clinical outcomes. Toward that goal, the characterization of devices to ensure their adherence to vendor claims or regulatory guidelines is necessary but not enough; we must move from compliance-based to performance-based quality assurance. New physics practices should aim to devise and implement new metrics that are reflective of the performance of new technologies as well as the expected clinical outcome [12]. For example, characterizing the performance of a system in terms of detection or estimation indices (as opposed to the more conventional physics quantities of resolution or noise alone) can directly speak to the capability of the technology to deliver an objective clinical goal. In this way, physics can offer a quantification that is evidence-based and that can enable the meaningful comparison and optimization of new technologies and applications.

1.2.5 Use Optimization

Having ensured the intrinsic capability of the technology, as its second goal, the physics practice uses those attributes to ascertain how the technology can best be deployed in clinical service to ensure the desired image quality and safety for a given patient. This speaks to the optimized use of the technology so that a desired clinical outcome can be targeted [13–18]. A significant component of this activity is protocol development and optimization, addressing specific clinical needs including dose optimization, adjustments for patient attributes, indication-specific image quality, and contrast agent administration.

1.2.6 Performance Monitoring

The combination of relevant assessment and prospective optimization stated above should ideally provide actual optimum image quality and safety. In reality, however, there are many factors that influence the actual outcome of the image acquisition including unforeseen conditions, technological variability, and human factors. This is partly addressed by the troubleshooting mandate of clinical physicists. But that action is sporadic and only address the most noticeable issues of the practice. The physicist should in addition analyze the output of the imaging operation to ensure adherence to targeted expectations [19–26]. Using aggregate curated data sets such as those currently used in dose monitoring, this analysis can ensure that the actual output of the imaging technology matches its promise, capturing both its inherent capability and its optimum use. This type of analysis can target both the quality and the consistency of the operation, helping to better understand and mitigate variability in the clinical operation, and to quantify the actual impact of new technologies. Medical physicists, due to their content expertise and numerical training, are uniquely qualified to undertake this data science-based analysis.

1.2.7 Technology Acquisition

Medical imaging has been and remains subject to perpetual technological innovation. This is evident across all modalities: wireless digital technology and cone-beam multi-dimensional imaging in radiography and fluoroscopy, 3D imaging in mammography, advanced reconstructions and spectral imaging in computed tomography (CT), new pulse sequences and functional applications in magnetic resonance imaging (MRI), 3D imaging and elastography in ultrasonography, hybrid imaging and molecular quantification in positron emission tomography (PET) and single phioton emission computed tomography (SPECT), just to name a few. Each new technology offers new features, a good number of which are founded on physical and technological foundations. Which system among an array of commercial offering, and which options of that system are best suited for a clinical setting? Clinical physicist, with their strong technical background, can provide crucial advice in the selection of a system and decisions about the array of features that it may provide. They can evaluate the comparative advantages of the new features, predict how the new features may deliver their claim, and how they can be integrated within the existing practice at the site. This provides crucial input on evidence-based purchasing, to be supplemented with additional consideration for wise selections, such as cost, from the other members of the healthcare team.

1.2.8 Technology Commissioning

Once a new medical imaging technology or system is installed, clinical physicists can play a vital role in their effective implementation in the clinic. New technologies cannot be assured to provide superior performance until their use is properly commissioned and optimized. A case in point is the transition from film to digital technology which led to a marked degradation of consistency across practice due to additional adjustment factors that were not optimized. Physics engagement is essential to ensure that well-intentioned and well-designed technologies are used effectively for the improvement of patient care.

Further, physicists can and do play an essential role in "commodifying the technology" so that the new addition does not compromise the consistency of care. The diversity of technology across a practice, while natural considering the evolving nature of the field, new innovations, and life cycle of systems (no institution can upgrade all its system all at once) creates a challenge to the consistency of image quality and dose across practice. While the consequent diversity is natural, it needs to be managed since an overarching hallmark of care is consistency. We cannot afford variability of care depending on what imaging room a patient is scheduled into. Good quality clinical physics can help manage and minimize this source of variability. Thus clinical physics can ensure wise selection as well as effective implementation of new technologies and applications consistent with the overarching new priorities of medicine (evidence, effectiveness, quantification, and value).

1.2.9 Manufacturer Cooperation

Considering the high innovation in the technology used in medicine today, the best practices are often enabled by a strong connection with the manufacturers that develop the technology. Best use of the technology requires understanding it well. Physicists, by expertise, tend to be best positioned to understand the technology. As such they are often ideal individuals from the institution to liaise with the manufacturer on the technical and operational features of the technology. Since they often have a perspective on the broad implication of the technology, they can also offer advice to manufacturers on how to best condition their products (e.g. making sure their image processing has adapted to the latest innovation in their detectors). They are also often best positioned to facilitate partnership to develop and advance new applications considering the nuances of the imaging systems that they can understand and communicate with the rest of the clinical team.

1.2.10 Translational Practice

A direct benefit of having a "scientist in the room" is the opportunity to improve the imaging practice through quality improvements, aka clinical scholarship. Many physicists engage and inform in research projects at healthcare institutions – a worthwhile added benefit of having physicists on staff. But beyond those, the scientific mind and the quantitative reasoning of the physicist can be put to use to address challenging elements of the clinical practice which by themselves might not even be considered "physics," but nonetheless can benefit from the scientific approach. Examples include optimizing workflows across a clinic, discrepancies in the exam coding and billing, or devising key performance indicators (KPIs). The improvements can include direct physics expertise as well, such a devising a new method to test magnetic resonance (MR) coils, keeping track of ultrasound transducers across a QC program, or image analysis methods for more efficient physics testing. For any of these projects, a clinical physicist can and should ensure the scholarship involved is extended to workable clinical implementation, as clinical scholarship is oriented not only toward generalizable knowledge and dissemination (as in regular scholarship) but dissemination to clinical practice for the ultimate benefit of the patient.

1.2.11 Research Consultancy

Clinical physicists can be catalysts and enablers for academic research. They can serve this function even though their primary mission is and should be clinical. Nonetheless, this is of primary relevance to academic healthcare institutions with a mission toward research. Meaningful and impactful research in medical imaging often requires an understanding of the imaging system deeper than that needed in clinical practice. Clinical physicists, by the virtue of their expertise, which always needs to remain current, are best positioned to provide the consultancy and sometimes crucial resources to enable academic research involving medical imaging. Obviously, this aspect of clinical physics should be put in balance with their primary focus, which should claim the majority of their effort; however, as good citizens of the institution, seasoned clinical physicists are able to manage their clinical responsibilities while providing limited but needed assistance toward academic pursuits.

1.2.12 Providing Education

Physicians, tasked with the interpretation of medical images, in addition to specialized medical competency, require technical competency. Physicists are the essential experts to provide the necessary training for physicians in terms of four required elements of physician technical competencies: (i) the foundations of contrast formation in a given imaging modality; (ii) the technological components that enable the acquisition of an image; (iii) the modality's operational parameters and their influence on image quality and patient safety; and (iv) how to practice imaging within the constraints of the imaging modality and the needs of the indication [27]. These elements are cornerstones of the physics competency expected from radiologists by the American Board of Radiology. Additional training in the effective use of new technologies, for either physicians or technologists is also necessary, so those individuals can be best empowered to focus on *their* direct mandate: patient care. Physicists are uniquely tasked and qualified to provide the needed education to such practicing clinicians.

1.3 Challenges to Effective Clinical Physics Practice

Quality practice of clinical physics can be challenging. The challenges are not insurmountable, as seasoned physicists and physics practices have been able to find practical ways to manage these challenges. However, mindfulness of these challenges can be informative as the discipline advances and quality educational methods are devised for the next generation of clinical physicists.

1.3.1 Scope of Competency

The first challenge is simply the magnitude of knowledge that a clinical physicist is expected to master to practice effectively in the clinic. This is not just traditional medical physics knowledge, which by itself is ever expanding thanks to the progressive nature of medical imaging; but further, a clinical medical physicist needs to have enough foundational clinical and associated peripheral knowledge to be effective clinically. For these peripheral areas, the physicist should have enough knowledge to be able to communicate across diverse clinical disciplines. Equally importantly, they should know, with confidence, what they know and what they do not know to be able to engage with the clinical process effectively. New topics that require expanded mastery include, but are not limited to, data science and artificial intelligence, process engineering, multi-factorial optimization, bio-informatics, radiomics, and radiogenomics.

Added to this list are the so-called soft skills of leadership and communication that have become essential for clinical practice. Good communication skills are essential for leading and working with clinical teams and for communicating with patients in matters related to dose or technical aspects of patient care. With those skills, clinical physicists should take ownership in closer collaboration with physicians and other healthcare professionals. Many physics outputs and services are currently oriented toward physicist "audiences." To fully harness the value of those services, the physicists should own an increasingly inter-disciplinary strategy to seek their full clinical impact, for which leadership and communication competences are needed alongside seasoned physics expertise. A clinical physicist should thus perpetually seek wisdom and mentorship in balancing the breadth and depth of these needed competencies for good practice.

1.3.2 Balancing Rigor and Relevance

Clinical imaging physicists are both scientists and care providers. As scientists they have been trained to seek perfection and seek reality, yet as practitioners they need to be equally aware of practical limitations and care delivery. The science that they pursue by itself is highly applied – not oriented toward generalizable knowledge, even though that is sometimes the case – but oriented toward applicable benefit to the patient. Maintaining this balance of scientific rigor and clinical relevance is a challenge. A perfect solution is often out of reach, due to lack of time, or money, or external support, but a solution is needed nonetheless. Navigating this landscape is yet another area where mindfulness, mentorship, and wisdom are needed for better practice.

1.3.3 Managing Surrogates

In clinical imaging physics we seek to assess and optimize the quality and safety of the practice toward the assumed eventual improvement of the care outcome. However, a direct relationship between our measures and the outcome is very difficult to ascertain given the diversity across the patients and confounding effects within the care process. Short of having conclusive evidence, we are left with surrogates (Figure 1.2). Within that space, measures that are more directly related to the quality and safety of care for the patient are likely most relevant. For example, organ dose and validated detectability indices are more closely related to the radiation burden and quality of a CT exam than computed tomography dose index (CTDI) and noise. However, more progressive surrogates such as organ dose are also more prone to estimation errors. Balancing the benefit of a high relevance of a metric and its limited approximation is a delicate choice that needs to be made on a situation by situation basis to ensure the most effective practice of clinical physics.

1.3.4   Integrating Principle- and Data-Informed Approaches

Most of physics is based on methodical principles and their logical conclusions. However, that can never be assumed to be without potential error, thus the reason for experiments. Applying the same to clinical medical physics, we may apply our knowledge of imaging devices and processes to devise their optimum use. However, the actual image data that they produce give us highly-relevant information about the effectiveness of our assumptions. A clinical physicist should be able to seamlessly integrate the principle-informed approaches of clinical physics with data-informed methods to ascertain and target the best practice. The current focus of healthcare on machine-learning and artificial intelligence provides ample resources toward that goal if physicists can learn to navigate and use these resources, and be a catalyst in their effective use in clinical care [28, 29].

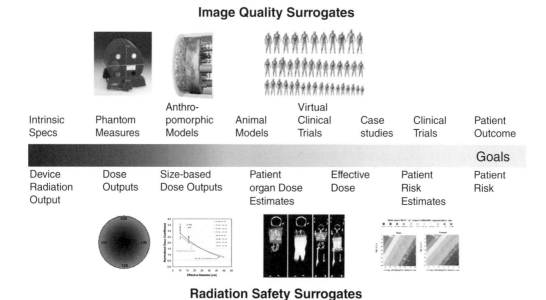

Figure 1.2   The spectrum of the surrogates of image quality (top) and radiation safety (bottom) (for radiation imaging modalities) to reflect the desire goals of the assessments (i.e. patient outcome and patient risk). Short of that knowledge, clinical physicists use reasonable surrogates along a spectrum. The ones on the left are easier to assess but relevance is inferred, while the ones toward the right tend to be more relevant but subject to estimation error. Balancing the two competing desires of relevance and robustness becomes a requirement of effective clinical physics practice.

1.3.5 Effective Models of Clinical Physics Practice

As outlined here and detailed in the chapters of this book, the values that clinical physics offer to clinical practice of medical imaging go well beyond compliance with current regulatory standards. However, that is not widely recognized within the healthcare enterprise today. Clinical physicists should secure justification for the contribution of their expertise to clinical practice. This call for a deeper investment in medical physics toward enhancing patient care comes at a time when radiologic interpretation duties consume even more time than before and National Institutes of Health (NIH) funding concerns and economic pressures in hospitals potentially pull physics and radiology apart. Many institutions are either not aware of this potential, or opt for the minimum of regulatory compliance. Some institutions, however, seem able to manage these pressures and effectively harness the value of physics in their practice. How? What are the best working models that can enable better concordance and integration of radiology and physics?

There are differences even among best practices, but all institutions that have managed to harness the full value of clinical physics in their practice toward improved patient care share certain common attributes:

1) There is high degree of consciousness at the leadership of the institution about the historical track record and value of medical physics.
2) Exemplary physicists have been able to go beyond the realm of theoretical possibility and demonstrate the value of physics within the clinical practice in practical ways.
3) The complementary nature of the expertise of the physician and the physicist is recognized and respected. A feature of civilized society is its ability to use professionals for its specialized needs. Such is the case for institutions that defer to physicists on issues that need physics solutions.
4) Funding for physics services is justified based on added value. At one institution, 2% of radiology revenue is allocated to radiological physics based on the track record that the investment has paid more than its share in ensuring the quality and safety of the operation, wise investment in equipment acquisition and replacement, and minimum liability for near misses.
5) In an era in which patients have choices, these institutions recognize that the distinction of a high-quality and high-safety operation can lead to greater market-share of healthcare services.

The above model of practice and justification of physics services in the imaging departments is based on the "in-house" model of physics practice. In recent years, there has emerged a steady and growing practice of consulting physicists that provide an essential service to the community. Providing physics services beyond meeting the regulatory compliance can readily be offered through these consulting practices provided that the clinical services are aware of the richness of physics contribution to clinical practice, as outlined in this chapter and detailed in the modality-specific chapters of this book. Encouraging physics-informed practices and adapting the practice models to meet the demand should be a high priority for the evidence-based and value-based practice of medicine. Indeed, the reimbursement framework itself needs to be modified to recognize the value of diagnostic clinical medical physics, both in quality of patient care and in cost savings due to improved efficiencies. Clinical physics should not be seen just as a cost center, but a central component of diagnostic imaging.

1.4 Conclusions

Medical imaging and interpretation continue to provide unprecedented value to healthcare. Innovative technologies offer enhanced opportunities for high-quality imaging care. These new clinical realities, however, require the utmost rigor in the effective use of technology in the drive toward high-quality, consistent practice of medical imaging that is patient-centered, evidence-based, and safe. Medical physics enables innovative precision care through the targeted clinical application of physical sciences. The relationship between medicine and physics is mutual and essential for the overall goal of medicine: fostering human health. In the current healthcare landscape of enhanced and diverse imaging options, optimized use of the technology cannot be assumed. Clinical physics can address this gap by extending beyond compliance testing toward intentional evidence-based and value-based use of the technology to serve clinical care.

References

1 Samei, E. and Grist, T.M. (2018). Why physics in medicine? *Journal of the American College of Radiology* 15 (7): 1008–1012.

2 Sackett, D.L. (1997). Evidence-based medicine. *Seminars in Perinatology* 21 (1): 3–5.

3 42 Code of Federal Register, Parts 412 and 495

4 45 Code of Federal Register, Part 170

5 42 Code of Federal Register, Parts 412, 413, and 495

6 Initial National Priorities for Comparative Effectiveness Research (2009). Committee on Comparative Effectiveness Research Prioritization, Institute of Medicine, The National Academies Press, Washington, DC.

7 Kessler, L.G., Barnhart, H.X., Buckler, A.J. et al. (2015). The emerging science of quantitative imaging biomarkers terminology and definitions for scientific studies and regulatory submissions. *Statistical Methods in Medical Research* 24 (1): 9–26.

8 Bae, J.-M. (2015). Value-based medicine: concepts and application. *Epidemiol Health* 37: e2015014.

9 NAM, Improving Diagnosis in Health Care (2015). *The National Academies of Sciences, Engineering, and Medicine*. Washington (DC): National Academies Press (US).

10 ACR Technical Standards (2018). https://www.acr.org/Clinical-Resources/Practice-Parameters-and-Technical-Standards/Technical-Standards (accessed January 20).

11 AAPM (2018). Medical Physics Practice Guidelines, https://www.aapm.org/pubs/MPPG/default.asp (accessed January 20).

12 Samei, E., Pawlicki, T., Bourland, D. et al. (2018). Redefining and reinvigorating the role of physics in clinical medicine: a report from the AAPM Medical Physics 3.0 Ad Hoc Committee. *Medical Physics* 45 (9): e783–e789.

13 Kalra, M.K., Maher, M.M., Toth, T.L. et al. (2004). Strategies for CT radiation dose optimization. *Radiology* 230 (3): 619–628.

14 Samei, E., Li, X., and Frush, D.P. (2017). Size-based quality-informed framework for quantitative optimization of pediatric CT. *Journal of Medical Imaging* 4 (3): 031209.

15 Zhang, Y., Smitherman, C., and Samei, E. (2017). Size specific optimization of CT protocols based on minimum detectability. *Medical Physics* 44 (4): 1301–1311.

16 Richard, S. and Siewerdsen, J.H. (2007). Optimization of dual-energy imaging systems using generalized NEQ and imaging. *Medical Physics* 34 (1): 127–139.

17 Prakash, P., Zbijewski, W., Gang, G.J. et al. (2011). Task-based modeling and optimization of a cone-beam CT scanner for musculoskeletal imaging. *Medical Physics* 38 (10): 5612–5629.

18 Winslow, J., Zhang, Y., and Samei, E. (2017). A method for characterizing and matching CT image quality across CT scanners from different manufacturers. *Medical Physics* 44 (11): 5705–5717.

19 Sanders, J., Hurwitz, L., and Samei, E. (2016). Patient-specific quantification of image quality: an automated method for measuring spatial resolution in clinical CT images. *Medical Physics* 43 (10): 5330–5338.

20 Trattner, S., Pearson, G.D.N., Chin, C. et al. (2014). Standardization and optimization of computed tomography protocols to achieve low-dose. *Journal of the American College of Radiology*. Mar; 11 (3): 271–278.

21 Ria, F., Wilson, J., Zhang, Y., and Samei, E. (2017). Image noise and dose performance across a clinical population: patient size adaptation as a metric of CT performance. *Medical Physics* 44 (6): 2141–2147.

22 Malkus, A. and Szczykutowicz, T.P. (2017). A method to extract image noise level from patient images in CT. *Medical Physics* 44 (6): 2173–2184.

23 Sodickson, A., Baeyens, P.F., Andriole, K.P. et al. (2009). Recurrent CT, cumulative radiation exposure, and associated radiation-induced cancer risks from CT of adults. *Radiology* 251 (1): 175–184.

24 Larson, D.B., Malarik, R.J., Hall, S.M., and Podberesky, D.J. (2013). System for verifiable CT radiation dose optimization based on image quality. Part II. Process control system. *Radiology* 269: 177–185.

25 Abadi, E., Sanders, J., and Samei, E. (2017). Patient-specific quantification of image quality: an automated technique for measuring the distribution of organ Hounsfield units in clinical chest CT images. *Medical Physics* 44 (9): 4736–4746.

26 Smith, T.B., Solomon, J.B., and Samei, E. (2018). Estimating detectability index in vivo: development and validation of an automated methodology. *Journal of Medical Imaging (Bellingham)* 5 (3): 031403.

27 Samei, E. (2016). Cutting to the chase: with so much physics "stuff," what do radiologists really need to know? *American Journal of Roentgenology* 206 (1): W9.

28 Sensakovic, W.F. and Mahesh, M.M. (2019). Role of the medical physicists in the health care artificial intelligence revolution. *Journal of the American College of Radiology* 16: 393–394.

29 Murdoch, T.B. and Detsky, A.S. (2013). The inevitable application of big data to health care. *JAMA* 309 (13): 1351–1352.

Part I

Radiography

2

Clinical Radiography Physics: Perspective

Ehsan Samei

Departments of Radiology, Medical Physics, Physics, Biomedical Engineering, and Electrical and Computer Engineering, Duke University Medical Center, Durham, NC, USA

Radiography is one of the most outstanding components of clinical imaging physics. As the modality that claims the most frequently performed examination, it has given rise to many meaningful engagements of physics in the clinical practice. Physicists apply rigorous testing methods to qualify x-ray tubes and detectors for adequate performance. Even so, most evaluations today still focus mostly on the technical specification of the technology and not the direct utility of the technology in clinical practice. The evolution of clinical physics in radiography from a technology focus (so called Medical Physics 1.0) to a more patient-centered focus (so called Medical Physics 3.0) has multiple faceted some of which are listed in Table 2.1. In this brief perspective we provide seven examples of how this evolution is taking shape.

2.1 Analogue to Digital

Radiography has experienced a change from analog to digital receptors. This change has provided significant potential for improved effectiveness of radiography in clinical practice. The separation of the processes of image acquisition, image rendition, and image display into multiple components enabled by the digital technology has provided an opportunity to optimize each component individually. But this task has not been fully claimed in the canon of clinical imaging physics today.

2.2 Detector versus Performance

Clinical physicists have devised methods to evaluate radiography detectors. This evaluation tends to be rigorous and may include advanced methods such as testing the modulation transfer function and the detective quantum efficiency (DQE). However, these evaluations tend to be limited to only the detector component of the system alone and do not speak to the performance of the system as a whole. For example, the modulation transfer function as measured only qualifies the resolution of the detector and not the resolution of the images expected from patient imaging as the focal spot blur is not included. The same applies to the DQE where the effect of the scatter and the anti-scatter grid is not incorporated. Thus, the signal-to-noise ratio that would be expected from a clinical

Clinical Imaging Physics: Current and Emerging Practice, First Edition. Edited by Ehsan Samei and Douglas E. Pfeiffer.

Table 2.1 Comparison of Medical Physics 1.0 and emerging 3.0 paradigms in radiography physics.

Radiography	1.0	3.0
Focus of MP's attention	Equipment, focused on individual systems and isolated performance	Patient, focused on consistency of care across practice
Image quality evaluation	Visual, subjective, in and through phantoms	Mathematical, quantitative, in and through phantoms and patient cases
Evaluation condition	Standardized techniques	Techniques most closely reflecting clinical use and variation across cases
MP "tools of the trade" for image quality evaluation	Visibility of dots/holes, line pairs, wire meshes	MTF, NPS, DQE, eDQE, SNR uniformity, noise component analysis, detectability
Routine QC	Individual checking of EI, Individual subjective evaluation of image quality	Continuous automated monitoring of EI and quality metrics, focus on trends and outliers
Patient dosimetry	ESE (ESAK), DAP	Organ dose, risk index
Image processing	Often ignored	Incorporated in quantitative evaluation and optimization
System evaluation	Focused on x-ray source and detector alone	Focused on the system as a whole including the anti-scatter technologies
Radiography applications	Focused on static radiography	Expansion to dual-energy, tomosynthesis, and other advanced applications
Protocols	Focused on maximum exposure for limited exam type	Comprehensive definition and oversight of optimum techniques across exams and body types

examination could not be directly predicted from the DQE measurements made on the detector alone (Figure 2.1) [1]. Updated physics methods are needed to address this, as physics tests are most relevant and meaningful when they can be of clinical predictive utility.

2.3 Post-processing

Post-processing is an ever present adaptive component of digital radiography. Post-processing markedly affects the quality of the images expected from a digital radiography system (Figure 2.2). Even so, the field of clinical imaging physics has hardly claimed that as a component of clinical physics practice. To date, there is no methodology to meaningfully ascertain the impact of post-processing on clinical images, to provide means to optimize post-processing toward targeted task performance, or make image rendering consistent across makes and models (Figure 2.3).

2.4 Advanced Applications

Digital technology has given rise to a series of advanced image acquisition applications. These include dual-energy imaging and tomosynthesis. While these applications have been adapted in certain clinics, clinical physics has lagged behind evaluating their performance or offering

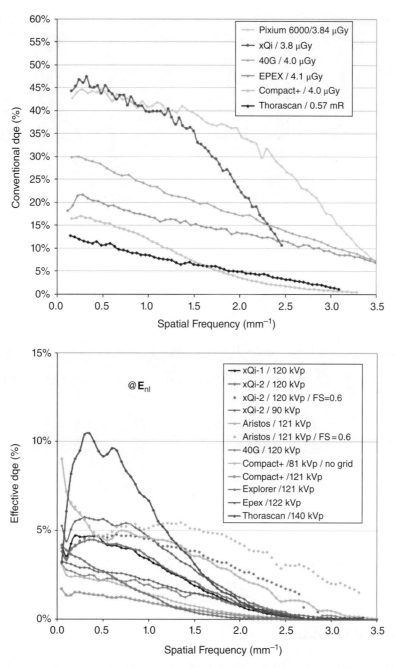

Figure 2.1 The DQE (left) and effective DQE (right) of select radiography systems demonstrating marked differences in the magnitude of the SNR expected from radiography systems when the impact of grid, focal spot, and anti-scatter grid is ignored (DQE) or incorporated (effective DQE) in the evaluation of the system.

cross-modality comparisons of their meaningful incorporation in the clinical practice. For example, both of the named advanced technologies offer means to reduce the anatomical clutter in images, which have been the bane of 2D projection imaging. But the main question is whether such reduction is sufficient to make these technologies effective enough in comparison to CT? One could imagine clinical applications for which the lower dose and cost of advanced methods can

Less equalization ⟶ More equalization

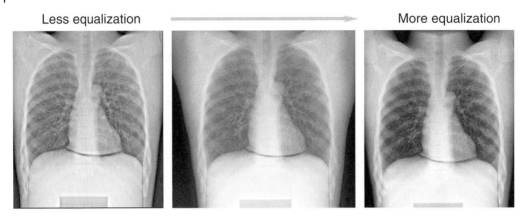

Figure 2.2 The profound impact of only one of the many adjustments through image post-processing on a singular radiograph.

Carestream   GE   Philips

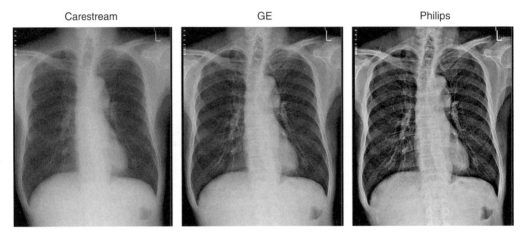

Figure 2.3 Marked differences in image rendering of a radiography of a chest phantom acquired on three different radiography systems.

make them better suited than CT in cost- and value-conscious healthcare. This is a question that should and can be answered by clinical physics expertise.

2.5 Protocol Definition

Apart from the technology, how we use the technology can have an impact on the resulting images. As such it is important to have robust and consistent techniques for radiographic imaging. States regulate the availability of technique charts in clinics. However, the current regulations only include select examinations and are primarily focused on maximum dose. Yet clinical physics can and should ensure consistency of techniques across systems of varying makes and models of diverse equipment performance, and further provide assurance by both safe and high-image quality operation. Even with a consistent system, the technique applied can affect image quality across patient examinations, and thus we need to address the definition and optimization of techniques across patient cohorts of differing sizes.

2.6 Consistency of Quality

Making image quality targeted and consistent across a clinical operation is by itself a necessary requirement of quality care. Different technology implementations offer differing image presentation while imagining should ideally be about the patient not the system. This necessitates enhanced image consistency to be as important as improved image quality. Traditionally, physicists test each radiography unit in isolation and pass/fail it based on its adherence to expected specifications. Equally, and perhaps even more importantly, clinical physics needs to speak to how that system can be consistently integrated within a clinical operation to provide consistent output. This necessitates system-wide adjustment and QC processes that include techniques and post-processing components as well, noted above.

2.7 Phantom versus Patient

Finally, the target of any healthcare activity should be the patient. Physics techniques often deploy phantoms – phantoms are in fact indispensable to evaluating and commissioning imaging systems. However, care should be exercised in not over-assuming the utility of the phantoms, as acceptable or superior system performance with phantoms may not guarantee patient performance. To make the phantom work more relevant, the phantom should be designed and used with the attributes of the patients (e.g. size and latitude) and the imaging technique in mind. The phantom results should ideally be related to patient cases as well. The best QC images are the clinical images themselves. Toward that goal, pioneering work has been done to extend physics evaluations to clinical cases [2]. This is a promising area that demands further attention and expansion to clinical practice.

These case examples highlight areas where clinical imaging physics can play a more impactful role in the use of radiography technology in clinical care. Some of these are further echoed in the following two chapters and as well can be recognized in the expanding practice of clinical physics in other imaging modalities. The point should also be stated that these potential areas are not only an opportunity for expanding the current territory of the discipline of medical physics, even though that might be the case; rather they are needed and essential for quality imaging practice and expected of a clinical operation that has been entrusted to provide a high standard of quality and acceptability toward the patients it cares for. Effective use of clinical physics is a requirement of value-based care.

References

1 Samei, E., Ranger, N.T., MacKenzie, A. et al. (2008). Detector or system? Extending the concept of detective quantum efficiency to characterize the performance of digital radiographic imaging systems. *Radiology* 249: 926–937.
2 Samei, E., Lin, Y., Choudhury, K.R., and Page McAdams, H. (2014). Automated characterization of perceptual quality of clinical chest radiographs: validation and calibration to observer preference. *Med. Phys.* 41: 111918.

3

Clinical Radiography Physics: State of Practice

David Gauntt

Department of Radiology, University of Alabama at Birmingham, Birmingham, AL, USA

3.1   Introduction

Radiography is the oldest of the radiologic imaging technologies and may have undergone more changes through its history than any of the other modalities. The most recent of these changes was the introduction of digital image receptors in the late 1980s, which was preceded by the development of high-frequency generators in the early 1980s. The adoption of these technologies was rapid and it is now difficult to find a clinically used system that is not a digital receptor coupled with a high frequency generator.

However, much of the current testing paradigm is based on techniques developed in the 1970s. In that decade, the state of the art included

- X-ray film and chemical processing
- Dual-screen film/screen image receptors
- Three-phase x-ray generators
- Ionization chambers for dosimetry

Consequently, the radiographic system comprised primarily the x-ray generator, x-ray tube, collimator, anti-scatter grid, the film and film/screen cassette, the film processor, and the light box or film changer. Stability and accuracy of the x-ray generator was a major concern; without the closed-loop control of the high-frequency generator, the tube voltage could vary with line current, aging of the circuitry, and a host of other variables. The weak link in the imaging chain was often the image processor, which did not always receive adequate attention from the physicist or the facility using it.

3.1.1   AAPM Reports

The American Association of Physicists in Medicine (AAPM) issued a number of reports describing Quality Control (QC) methods. These are summarized in Table 3.1. The first report describing QC of digital imaging equipment was published in 2006, the same year as the last report on film processors. The first comprehensive report on QA methods for digital radiography (Report 150) has been in development for a number of years.

Clinical Imaging Physics: Current and Emerging Practice, First Edition. Edited by Ehsan Samei and Douglas E. Pfeiffer.
© 2020 John Wiley & Sons, Inc. Published 2020 by John Wiley & Sons, Inc.

Table 3.1 AAPM reports on testing of radiographic equipment.

Report	Year	Title
4	1977	Basic Quality Control in Diagnostic Radiology [1]
14	1985	Performance Specifications and Acceptance Testing for X-Ray Generators and Automatic Exposure Control Devices [2]
74	2002	Quality Control in Diagnostic Radiology [3]
		Note: this report covered QC of all imaging modalities, including computed radiography but no other forms of digital radiography.
93	2006	Acceptance Testing and Quality Control of Photostimulable Storage Phosphor Imaging Systems [4]
94	2006	Validating Automatic Film Processor Performance
116	2009	An Exposure Indicator for Digital Radiography [5]
151	2015	Ongoing Quality Control in Digital Radiography: The Report of AAPM Imaging Physics Committee Task Group 151 [6]

3.1.2 ACR Technical Standard

The American College of Radiology (ACR) has issued technical standards for medical physics performance monitoring of various imaging modalities, including radiography. These standards are intended to be guidelines and not rigid specifications or requirements.

The document "ACR Technical Standard for Diagnostic Medical Physics Performance Monitoring of Radiographic and Fluoroscopic Equipment" was most recently revised in 2011 [7]. It includes

- A definition of the requirements for a Qualified Medical Physicist (QMP)
- A list of the tests that should be performed on radiographic equipment annually by a QMP
- A list of the tests that should be performed more frequently as part of a continuing QC program under the supervision of a QMP
- A statement that Acceptance Testing should be more comprehensive than annual testing.
- A statement of the need for appropriate written reports and follow-up by the QMP.

In addition, it includes a section titled "Radiation Safety in Imaging" that briefly describes the philosophy of radiation management in radiography and fluoroscopy, including

- The use of nationally developed guidelines in selecting protocols
- The need for all appropriate personnel (physicists, radiologists, technologists) to understand the nature and risks of ionizing radiation.
- The need to adjust exposure techniques to accommodate different body habitus.
- The need to estimate patient exposure for routine exams of typical patients annually, and to compare the patient exposure to national norms.

3.1.3 Current QC Regulations and Procedures

In the United States, the manufacture of all medical devices is regulated by the Food and Drug Administration (FDA). In particular, the FDA specifies performance standards for all radiographic systems at the point of sale to the customer. Use of the systems is not regulated by the FDA; however, most individual states issue regulations specifying the ongoing performance of radiographic systems, and typically prescribe an annual testing regimen to be performed or overseen by a QMP who ensures that the system meets the state regulations. Typically, any system that meets the FDA standards will meet the state regulations, so often the QMP will compare the performance of the systems to the FDA regulations.

The sole exception to this regulatory framework is mammography, for which the equipment performance and testing regime are strictly regulated by the FDA, under the authority of the Mammographic Quality Standards Act (MSQA). Mammography is covered in a separate chapter of this book.

3.2 System Performance

The tests described below cover only those that would be performed by a QMP and does not include the continuous QC that should be performed by a technologist, nor does it include testing specific to obsolete technologies (film processors, single phase generators, etc.).

The following table is based on work by AAPM Task Group 150 and is a list of QC tests that are typically performed on radiographic equipment. For each test, the table describes whether the test is mandatory (required by regulation) (Man), recommended (Rec), or optional (Opt). The table includes tests commonly performed, tests that may soon become standard practice, and tests that are specific to digital systems.

The following are descriptions of tests selected from Table 3.2.

3.2.1 Intrinsic Performance

3.2.1.1 Integrity of Unit Assembly
This is a simple test, typically verifying that cable insulation is not cracked, interlocks are working properly, and safety measures are in place and working properly [7–9].

3.2.1.2 Beam-on Indicators and Controls
This test simply verifies that when an exposure is started, the appropriate visual indicators are activated, and that when the exposure switch is released prematurely the exposure terminates [9].

3.2.1.3 KERMA-Area Product
This test is more generally performed in Europe than in the United States. For a given exposure technique, the air kinetic energy released per unit mass (KERMA) and field size are measured at the same distance from the focal spot, and the product compared to the KERMA-area product (KAP) value displayed by the acquisition workstation [10].

3.2.1.4 Light Field Illumination
The illuminance of the light field is measured at the center of the light field at a specified distance from the focal spot and is compared to the specifications of the FDA [8].

3.2.1.5 Light Field/Radiation Field Congruence
This test verifies that the edges of the light field adequately match the edges of the radiation field. Typically, radiopaque markers are placed at the edges of the light field, an exposure is acquired, and then the shadows of the markers on the image are inspected [3, 9, 10].

Table 3.2 QA tests for digital radiographic systems.

QA Test	Acceptance Test	Performance Test	QA Test	Acceptance Test	Performance Test
X-RAY GENERATOR					
Aluminum half-value layer (HVL)	Man	Man	Tube voltage accuracy	Man	Man
Exposure timer accuracy	Man	Man	Tube voltage waveform	Rec	Opt
Exposure reproducibility	Man	Man	Focal spot size	Rec	Opt
mR/mAs linearity	Man	Man	Tube output	Man	Man
SYSTEM TESTS					
Exposure Indicator Test	Man	Rec	System spatial resolution	Rec	Rec
Distance Calibration	Man	Opt	Patient Equivalent Phantom Test	Rec	Opt
X-RAY COLLIMATOR					
Radiation/light field congruence	Man	Man	Positive beam limitation	Rec	Rec
Light field illuminance	Rec	Opt	Mechanical inspection	Rec	Rec
Collimator dial accuracy	Rec	Rec	Additional filtration	Rec	Opt
SID accuracy	Rec	Rec	Off-focus radiation	Rec	Opt
Rad field/receptor congruence	Rec	Rec			
GRID					
Grid Uniformity and Artifacts	Man	Man			
AUTOMATIC EXPOSURE CONTROL SYSTEM (AEC)					
Reproducibility	Man	Man	Density selector	Man	Man
Minimum response time	Rec	Opt	Tube voltage tracking	Man	Man
Sensitivity calibration	Rec	Rec	Patient thickness tracking	Man	Man
Sensitivity selector	Rec	Opt	Field of view compensation	Rec	Opt
Cell Selection	Man	Opt	Backup timer	Man	Man
Cell balance	Man	Man			

IMAGE RECEPTOR FLAT FIELD

Test		
Detector Response	Rec	Opt
Signal Nonuniformity	Rec	Opt
Noise Nonuniformity	Rec	Opt
Signal-to-Noise Nonuniformity	Rec	Opt
Minimum Signal-to-Noise	Rec	Opt
Anomalous Pixels/lines	Rec	Rec
Correlated image artifacts	Rec	Opt
DQE	Opt	Opt
Large Signal Capability	Rec	Opt
Visual Inspection	Rec	Rec

IMAGE RECEPTOR WITH TEST OBJECT

Test		
MTF	Opt	Opt
Spatial Resolution	Rec	Rec
Spatial Resolution Nonuniformity	Rec	Opt
Contrast/Noise Ratio	Rec	Rec

IMAGE PROCESSING

Test		
Setup of image processing	Rec	N/A
Evaluation of changes to image processing	N/A	Opt

INTEROPERABILITY

Test		
DICOM Modality Worklist configuration	Opt	Opt
DICOM Modality Worklist Information Display	Opt	Opt
DICOM Modality Worklist Information Accuracy	Opt	Opt
RIS (Procedure) Code Mapping	Opt	Opt
Received Image Appearance	Opt	Opt
Propagation of Image Annotations and Orientation/Laterality	Opt	Opt
Physical Measurement Consistency	Opt	Opt
Propagation and Display of Image Metadata	Opt	Opt
Proper Image Compression Settings	Opt	Opt
Patient Information Editing	Opt	Opt
Downtime procedure validation	Opt	Opt

3.2.1.6 Collimation and Radiation Beam Alignment

This test is based on the FDA regulations, and is done to verify that the radiation field does not excessively extend past the edges of the image receptor, and that the radiation and light fields are reasonably well aligned [7, 8].

3.2.1.7 Automatic Exposure Control (AEC) System Performance

This test is done to assure that image receptor dose is always appropriate when under automatic exposure control. The details of the test vary significantly between film/screen systems and digital systems. Since film/screen systems are affected by reciprocity law failure (i.e. a 100 mAs exposure taken in 1 ms will darken film more than a 100 mAs exposure taken in 1000 ms), the test verifies that film optical density remains constant as acquisition conditions change under AEC operation. With digital systems, it is necessary to ensure that the exposure indication provided by the system is maintained within an acceptable range as kVp and phantom thickness are varied [7]. The deviation index is being incorporated by more manufacturers as a method for ensuring appropriate control of exposures (Shepard SJ, July 2009).

3.2.1.8 kV Accuracy and Reproducibility

Ensuring that the tube voltage is accurate and stable is necessary because errors in tube voltage can both affect the image contrast and make tube output calculations based on tube voltage inaccurate [7].

In the 1970s, testing tube voltage accuracy was critical and difficult. The output voltages of single-phase and three-phase generators were sensitive to changes to line voltage, and the user was responsible for adjusting a manual compensation setting. The voltage could be measured only by connecting the generator to the x-ray tube though an external high-voltage tank that contained a precision voltage divider; measuring the voltage on the divider provided a direct measurement of the voltage on the tube. During this time, some non-invasive measurement techniques were developed that assisted in performing this task.

By the 1990s, high-frequency generators were in widespread use. These systems use closed-loop feedback that compensates for most errors that could affect the tube voltage. In addition, the development of non-invasive kV meters allowed the physicist to make an indirect measurement of the tube voltage simply by placing a sensor in the radiation field. Thus, the test has become much easier and fails much less often.

3.2.1.9 Focal Spot Size

The size of the x-ray focal spot has an impact both on the tube lifetime and on the system spatial resolution. If the focal spot is too small, the target track on the anode can overheat and be damaged; if the focal spot is too large, geometric unsharpness can degrade the spatial resolution.

Tests of the focal spot size have historically been based on National Electrical Manufacturers Association (NEMA) standard XR-5 [11], which prescribed procedures to measure the focal spot size, both using star patterns and slit cameras. This standard also specified tolerance of the focal spot size, typically allowing the focal spot size to be 50–100% larger than the specified size and yet remain within industrial standards. This standard was recently retired, and has been replaced by IEC standard 60336:2005 [12].

The most common test of the focal spot size is to acquire a magnified image of a star pattern, determine the locations in the image where the lines are blurred to invisibility, and calculate the focal spot size based on equations given in XR-5. One challenge in performing this test is selecting the appropriate radiographic magnification to use. If the magnification is too small, no blur is visible. If the magnification is too large, the blur radius corresponds to the second zero crossing of the modulation transfer function (MTF) rather than the first, and the focal spot size estimate is too small by approximately a factor of two. The lower limit on acceptable magnification is tighter in digital image receptors than with film/screen cassettes or industrial film, due to the lower inherent spatial resolution.

3.2.1.10 Beam Quality Assessment (Half-Value Layer)

The aluminum half-value layer (HVL) of a beam, the amount of aluminum required to reduce the exposure by 50%, is affected both by the amount of filtration in the beam and, minimally, by tube aging. Thus, this measurement is useful because insufficient filtration will result in excessive skin dose to the patient, and because an increase in HVL can indicate that a tube is nearing the end of its useful lifetime [7].

The HVL can be measured using an ionization chamber simply by determining the amount of aluminum required to reduce the measured air KERMA by 50% for identical technical factors. In recent years, radiologic multimeters have become common; these devices will indirectly measure the air KERMA, tube voltage, and HVL in a single exposure.

3.2.1.11 Tube Output Versus kVp

The output exposure of the tube is measured at a specified distance from the focal spot at various tube voltages. The ratio of the output exposure rate to tube current is calculated and recorded. The results are used in patient dosimetry, and also compared to previous measurements and/or typical results (e.g. Table III of AAPM Report 25 [9]).

3.2.1.12 Grid Alignment

A misaligned anti-scatter grid will have suboptimal primary radiation transmission, resulting in reduced contrast-noise ratio and increased patient dose. The primary transmission can vary across the image, which in chest radiography can mimic pathology. The conventional test for grid alignment is based on the FDA requirement that the central ray of the x-ray field be normal to the patient table. However, this test is not sensitive to errors such a lateral offset of the grid, or a tilt caused by an error in installation. AAPM Task Group 150 is expected to recommend grid alignment tests that can detect these errors.

3.2.1.13 Linearity of Exposure Versus mA or mAs

The tube output per time should be directly proportional to the tube current (mA), and the integrated tube output should be directly proportional to the current-time product (mAs). In practice, this can fail on vintage equipment for short exposures due to overshoot or undershoot of the tube current curve, and for long exposures due to excess discharge of supply capacitors. Similarly, the mechanism for setting the tube current can be non-linear, causing an error in the tube output rate as the tube current is changed. Thus, it is necessary to measure the tube output for a variety of tube currents and exposure times, and verify that the tube output is proportional to the current-time product. Modern high frequency generators rarely, if ever, demonstrate exposure non-linearity [7].

3.2.1.14 Exposure Reproducibility

In the film/screen era, exposure reproducibility was a critical test. If the dose to the image receptor was significantly higher or lower than desired, the film would be overexposed or underexposed, possibly requiring a repeat of the exam. Thus, a standard test was to measure the tube output for a set of repeated exposures under identical conditions, often with AEC operation [7].

The test is less critical with digital image receptors due to the high dynamic range of the receptor; however, excessive tube output variation still can be a symptom of system failure. Due to the feedback mechanisms in high frequency generators, few failures are discovered clinically.

3.2.1.15 Timer Accuracy

In older equipment, the exposure was terminated electronically or mechanically after a preset time. The components used in these circuits were prone to failure. Devices measured the time of an exposure by counting pulses or detecting the rising and falling edges of the exposure. These measurements were compared to the value displayed by the acquisition unit and/or the value set by the operator. Digital components of modern generators yield few timer accuracy failures [7].

3.2.1.16 Equipment Radiation Safety Functions

In radiographic units, two systems are used specifically for patient radiation safety: the positive beam limitation (PBL) system and the backup timer [3, 7, 9].

The PBL device senses the size of the image receptor and constrains the collimator to keep the radiation field within its sensitive area. This is tested partly by the collimation alignment test (see Section 3.2.1.6), but also by verifying that the size of the light field changes appropriately as different image receptors are placed in the Bucky. For integrated digital systems, there is often a field size control that will determine the active area of the detector; the light field size should vary in response to changes in this control.

The backup timer is used to ensure that the exposure will last no longer than a predetermined fixed time (typically several seconds), even when there is an electronic failure in the manual timer or the AEC system, or there is an unexpected radiopaque object in the beam during AEC operation.

3.2.1.17 Patient Dose Monitoring System Calibration

Film/screen systems provided almost immediate feedback to the technologist when excessive or insufficient radiation was used in an exam: the film would be overexposed or underexposed. However, the advent of digital image receptors has partially decoupled image quality from patient dose. While insufficient dose to the image receptor will result in lower image quality by increased noise, excessive dose will result in improved image quality so long as the dose is not so high that the detector saturates. The ranger over which the detector signal remains linear with incident exposure is very large, covering several orders of magnitude. Over much of this range, the change in noise properties may be imperceptible and the image quality only improves until detector saturation is reached [7].

Consequently, digital imaging systems generally provide a measure of the detector dose; these can be used to identify situations where patient dose is excessively high. This is useful only if it is monitored through a continuous quality program, and if the dose indicator is behaving properly. Thus, it is the responsibility of the QMP to ensure that there is a system in place to monitor the dose indicators, and to verify that the dose indicators are working properly.

3.2.2 Qualimetry

3.2.2.1 Image Artifacts

For this test, an image is taken of a flat-field image and examined for artifacts. With film/screen imaging, image interpretation was fairly easy; an artifact was either visible or invisible. With digital imaging, the visibility of most image imperfections can be adjusted by changing the display contrast (e.g. through the window width setting). With inappropriate settings, most malfunctioning image receptors can be made to pass, and any working image receptor can be made to fail. AAPM Report 150 is expected to provide recommendations in adjusting window settings for appropriate artifact tests in digital systems. Of greatest importance is to ensure that artifacts neither mimic pathology in an image nor mask it, making correct interpretation of the image difficult or impossible [7].

3.2.2.2 Digital Image Receptor Performance

Some manufacturers of digital radiographic systems provide automatic tests involving custom radiographic test objects to validate the proper performance of the image receptor, testing characteristics such as uniformity, spatial resolution, and contrast to noise ratio. AAPM Report 93 provides recommendations for vendor-independent tests of computed radiographic image receptors. However, the AAPM has never issued a report on testing flat panel digital image receptors. The need for such a report formed the impetus for forming AAPM Task Group 150, and description of tests for flat panel detectors is expected to form a considerable part of AAPM Report 150 [7].

3.2.2.3 Video and Digital Monitor Performance

Most monitor testing involves qualitative analysis of a test pattern (such as the Society of Motion Picture and Television Engineers [SMPTE] test pattern or the TG18-QC test pattern), which provides a set of regions of different luminance, plus spatial resolution (line pair) test regions. The most typical tests using this pattern are measurements of maximum and minimum luminance, verification that all displayed gray levels are distinct, and measurement of the limiting resolution. These tests were originally developed for analog cathode ray tube (CRT) displays, but continue to be useful for digital displays [7, 13].

In 2005, AAPM Task Group 18 released AAPM Online Report 3, which describes test procedures and recommended action limits for digital display monitors, both secondary (acquisition) and primary (diagnostic) displays. A major innovation was the recommendation that displays be compliant with the DICOM Grayscale Standard Display Function (GSDF), which is intended to improve perceptual linearity of the displayed images and maintain consistency between monitors.

3.2.3 Radiometry

3.2.3.1 Entrance Skin Exposure

The medical physicist should determine the entrance skin exposure for various routine procedures and compare them to established diagnostic reference levels [14]. This is typically done by measuring the ratio of exposure rate to tube current at a variety of tube voltages, determining the tube voltages and current-time products for the procedures (either using a technique chart, review of actual patient exams, or using anthropomorphic phantoms), and then calculating the entrance skin exposure. For exams controlled by AEC systems, anthropomorphic phantoms or phantoms with standard tissue equivalence can be used [15].

3.3 Testing Paradigm and Clinical Implementation

Facilities generally should follow a three phase testing paradigm, as outlined in the 2011 ACR document "ACR Technical Standard for Diagnostic Medical Physics Performance Monitoring of Radiographic and Fluoroscopic Equipment" [7]. These phases include acceptance testing, periodic (usually annual) QC testing, and continuous quality testing. Continuous quality testing may involve tests to be done on a daily, weekly, monthly, or quarterly basis.

The first two phases, acceptance testing and periodic testing, are done by a QMP, while continuous quality testing is generally done by a technologist.

Table 3.2 (above) provides examples of when different tests may be performed. Note that when major components of a system are replaced (e.g. x-ray tube, image receptor, software upgrade), it is important to perform the appropriate subset of acceptance tests.

3.4 Med Phys 1.5

The continuing changes in radiographic QC are driven largely by the widespread adoption of digital imaging technologies coupled with the improved dependability of high frequency, digitally controlled generators. Tests that have been modified or created in response include five broad categories:

1) Generator performance tests
2) Tests of the digital image receptor performance
3) Tests that make use of the dynamic range or the quantitative nature of digital image receptors
4) Digital image processing evaluation
5) Verification of the interface between the digital radiographic system and the digital environment – that is, the radiology informatics system (RIS) and picture archiving and communications system (PACS) systems.

3.4.1 Generator Performance Tests

As has been alluded to above, improved generator design and performance are causing many of the historically performed and regulatorily driven tests of the generator performance moot. Many aspects of the generator, such as mA/mAs linearity, kVp accuracy and timer accuracy have very low probability of failure once a system has been confirmed to have been installed and calibrated correctly. A failure of one of these tests is typically combined with some much more catastrophic, and more obvious failure that would be observed during clinical use of the unit rather than during annual performance evaluation.

3.4.1.1 Tests of the Digital Image Receptor Performance

To date, most tests of the digital image receptor have been vendor provided tests. However, there is merit in the ability to perform quantitative tests independently of the vendors. A significant challenge in performing such tests is the amount of processing that that a digital image undergoes between acquisition and storage; which may make it difficult or impossible to use these images to evaluate the behavior intrinsic to the digital detector. To meet the needs of the medical physicist, NEMA has released standard XR-29-2015 [16], providing for the export of "Original Data" images ("For Processing" images in DICOM terminology). These are images with a minimum amount of processing (typically gain and offset correction only), so the pixel value has a well-defined relationship to the detector dose; this is necessary for quantitative analysis to be physically meaningful.

3.4.1.2 Tests that Make Use of the Digital Image Receptor

Some useful tests were not routinely performed because of the difficulty in accomplishing them with film/screen cassettes. One such example is the test of off-focus radiation. This is radiation from parts of the x-ray anode other than the focal spot that can contribute to an overall reduction in contrast to noise ratio. Off-focus radiation can be removed from the beam by the use of a small precollimator close to the focal spot. However, it may be possible to accidently omit this precollimator when a new tube is installed. This condition can be detected by acquiring a pinhole radiographic image of the anode. The small dynamic range of film/screen cassettes made this impractical; however, the test is fairly simple with a digital detector.

On the other hand, the use of digital image receptors has made the measurement of focal spot sizes using a star pattern more difficult; this is because digital image receptors generally have poorer spatial resolution than film/screen cassettes, and much poorer spatial resolution than direct film. If the radiographic magnification of the star pattern is inadequate, the blur pattern may be hidden by the intrinsic spatial resolution of the image receptor leading to an overestimate of the focal spot size. This may be prevented by increasing the magnification; however, if the magnification is too large the first blur radius may be larger than the radius of the image of the star pattern. If the lines are not resolved at all, an estimate of the focal spot size is impossible; if the lines are resolved up to the second blur radius, the focal spot size will be overestimated by a factor of two.

3.4.1.3 Tests of the Digital Network Interface

Interoperability tests are an important part of the acceptance test of the modern digital radiographic system. In a new installation, these may be the tests most likely to fail an acceptance test, due the large number of problems (in the system and in the network) that can cause interoperability failures.

Typically, this involves testing the connection to the Radiology Information System, and thus ensuring that the acquisition workstation displays ordered patient exams appropriate to the system, and does not display ordered exams that are inappropriate (e.g. different modality or different facility). It is also important to verify that images are sent to the PACS system properly after an exam has been performed. Specific attention should be paid to the integrity of the processed image on the PACS to ensure that all lookup table references have been transmitted and interpreted properly.

References

1 AAPM (1977). *Report 4*. AAPM.
2 AAPM (1985). *Report 14*. AAPM.
3 AAPM (2002). *Report 74*. AAPM.
4 AAPM (2006). *Report 93*. AAPM.
5 AAPM (2009). *Report 116*. AAPM.
6 Gray, J.E., Archer, B.R., Butler, P.F. et al. (2005). Reference values for diagnostic radiology: application and impact. *Radiology* 235 (2): 354–358.
7 ACR (2011). *ACR Technical Standard for Diagnostic Medical Physics Performance Monitoring of Radiographic and Fluoroscopic Equipment*.
8 *Code of Federal Regulations 21CFR1020.31*(n.d.).
9 AAPM (1988). *Report 25*. AAPM.
10 NEMA (1992). *Standard XR 5–1992 (R1999)*. NEMA.

11 Shepard, S.J., Wang, J., Flynn, M. et al. (2009). An exposure indicator for digital radiography: AAPM Task Group 116 (executive summary). *Medical Physics* 36 (7): 2898–2914.

12 IPEM (2005). Report 91. IPEM.

13 AAPM (n.d.). *Online Report 03*. AAPM.

14 *IEC 60336:2005* (2005).

15 AAPM (1990). *Report 31*. AAPM.

16 AAPM. (2015). *Report 151*.

17 Gray, J., Archer, B., Butler, P. et al. (2005). Reference values for diagnostic radiology: application and impact. *Radiology* 235 (2): 354–358.

18 NEMA (2016). *NEMA Standard XR-30*. NEMA.

4

Clinical Radiography Physics: Emerging Practice

Jered Wells

Clinical Imaging Physics Group, Duke University, Durham, NC, USA

4.1 Philosophy and Significance

As the oldest and most common of imaging modalities, radiography is ubiquitous in the practice of medical imaging. Its unique combination of speed, high resolution, and cost-effectiveness is so far unrivaled by other modalities. Radiography can also be seen as one of the most heterogeneous modalities in modern medical imaging due in no small part to its many varied applications, but also to the inconsistency with which clinical radiographic care is delivered. Despite its rich history, prevalence, and apparent simplicity, radiographic projection imaging is fraught with nuance, intricacy, and variability that complicate clinical utilization, testing, troubleshooting, and optimization. These challenges have exposed a great need for more comprehensive, relevant, and clinically integrated physics support.

4.1.1 The Clinical Relevance of Physics Testing

Historically, the *modus operandi* of physics support for radiographic installations has been centered on the assurance that imaging systems perform adequately from a purely mechanical perspective. This level of support is also the focus of the majority of state and federal regulations. There is actually some evidence that modern radiographic equipment, in an effort to explicitly ensure regulatory compliance and safety, may in fact be over-tested [1]. For example, radiation output reproducibility has an exceedingly low rate of failure on modern x-ray equipment. On the other hand, tests of automatic exposure control (AEC) performance, which is central to the use of these systems, fail much more frequently. As modern and more stable equipment replaces older systems, mismatches between equipment testing and failure frequency results in suboptimal physics QA effort and possibly missed opportunities for impending failure detection. Newer technologies with notably lower compliance failure rates for basic output testing may fail in new ways which conventional tests do not adequately predict or even detect.

While federal and most state regulations cover many aspects of exposure-centric radiographic performance, there are some aspects of modern digital system performance standards that are inadequately mandated or absent altogether – image quality is a principle example. Organizations such as The National Institute for Occupational Safety and Health (NIOSH) rely on enhanced

Clinical Imaging Physics: Current and Emerging Practice, First Edition. Edited by Ehsan Samei and Douglas E. Pfeiffer.

performance standards (Appendix A of 20 CFR 718.102) for images designated for evaluation and diagnosis of pneumoconiosis (a.k.a. asbestiosis, silicosis, and coal workers' pneumoconiosis or "Black Lung Disease"). However, generalization of these image quality requirements for all radiographic systems has not been observed, and the specific requirements may not be applicable to all (i.e. non-chest) radiographs. Additional attempts at establishing enhanced performance standards in radiography by the American College of Radiology (ACR) have been discontinued largely due to the difficulties posed by the aforementioned variability in the radiography landscape. This presents an opportunity for physicists to develop more relevant tests and tools for interrogating those system features that have a greater overall impact on clinical image quality and care, areas where opportunities for optimization are often missed due to an over-reliance on outdated regulations and compliance requirements.

4.1.2 Physics Support and the Clinical Need for MP 3.0

As clinical physics support transitions from compliance assurance to an operational resource, a balance between what is practical and what is actually useful must be achieved. The standard for physics service has been equipment focused for some time, but adequate mechanical performance does not always translate directly to adequate delivery of patient care. On the one hand, system components should be tested in isolation such that no single part exceeds predetermined bounds deemed clinically tolerable. This is the essence of medical physics 1.0 (MP 1.0) and will continue to be an important precursor to MP 3.0 support. At the same time, the adequacy of individual sub-systems does not necessarily ensure high quality of the radiographic deliverable – an x-ray image of diagnostic quality at a reasonable dose. This is the major challenge set before the MP 3.0 consultant: what *quantifiable* indications are most significant, and how can they be used to create *positive* clinical change?

Moreover, MP 3.0 has an even greater mandate in radiography to approach the challenge of ensuring not only the quality of care, but also the consistency with which this quality is delivered. Achieving "high quality" means little if excessive uncertainty and inconsistency cause provider and patient confidence to waver. Therefore, successful implementation of the MP 3.0 mindset will require medical physicists to bridge the knowledge gap between physicists, physicians, technologists, administrative staff, and patients. These previously siloed entities will need to share their expertise in the formation of more comprehensive solutions toward the integration of new technologies into new and existing imaging enterprises. With these challenges in mind, radiography is a modality ripe with opportunity to embody the ethos of MP 3.0.

4.2 Metrics and Analytics

4.2.1 Intrinsic Performance

MP 1.0 has historically done a good job assuring proper performance of the mechanical core of x-ray units. Annual physics testing of radiography machines can help to isolate problems with individual sub-systems or components which may otherwise go undetected during normal clinical use and regular preventative maintenance. However, even if each individual component of an x-ray imaging system is performing to specification, this does not necessarily ensure optimality of machine use, technique prescriptions, or image outcomes. The following examples highlight these points and provide recommendations for implementing impactful changes in the clinical operation.

4.2.1.1 HVL

The minimum half value layer (HVL) test is a common MP 1.0 task as it is a regulatory requirement for system performance. The regulation is designed to prevent the utilization of excessively soft beams with a preponderance of low-energy photons which contribute to patient dose rather than the formation of a diagnostic image. To meet regulatory requirements, HVL can be increased through the addition of "spectral filters" in the x-ray beam. This often takes the form of small thin aluminum sheets added between the tube output port and collimator assemblies to ensure a passable minimum HVL. Further beam hardening can also offer some dose-saving benefits. In adult lung imaging, additional filtration (e.g. 0.2 mm Cu) is merited to reduce entrance skin exposure (ESE) without significant loss of image quality [2]. While sophisticated manipulation of kVp and beam filtration can be performed to optimize the image quality-dose tradeoff, it is left to the realm of MP 3.0 to validate and verify that appropriate kVp and filter combinations are deployed across the radiographic protocol space. Some machine databases may automatically cycle extra filtration into the beam, and it is important to survey at least some protocols to get a sense of filter appropriateness on the basis of patient size and habitus, anatomical region, and diagnostic task. In the case of extremity and bone imaging, much of the photon flux responsible for providing bone contrast in the photoelectric range of energies is attenuated by added beam filtration. Both newborns and geriatric patients tend to have low bone mineralization resulting in lower bone contrast relative to older children and adults. Therefore, despite the dose-saving benefits, adding beam filtration to some pediatric and geriatric bone studies may be ill-advised due to unacceptable image quality detriment.

4.2.1.2 Automatic Exposure Control

The AEC is a useful tool for providing consistent detector exposure, and it merits special attention for its critical role in the imaging chain. Chapter 3 nicely outlines a quality assurance program for intrinsic performance of the AEC system. Assuming adherence to this plan, the opportunity for MP 3.0 is in the application of AEC in the clinical workflow. Even a perfectly tuned AEC system, if used incorrectly, can result in suboptimal image quality. It is in the clinical interest that physics support of devices with AEC include some education for technologists about the hardware and how it can be best adapted to the diagnostic demands specific to individual imaging protocols and utilized on systems with different detector technologies. More discussion and an example on this topic can be found in Section 4.2.3.

4.2.1.2.1 AEC Speed Settings The concept of "speed" may be an antiquated term to those unfamiliar with screen-film imaging. Film speed is a measure of film sensitivity to radiation. Although many factors can affect film speed, it is primarily related to the size of silver halide film grains, emulsion thickness, and the presence of radiosensitive dyes. As a result, the term film speed is related not only to dose, but also resolution and image density as well. This was paired with intensifying screens that had their own speed, dependent upon phosphor crystal compound, phosphor crystal size, phosphor thickness, and reflective layers.

Modern digital imaging systems have largely decoupled resolution and image grayscale density effects from dose, and as such, it may not be appropriate to assign a "speed" to digital systems [3]. However, AEC target exposure continues to be characterized in terms of its speed-equivalent setting on some systems. Put simply, the speed of a detector can be equated to target detector exposure (in accordance with ISO 9236 standards) using the equation $S = 1000/K_S$ where S is speed as a function of incident air kerma K_S defined in units of μGy [4, 5]. Although this equation is in some ways an over-simplification of the concept of film-screen system speed, it is adequate to bridge the historic concept to the modern need to maintain proper target detector exposure.

Using the above definition, speed equivalence can be assigned to modern digital detectors. In general, most computed radiography (CR) devices should be exposed at roughly 200 speed-equivalent while most CsI-based digital flat panel detectors (FPDs) provide adequate images at approximately 400 speed-equivalent. One way to validate and fine tune exposure speed equivalency assignments can be achieved by obtaining the detective quantum efficiency (DQE) of the detector in question and comparing its DQE(0) to the DQE(0) and speed-equivalence of other clinically deployed AEC and detector combinations that deliver acceptable image quality. Under the assumption of detector linearity, a simple equation relating speed and target exposure of two detectors can be derived as $S_2 = S_1 X_1 / X_2$ or, in terms of DQE, $S_2 = S_1 DQE_2(0)/DQE_1(0)$. Such considerations are paramount as facilities upgrade older CR devices to more radiosensitive digital FPDs.

4.2.1.2.2 Protocols Protocol-specific modification of the AEC has important clinical consequences. For instance, consider the different demands of scoliosis imaging. A post-surgical diagnostic image of hardware installation requires high contrast-to-noise ratio (CNR) to detect infection or malfunctions (breaks) associated with bone screws set in the vertebral bodies. By comparison, the minimum image quality thresholds for back brace fitting and Cobb angle measurement are far lower since the detail of interest is the gross curvature of the spine, which can be adequately visualized at substantially lower exposure. The AEC speed may, therefore, be modified according to the image quality requirements of the diagnostic task.

Another protocol-specific consideration related to AEC use is the differential activation of photocells. The AEC photocells in general radiography are commonly arranged according to the schematic in Figure 4.1. This arrangement allows exams of variable anatomy and field size to be imaged appropriately. For instance, adult anterior–posterior (AP) and posterior–anterior (PA) lung images are typically acquired with cells 1 and 2 active in order to achieve the target detector exposure and image quality within the anatomy of interest – the lungs. Activation of cell 3 in this instance would increase the exposure, perhaps unnecessarily, as it compensates for reduced penetration through the mediastinum. On the other hand, if the interpreting physician requires good coincident visualization of the mediastinum and lungs, it may be appropriate to activate all three cells simultaneously so long as the exposure is not so high as to cause signal saturation in the more radiolucent lung regions. The vast majority of other AEC exams are acquired with only cell 3 active, although

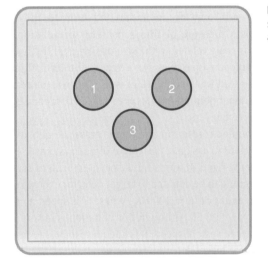

Figure 4.1 Typical AEC cell arrangement superimposed on a wall Bucky schematic. Similar arrangements can also be found in table Buckys.

images of larger patients with larger field of view (FOV) may benefit from simultaneous activation of all three photocells to achieve a more appropriate exposure over the larger active area of the detector. Whatever the case may be, the anatomy of interest should always completely overlap the active AEC cells in order to deliver an image with appropriate signal to noise ratio (SNR) in the target regions (see Section 4.4.1.1).

4.2.1.2.3 AEC Artifacts All MP 1.0 and 3.0 AEC testing recommendations up to this point have regarded some assessment of the intrinsic performance of the AEC cell response. Ensuring adequate AEC cell response implies adequate detector exposure, which in turn implies diagnostically acceptable quantum mottle manifesting as image noise. However, it is possible for the AEC photocells to negatively impact image quality by actually appearing in patient images. Figure 4.2 demonstrates how the opacity of some photocells can cause artifacts in images, especially images of smaller anatomy or anatomy with low inherent contrast. The threshold at which the photocell artifact becomes unacceptable may be determined by the physicist with conventional measures of image uniformity. However, this should be paired with understanding the interpreting radiologist's ability to ignore such artifacts, the degree to which artifacts appear in actual clinical images, and what level of artifact is generally achievable in practice.

4.2.1.3 Exposure Indicator

The exposure indicator (EI) is a necessary quality control (QC) tool in modern digital radiography [6]. Whereas film sensitivity and darkening used to limit radiographic exposures to a narrow acceptable range, the wide detector latitude and availability of post-processing afforded by digital receptors have transformed radiographs obtained with otherwise unacceptable techniques into images of diagnostic quality. In one sense, EI is a surrogate measure for film darkening as it is based primarily on the average pixel gray scale response of "raw" pixel values, which is in turn proportional to incident detector exposure. However, in practice, EI has a more useful interpretation as an index for tracking the relative noise present in a digital radiograph. This makes EI one of

Figure 4.2 AEC photocells appear on a flat field table Bucky image. Window and level were set to highlight the artifact.

the few tools widely available for the *objective* monitoring of image quality outcomes in digital radiography.

Despite its importance to clinical radiography practice, EI has received little regulatory attention and even within the testing protocols of many medical physicists. Historically speaking, the variety of vendor-specific EI formulations has been immense. Only recently have standardized recommendations become available by the American Association of Physicists in Medicine (AAPM) and the release of IEC 62494 [7]. However, without regulatory oversight of EI compliance to existing standards, it is left to the physicist to recommend and enforce compliance and make the proper recommendations for EI conformance to achievable norms. When possible, this may include upgrading or switching equipment settings to report the International Electrotechnical Commission(IEC)-compliant value to standardized EI reporting across an imaging enterprise. In general, regardless of EI formulation, it is important for EI to be properly calibrated and ensure its utility as a reliable indicator of image quality and an indicator of patient dose appropriateness.

4.2.1.3.1 *Factors Affecting EI Accuracy*

To maximize the clinical utility and operational consistency in EI interpretation, one must first ensure that EI is properly calibrated on all digital radiography units. In general, EI accuracy to within 10% error is achievable while EI error exceeding 20% suggests that recalibration may be necessary. There are a number of reasons to suspect that the EI may be delivering inaccurate readings. Detector sensitivity and pixel value response may drift over time leading to concurrent drift of the EI accuracy, but outright EI miscalibration is also a possibility.

One common source of EI error and miscalibration is improper management of scatter radiation. Specifically, IEC 62494 requires that EI calibration exposure readings be made with backscatter rejection practices [7]. If, for instance, the EI is calibrated using an ion chamber (IC) in direct contact with the image receptor, the exposure reading will be higher than expected – generally by about 25–30%. Unfortunately, some units calibrated to manufacturer specifications are subject to this type of systematic calibration error [8]. Because the backscatter radiation is detected only by the (unshielded) IC and not the detector itself, this leads to over-reporting of the EI, which in turn may prompt unnecessary changes to acquisition technique factors in clinical practice. Figure 4.3 illustrates that, when using an unshielded IC device, it is important to use an air gap to reduce the amount of backscatter radiation reaching the dosimeter (in conjunction with any necessary inverse square corrections). By contrast, lead-backed solid state (SS) dosimeters are designed to reject backscatter radiation incident on the back of the dosimeter. Therefore, it is not necessary to implement an air gap when using shielded dosimeters. This discrepancy highlights the importance of understanding not only vendor protocols and claims, but also the impact that different dosimetry devices have on the final measurements used to calibrate values such as EI [9].

Apart from gross miscalibration, EI reporting failures can manifest for a number of reasons, some outside the control of clinical staff. EI performance, because of its inherent dependence on the detector radiation response, may change as a function of kVp, beam hardness, etc. This in turn can affect the reported EI and recommended EI ranges in clinical images. EI computation is also highly anatomy-dependent, relying heavily on image segmentation, histogram analysis, and region of interest (ROI) definition. Segmentation errors are a principle source of misleading EI reporting. The misidentification of target anatomy and histogram analysis errors can yield unacceptable EI values for otherwise acceptable images, and *vice versa*. Other variables such as hardware in the FOV, grid use, collimation, shuttering, patient positioning, and modification of technique factors all may impact the reported EI, and it is for these reasons that EI should be used with a degree of

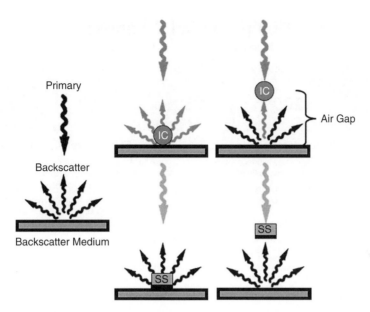

Figure 4.3 Illustration of exposure measurements involving primary and backscattered radiation measured using an unshielded ion chamber (IC) versus a lead-backed solid state (SS) device. Radiation colored in red and blue represents signal detectable by the IC and SS devices, respectively.

caution. Awareness of these variables and their potential impact on image quality indicators can ultimately improve the clinical utilization of EI.

4.2.1.3.2 EI and Clinical Consistency Regardless of the EI formulation used, compliance from an MP 3.0 perspective means first ensuring that EI is being reported accurately as a function of detector exposure so that it can be used in a manner sufficiently similar to the IEC standard. Only then can it be used to improve consistency in patient care. In practice, technologists must be educated on how to use EI as a tool to discriminate between acceptable and unacceptable images and technique factors. Figure 4.4 provides a sample clinical posting that can be used to provide target EI exposure levels consistent with the radiographic technology in addition to a range of acceptable EI values to improve clinical consistency in the quality of imaging deliverables. With appropriate adaptation, this chart can be amended to suit any EI formulation.

The use of EI as a noise index provides an opportunity to establish an image quality standard for digital radiography rather than establishing a clinical standard based on target detector exposure. This proposal acknowledges that different clinical detection tasks such as nodules, fractures, and foreign bodies do not necessarily require the same target detector exposure to produce a diagnostic image. This implies that the target EI value may change in a protocol-dependent manner. The AAPM and IEC have developed the deviation index (DI), which is promoted as a useful metric for these kinds of situations. The DI provided feedback based on the how close the EI of an image is to the target EI for that imaging protocol. It provides a static target index in the landscape of variable target detector exposures [6, 7]. For units equipped with DI and protocol-specific target EI definitions, the image quality requirements for adequate visualization of different diagnostic tasks can be used as justification for increasing or decreasing the target detector exposure on a protocol-by-protocol basis. Because of advancements like DI, physicists have additional opportunities to make impactful contributions toward the more efficient use of medical radiation in projection radiography.

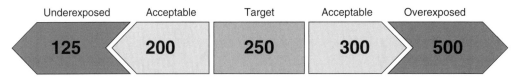

Philips Digital Diagnost
Exposure Indicator (EI_s) Ranges

Underexposed	Acceptable	Target	Acceptable	Overexposed
125	200	250	300	500

EI is below 125 (underexposed)

- **FOR PEDIATRICS**, if image quality is unacceptable, try adjusting image processing settings first.
- **FOR ALL PATIENTS**, if image quality cannot be recovered (e.g. image is too noisy or grainy; relevant anatomy not visible), repeat at higher dose–doubling mAs will double the EI.
- Example: EI = 63 → Increase mAs by 4x and **REPEAT ONLY IF IMAGE QUALITY IS UNACCEPTABLE**

EI is above 500 (overexposed)

- Take a repeat image at lower dose **ONLY** if the relevant anatomy is "clipped" or "burned out"– halving the mAs will halve the EI.
- Example: EI = 1000 → Decrease mAs by 4x and **REPEAT ONLY IF IMAGE QUALITY IS UNACCEPTABLE**

The exposure indicator (EI) provides an estimate of how much radiation exposure has reached the image receptor – **not patient exposure!** And remember that EI is to be used as a guide - **not an absolute indicator of image quality**. As such, images should not be repeated based on EI values alone, but rather upon assessment of image quality and the clinical utility of images. Also note that EI **may vary according to patient centering, imaging technique (mAs, kVp, collimation, filtration, etc.), anti-scatter grid use, anatomical region, images shuttering, etc.**

Figure 4.4 Sample exposure indicator reference sheet for clinical deployment.

4.2.2 Qualimetry

In the spirit of MP 1.0, individual component performance must be assured. Radiography is fortunate to be a modality of considerable technical development in the way of advanced analytical methods for assessing systems and image quality. Frequency-based image quality metrics such as modulation transfer function (MTF), noise power spectrum (NPS), and DQE are well-established and accepted metrics in the field and are useful for characterizing the detector response to radiation. Measured in accordance with IEC 62220-1-1 specifications [10], these metrics effectively summarize the idealized detector response to a flat field phantom (i.e. filter) placed near the x-ray source. While the MTF, NPS, and DQE can be very useful for characterizing the image quality *potential* of the system, they are often of limited utility in the characterization of system performance as a whole, especially under non-ideal clinical conditions.

While baseline performance analysis is important, the quality of clinical outcomes is not necessarily assured despite the adequacy of the individual components tested in isolation. Confounding factors such as image processing, scattered radiation, and the influence of anatomical variability on image quality are often ignored in exchange for testing simplicity. The addition of ancillary equipment (e.g. antiscatter grids) to the workflow, image processing, and the natural variability within the patient population itself only adds to the uncertainty of image quality outcomes. Ultimately, it is the performance of the imaging system as an integrated whole that yields the deliverable – a medical image of adequate diagnostic quality. It is therefore necessary to design tests and robust metrics that examine the system performance as a whole, and in turn, apply objective numerical analysis of the results to meaningfully modify system performance, prescriptions, and clinical outcomes to suit diagnostic needs.

4.2.2.1 Phantom-Based Image Quality

Image quality phantoms can provide more comprehensive and clinically relevant alternatives to overly idealized MP 1.0 analyses. In the field of imaging physics, phantoms are objects that can be

Table 4.1 Examples of radiography phantoms.

Phantoms	Pros	Cons	Examples
Flat Field	• Simple • Filters are small and easy to transport • Large analysis area	• Inadequate (fine) detail • Not recommended for image processing analysis or optimization	• RQA filtration (e.g. 21 mm Al) [11] • Material slabs (e.g. acrylic or polyethylene)
Geometric	• Generally simple IQ analysis (e.g. CNR) • Different modules for targeted IQ analysis	• Unrealistic (fine) detail • May require custom software for more efficient and objective QC	• LucAl Phantom [12] • Line pair and edge (MTF) test tools • Wire mesh patterns • Contrast-detail arrays • DIGI-13 test device • "Duke" Phantom [13, 14]
Anthropomorphic	• Closely emulate patient anatomy • Good for subjective (e.g. radiologist) assessment	• Expensive • Can be large/heavy • Conventional IQ measures (e.g. CNR) can be difficult	• "Real bone" or "true bone" phantoms • Kyoto Kagaku phantoms

imaged to evaluate, analyze, or optimize the performance of imaging devices by emulating some property of the subject imaged with the device in regular practice. Table 4.1 provides a brief overview of radiographic phantom options organized into three distinct classes: flat field, geometric, and anthropomorphic phantoms. Each phantom class has several distinct benefits and drawbacks regarding its use as a patient surrogate. MTF, NPS, and DQE analyses take advantage of the overall simplicity of flat field phantoms (i.e. filters) to provide a means for convenient and repeatable assessment. Flat field phantoms can also be paired with advanced analytical measures such as the effective DQE (eDQE), which incorporate factors such as acquisition geometry to produce more clinically relatable measures of overall system performance [15]. Geometric phantoms are developed as more detailed alternatives to flat field phantoms by making use of simple geometric shapes that approximate the look of specific imaging tasks or patient anatomy. They may also be outfitted with modules from which the user can make subjective or objective image quality assessments, such as high contrast resolution from line pair phantoms or low contrast resolution from contrast detail phantoms. The most detailed class of phantoms tend to be anthropomorphic phantoms that closely emulate the look of patient anatomy either through use of actual human tissue (e.g. bones) or intricate models manufactured from tissue-equivalent materials.

No matter the phantom used, there is a persistent need to ensure that results derived from their use are sensitive to and correlate sufficiently with patient imaging outcomes. This is, after all, the fundamental purpose of phantom imaging. If, for instance, AEC performance is to be assessed, flat field phantoms are generally sufficient for this purpose. On the other hand, if technique factors and image processing are to be optimized, anthropomorphic phantoms may be necessary. Image processing optimization is a particularly onerous problem due primarily to the context-dependent performance of nonlinear processing components [16]. For this reason, flat field and even geometric phantom results do not tend to correlate well with some aspects of clinical image quality outcomes – texture-based analysis being principle among them. For these reasons, the MP 3.0 physicist should determine the appropriate phantom to use for the application under consideration.

The physicist is further tasked with using an appropriate metric for analysis. CNR is one of the most common metrics favored for its simplicity and good correlation with object conspicuity. However, CNR does have notable shortcomings that are important to acknowledge: it is not sensitive to the effects of noise texture, resolution, object size, object shape, and observer-based object visualization. Knowing these limitations can help to appropriately frame the conclusions drawn from phantom imaging.

Despite their challenges and shortcomings, phantoms and their associated metrology will continue to serve an important role as part of robust QC programs that, under the supervision of an MP 3.0 physicist, can be used to assure consistency across the radiography enterprise [17, 18]. When necessary, physics should be able to defend the use of conventional metrics for phantom analysis, and when conventional metrics prove to be inadequate, research and deploy newer, more appropriate metrics to better inform clinical practice. Regardless of application, the use of phantoms in radiography should ultimately generate *quantifiable* data that can be used toward the *objective* assessment and optimization of radiographic image quality and patient care.

4.2.2.2 Patient-Based Image Quality

Much of physics testing is performed to emulate certain aspects of the clinical application. This has implications on the selection of technique factors, imaging geometry, and phantoms used in routine practice as physicists attempt to *prospectively* interpret how a machine will perform when the time comes to actually image patients. Despite the effort spent mimicking various aspects of the patient imaging scenario, the patient images themselves are the *de facto* "gold standard" for QC in practice. Ongoing QC monitoring of patient image quality on an image-by-image basis is of course constrained by the burdensome nature of sifting through and analyzing dozens, hundreds, and perhaps even thousands of radiographic examinations on a regular basis. But it stands to reason that, despite the many efforts to assure quality through emulation of the clinical practice, patient image outcomes will always differ from, yet ultimately determine the acuity, of any predictive efforts.

Some work has been done to migrate from more phantom-centric methods toward patient-based qualimetry in radiography [19, 20]. These efforts have focused primarily on chest radiography for a number of reasons:

- chest radiography is common
- there are many indications for chest radiography
- images are acquired in ideal (dedicated radiography suites) and non-ideal (bedside) environments
- patient size, habitus, anatomy, and positioning vary widely
- disease state has great impact on the ideal imaging technique
- chest radiography is challenging.

Development of a robust and effective patient image-based QC program requires a number of special provisions and automation. Images must first be made available for analysis, which usually requires communication with a picture archiving and communications system (PACS). Data integrity checks should then be implemented by sorting and filtering exams on the basis of series description, patient position, etc. These types of programs often require some form of segmentation and ROI definition to guide the analysis. An example of automated ROI definition is illustrated in Figure 4.5. Finally, data must be analyzed, often with customized metrics specific to the task being measured. The aforementioned work in patient-based chest radiography employs bandpass filtration to isolate image features specific to a list of image quality metrics that correlate with characteristics inherent to a quality chest radiograph. Macroscopic and microscopic

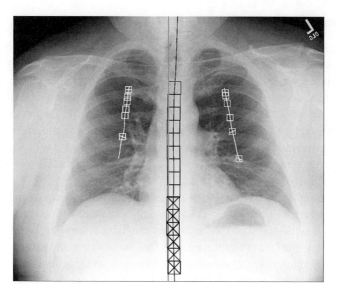

Figure 4.5 Automated ROI definition for patient-based chest image quality assessment.

Table 4.2 Patient-based chest image quality metrics correlated to observer preference.

Macroscopic Metrics	Microscopic Metrics
Lung Gray Level	Lung Detail
Rib-Lung Contrast	Lung Noise
Mediastinum Alignment	Rib Sharpness
Sub-Diaphragm-Lung Contrast	Mediastinum Detail
Sub-Diaphragm Area	Mediastinum Noise

image features shown to correlate strongly with radiologists' perceptions of chest image quality are outlined in Table 4.2.

This type of advanced qualimetry is emblematic of the "high risk/high reward" work that is an example of an MP 3.0 approach. Analysis of *in vivo* chest image quality results across a healthcare enterprise can uncover systematic differences in the quality of images from different devices, clinics, vendors, operators, and patient populations. Identification of significant image quality differences can, in turn, guide the next steps in an appropriate, measured, and scientifically-informed response. Such a QC program extends beyond analysis of parameters and components *intrinsic* to the imaging system; it begins to account for *extrinsic* factors. These extrinsic factors can significantly impact image quality, perhaps even more so than system components investigated during conventional physics testing. The relative impact of factors such as system performance and variability, technologist training, patient positioning, and body habitus can begin to be understood under this framework. Although exhaustive, this type of exercise is needed to ensure optimal utility and management of clinical devices, radiation, personnel, time, and resources.

4.2.3 Radiometry

Radiographic imaging is ubiquitous in medical imaging. It is used frequently for its speed in emergency situations, to monitor patients in recovery, and for screening, notably in mammographic and dental imaging. While radiographic imaging generally carries a low radiation burden, it can range from microsieverts to several millisieverts or more.[1] To this end, some states mandate adherence to established diagnostic reference levels (DRLs) for ESE derived from the literature [21] to provide guidelines for the safe practice of radiography.[2] By contrast, some professional societies take the position that single medical x-ray procedures with effective dose below 50 mSv may have risks too low to be detected. The value of tracking cumulative patient dose is questionable [22], and there are good reasons to *not* track cumulative patient dose, namely patient misperception of radiation risk.

It is also the position of some professional societies that "medical imaging procedures should be appropriate and conducted at the lowest radiation dose consistent with acquisition of the desired information."[3] This is consistent with the "as low as reasonably achievable" (ALARA) principle that has become pervasive in the field of medical imaging.[4] To complicate matters further, there is a distinctive lack of regulatory enforcement of image quality standards, as care providers determine for themselves the adequacy of image quality performance as part of the practice of medicine. Fortunately, medical physicists are uniquely equipped with the skills and understanding to maintain compliance with these mandates. If necessary, the MP 3.0 physicist may even justify the need to exceed established regulatory dose compliance levels. Further, medical physicists should contribute at the legislative level for common sense reform of radiation safety and healthcare laws consistent with the recommendations of healthcare professionals and the need for quality diagnostic imaging in the field.

4.2.3.1 Entrance Skin Exposure

ESE is initially presented in this text as an MP 1.0 concept. While its computation is straightforward, a few simple adaptations of its interpretation can carry this measure of patient exposure forward into an MP 3.0 operation. To do so, it must be understood first and foremost that patient and system-specific *target ESE is not a scalar*: it is a function of several variables such as:

- patient size
- patient composition and disease state
- imaging geometry
- ancillary equipment
- detector technology
- imaging task.

Patient size (thickness) and composition are principle determinants of technique and ESE. Imaging geometry, including aspects such as source-to-image distance (SID), air gap, and field size, will affect the scatter fraction and ultimately the total exposure reaching the detector. Ancillary equipment such as antiscatter grids can dramatically impact image quality and dose. Detector technology, as indicated metrics such as DQE, determines the requisite detector dose to achieve an image of diagnostic quality. Finally, the imaging task is the principle determinant of target image quality and radiation dose required to achieve optimal diagnostic utility. Even identical views of

---

1 https://www.radiologyinfo.org/en/info.cfm?pg=safety-xray.
2 Rules and Regulations – Title 25, Texas Administrative Code §289.227(j).
3 https://www.aapm.org/org/policies/details.asp?id=318&type=PP.
4 https://www.nrc.gov/reading-rm/basic-ref/glossary/alara.html.

the same body region, when imaged for different diagnostic purposes, can have drastically different dose implications. Lung images, for instance, require relatively little dose for adequate visualization, whereas the ribs generally require much higher dose owing to the need for lower kVp to achieve better contrast of the bony detail.

Therefore, rather than simply computing ESE, the clinical utility of this simple measure can be dramatically improved by understanding what constitutes an appropriate ESE as a function of the aforementioned variables. It is not the diagnostic goal to deliver a targeted amount of radiation to the patient. Rather, radiation exposure in radiology is the means to an end – a diagnostic-quality image. This simple fact is a suitable rationale for increasing the ESE as needed for protocols with suboptimal image quality.

4.2.3.2 Dose (Kerma) Area Product

An alternative measure of patient radiation exposure is the dose area product (DAP) – also referred to as kerma area product (KAP). As the name implies, it is the product of radiation dose (to air) and the cross-sectional area of the radiation beam. One major advantage of DAP over ESE is its insensitivity to distance from the x-ray source. Due to the combined effects of the inverse square law for radiation intensity and the proportionality of radiation field coverage area to the square of point source distance, DAP is (relatively) constant with respect to radiation (point) source distance. DAP also has the benefit of being easily translatable to effective dose. Lookup tables provided by Wall et al. provide the means to do just that on a patient-by-patient basis with respect to exam type, view, patient age, and sex [23]. While ESE is translatable to a DAP-like quantity, the calculation requires additional assumptions, measurements, and estimations related to patient thickness, field size, and image acquisition geometry. For these reasons, DAP poses significant benefits over ESE, and the assurance of its accuracy as part of the MP 1.0 canon can lead to meaningful patient radiation risk data gleaned from DAP analysis.

4.2.3.3 Radiometry Caveats

Notwithstanding the benefits offered by DAP and ESE, it behooves the physicist to understand the limitations of both measurements. Modification of beam quality, either by changing the kVp, beam filtration, or both, may impact the interpretation of what constitutes an appropriate ESE or DAP. Furthermore, adequate knowledge of machine output and calibration are necessary for accurate radiometry. The tube output measurements recommended in the Radiography 1.0 chapter may drift over time or after service (e.g. tube change), and ESE estimates should be adapted accordingly. For system-reported DAP, accuracy must be verified if it is to be used as a metric for dose monitoring in radiography with particular note to DAP accuracy as a function of both kVp and beam filtration. The actual patient organ dose implications of changing kVp, beam filtration, and imaging geometry should also be investigated to provide some assurance of dosimetry reliability in the clinical deployment.

4.3 Testing Implication of New Technologies

4.3.1 Hardware

4.3.1.1 Digital Dosimeters

Amid the push toward a MP 3.0 mindset, a strong MP 1.0 core has played, and will continue to play, an important role in radiography quality assurance. Although many technological advancements have propelled radiographic imaging through the past century, many of the standard MP 1.0 tests continue to reveal information critical to maintaining high standards of patient care. The value of these tests can be further enhanced by introducing new dosimetry technologies to the physics workflow. Digital dosimeters can offer deeper insight into the intricacies of system performance while also adding a level of convenience in data collection. Simultaneous assessment of many beam characteristics along with computerized data acquisition have streamlined the testing process over manual data reading and entry. As discussed in Section 4.2.1.3.1, Factors Affecting EI Accuracy, lead-backed SS dosimeters are largely immune to backscatter contamination – an added benefit over ICs that must be carefully positioned to mitigate the effects of backscatter. The availability of kVp and exposure waveforms can also provide a valuable temporal component to data analytics. Figure 4.6 shows two instances of tube output testing with a digital solid-state dosimeter. The two instances show repeated measurements at fixed kVp and mAs and the appearance of a random "double pulse" in the second acquisition. This resulted in doubling of the exposure and elongation of the measured beam duration. While this problem may have also been noted using older dosimetry equipment, the extra information afforded by the digital dosimetry system helped in the root cause analysis effort. It quickly revealed a tomography switch had been erroneously activated during generator service. In this instance, a repair order was completed within 25 hours and was likely accelerated by the availability of additional troubleshooting information that helped to specify the exact source of the problem.

4.3.1.2   (Digital) Detectors and Backscatter Radiation

Even in the age of advanced digital FPDs, backscatter radiation and its deleterious impact on image quality continues to provide imaging physicists with opportunities for clinical quality improvement. Thus far, discussion in this chapter has twice made mention of lead-backed digital dosimeters and their benefits (see Sections 4.2.1.3.1 and 4.3.1.1). Digital image receptors are no exception to the benefits afforded by lead backing, and they are also no exception to the pitfalls of its omission. Figure 4.7 contains a clinical example of the consequences of removing lead backing from the design of a digital FPD in an effort to reduce its weight. Because the lead backing is no longer present to absorb stray radiation, the electronic components behind the radiosensitive plane of the detector cast a shadow in the clinical image. In the spirit of Figure 4.3, Figure 4.8 illustrates the etiology of this "backscatter artifact."

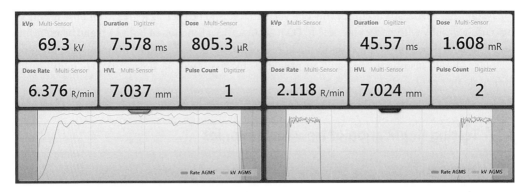

Figure 4.6   Random "double pulse" measured from radiographic tube output testing at RQA5 beam quality. Two sequential acquisitions with identical technique exhibit expected performance (left) and an unexpected "double pulse" with double the dose (right).

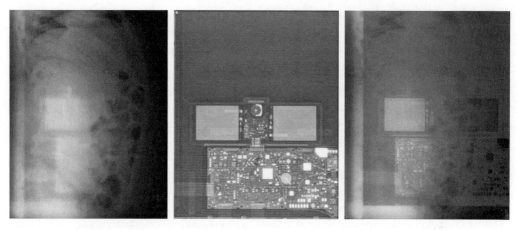

Figure 4.7 Root cause analysis of "backscatter artifact." Cross-table lateral abdomen image (left) containing "backscatter" artifact. Image of the same wireless digital detector (center) exposed through its backside revealing the detector battery and electronics. Registration of the left and center images (right) showing that image artifacts correlate well with the image of the detector electronic components.

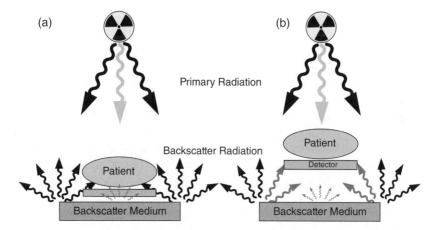

Figure 4.8 Illustration of primary and backscatter radiation detection. Primary radiation incident on the patient and detector is indicated in green while backscatter radiation incident on the detector is indicated in red. (a) Images acquired with the backscatter medium immediately posterior to the detector encounter very little backscatter radiation. (b) Introduction of an air gap behind the detector combined with poor collimation allows excess backscatter to reach the detector resulting in excessive "backscatter" artifact.

Several factors may exacerbate backscatter artifacts:

- **Inadequate (absent) detector backing** – As demonstrated in Figures 4.3, 4.7, and 4.8, the absence of lead backing allows excessive backscatter radiation to reach the detection medium in both dosimeters and image receptors alike.
- **Poor x-ray field collimation** – Figure 4.8 illustrates that poor collimation, directly exposes objects behind the radiographic detector, and can produce large amounts of backscatter radiation that subsequently reaches the back of the image receptor.
- **Poor imaging technique** – Poor technique, especially when combined with poor collimation, can increase the likelihood of backscatter artifact. A very intense backscatter field and subsequent artifact may gain prominence in an image of underexposed patient anatomy.

- **Imaging geometry** – Like other digital detectors, wireless FPDs require regular calibration. If the calibration geometry is not sufficiently similar to that encountered in clinical application, differences in the backscatter radiation field may result in artifacts.

Figure 4.9 shows how the application of lead backing to the wireless digital FPD can reduce the appearance of backscatter artifacts. Based on the physicists' recommendations, this vendor eventually incorporated lead backing into the design of the commercially-available product. This example demonstrates the importance of a solid understanding of fundamental radiation physics. It also demonstrates the potential insufficiency of MP 1.0 tests insofar as they do not always adequately emulate the broad spectrum of clinical imaging scenarios. It would of course be impractical for physicists to test for every eventuality, but this example does expose a gap between the current state of clinical imaging physics practice in radiography and where the field could advance. Combining a rich foundation in radiation physics knowledge with the MP 3.0 mindset can help the imaging physicist to quickly design the correct experiments to troubleshoot and accurately diagnose clinical image quality problems (like backscatter artifacts) with high impact on the delivery of patient care.

4.3.1.3 Clinical Relevance of Physics Test Parameters

While physics testing of system performance characteristics such as exposure reproducibility are mandated, the specific technique factors at which these tests are performed are not. For example, exposure linearity testing is a standard part of any physicists' canon of tests as it is governed by federal regulation per 21 CFR 1020.31(c)(1), but the test may be performed at any number of available combinations of technique settings, some of which may routinely pass inspection and others that may periodically or chronically fail to meet performance standards. It is then left to the discretion of the physicist to decide if a failure at any setting constitutes a failure of the entire system or if a pass at any setting constitutes a pass of the system as a whole. While the former is certainly the more conservative approach, there may be scenarios where more leniency is appropriate. This quandary raises two important questions: which technique factor(s) best represent the performance of the system in clinical practice, and does enforcement of performance standards at these particular settings adequately ensure high clinical quality for the system as a whole?

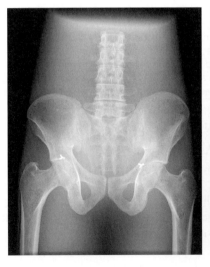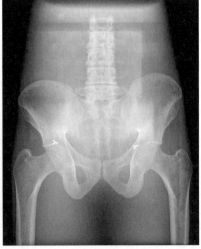

Figure 4.9 Lead backing reduces the appearance of backscatter artifacts in images of a pelvis phantom. Poor x-ray field collimation can result in excessive backscatter artifacts (left). The introduction of lead backing to the detector (right) can mitigate image quality detriment due to backscatter.

Fortunately, the move to digital imaging technologies permits easy auditing of the clinical operation. Using data collected from a dose monitoring system, Figure 4.10 and Table 4.3 were generated to interrogate the radiographic technique factors and demonstrate several notable clinical trends. The predominance of higher kVp imaging is consistent with the high chest imaging

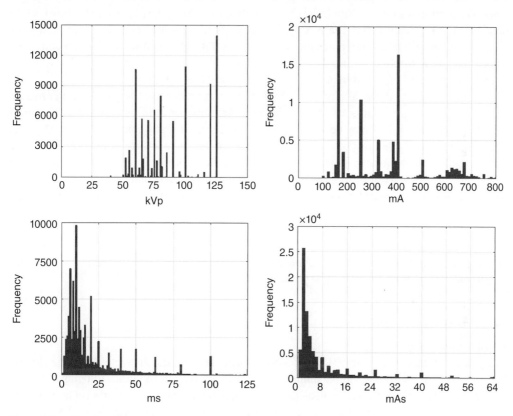

Figure 4.10 Distributions of technique factors across (digital) radiography data collected over four months ($N \approx 95\,960$). Less than 5% of all values exist beyond the charted area for each plot.

Table 4.3 Prevalence of the most common (digital) radiographic technique factors from Figure 4.10. Note that all values represent histogram bin centers rounded to the nearest integer (nearest 10 in the case of mA).

Prevalence	kVp	mA	ms	mAs
1	**125** (15%)	**160** (21%)	**10** (10%)	**2** (27%)
2	**100** (11%)	**400** (17%)	**6** (7%)	**3** (14%)
3	**60** (11%)	**250** (11%)	**8** (6%)	**4** (9%)
4	**120** (10%)	**320** (5%)	**20** (5%)	**1** (6%)
5	**80** (8%)	**380** (5%)	**12** (5%)	**5** (5%)

prevalence.[5] *A priori* knowledge of recommended radiographic technique factors (120 and 125 kVp for standard adult chest series and 100 kVp for portable adult chest images) also supports these findings. The survey of mA stations shows a clear multi-modal distribution which overlaps a more continuous distribution of x-ray tube current settings. The multi-modal distribution consists primarily of mA stations which are preset by two vendors for all manual and AEC imaging while the continuous distribution is derived from mAs and ms values reported by a third vendor that does not explicitly define the mA by default prior to exposure. The positively-skewed ms distribution shows a clear preference for fast exposures. Finally, the mAs distribution and prevalence table show that more than half of all clinical radiographs are obtained using less than 5 mAs, and over 90% of all radiographs are obtained using less than 32 mAs.

Taking into account the wealth of data afforded by a comprehensive dose monitoring program, regular physics testing parameters can be adapted to be more consistent with the regular clinical operation. On one hand, it may be worth running the gamut of many combinations of kVp, mA, and ms settings in the interest of more comprehensive acceptance testing. On the other hand, as part of regular annual quality assurance testing, the physicist may opt to make more efficient use of system downtime by testing a select subset of common parameters that adequately characterize system performance. Regardless of the testing specifics, it is important to (i) understand how the systems and settings are used clinically, (ii) understand what techniques are generally achievable by the system in question consistent with manufacturer recommendations and performance limits, (iii) make efficient and effective use of clinical time, and (iv) ensure that both passes and failures adequately represent anticipated clinical system performance and not the response to obscure technique combinations found only in physics testing.

4.3.2 Acquisition Methods

4.3.2.1 Dual-Energy

The primary use for dual-energy (DE) imaging in radiography is the distinction of bone attenuation from that of soft tissue. Some applications of DE subtraction in chest radiography include discrimination of calcified nodules, detection of vascular disease, and classification of bony lesions, among other uses. Another niche application is DE x-ray absorptiometry (DXA or DEXA) for the estimation of bone mineral content (BMC) and bone mineral density (BMD) in patients at risk of osteoporosis or other bone loss conditions. In the assessment of either application, it is important to understand how the two beam energies are achieved. In digital DE subtraction systems and some DXA systems, two independent pulsed x-ray beams with distinct energies are achieved by fast kV switching. Other DXA manufacturers elect to use a K-edge filter to produce single x-ray beams with two distinct energy peaks distinguished through the use of energy-discriminating detectors (e.g. cadmium zinc telluride). Regardless of DE method, these systems require special exception during testing for accurate physics assessment. For systems with fast kV switching, this may involve forcing the machine to emit single energy pulses in service mode. For systems with K-edge filtering, assessment may be more complicated due to the atypical shape of the x-ray spectrum. Even more forethought should be exercised with regard to how the results of physics testing can be extrapolated to affect a meaningful clinical change. DE radiography requires optimal quality of standard, soft-tissue, and bone images for interpretation to complete the diagnostic task. By

---

5 Chest imaging prevalence of 46–48% estimated from data in DICOM field (0018,0015) Body part Examined and confirmed by keyword search of DICOM field (0008,1030) Study Description

contrast, DXA is a quantitative modality necessitating high accuracy and precision of select numerical indicators of patient health. Therefore, as far as DE imaging is concerned, the application of the technology strongly indicates the need for an MP 3.0 approach to assessment.

4.3.2.2 Tomosynthesis

Typical medical physics testing may pass a system based on the independent performance of individual components, but fail to deliver an adequate evaluation for a specialty imaging product such as tomosynthesis. Both conventional tomography and digital tomosynthesis units require precise tube movement to reliably produce a sharp in-plane image or reconstruction of the target anatomy. Static baseline system geometry tests required by state and federal regulations are insufficient to ensure that the dynamic geometry requirements of tomographic image acquisition are met. Therefore, to assure quality beyond compliance, the MP 3.0 physicist should consider the value of dynamic geometry tests for tomosynthesis. Specialty phantoms are available for this type of testing [24]. Alternatively, the physicist may develop their own device or software for quality assurance.

Physicists should also advise and alert clinical personnel of potential problems with specialty technologies like tomosynthesis and formulate an appropriate response plan if issues do arise. Namely, the effects of patient motion are accentuated by the longer acquisition times; for example, the inability of some patients to maintain a breath hold for the length of time required. Because of the of potential for patient noncompliance, it is important to establish specialty retake/reject policies associated with procedures such as tomosynthesis and other specialty imaging protocols, especially those with a higher dose burden. Pediatric, geriatric, and inpatient populations may be particularly susceptible to compliance issues due to the long imaging times associated with tomosynthesis scans – up to several seconds in some cases. Technologists, physicians, and physicists should collaborate and rationalize the tradeoffs between indications for specialty imaging protocols, their benefits, drawbacks, risks, and alternatives in order to establish an acceptable standard operating procedure such that the patient is best served by the available technology.

4.3.3 Image Processing and Analysis

The following three examples detail opportunities in which clinical medical physics is uniquely positioned to provide much needed support and advice in the way of radiographic image processing. By drawing on basic radiography physics principles and image quality analytics, physics support can yield impactful changes in the image processing workflow.

4.3.3.1 Image Processing Management

Image processing management, especially in a multi-vendor or multi-model environment, is formidable. Not only do different vendors have unique algorithms with unique parameter inputs, but different software releases and system models within the same vendor universe may contain changes that break image processing continuity. While access to tabulated image processing settings is mandated by NEMA/MITA XR 30-2016, individual vendor compliance with this mandate is unreliable, and the format of vendor-specific image processing variable output is irregular [25]. This level of inconsistency within the clinical environment can lead to large discrepancies in the "look" of images across the imaging enterprise. Figure 4.11 shows an example of image processing differences spanning a variety of vendors and x-ray imaging system models. Although the same anthropomorphic phantom has been imaged on each of four digital mobile radiography systems with comparable techniques and baseline detector performance characteristics, image processing discrepancies are largely responsible for disparities in gray level, equalization, and contrast detail

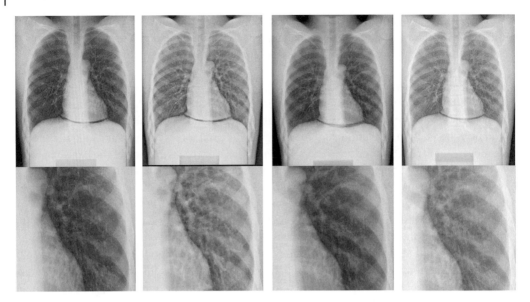

Figure 4.11 Chest phantom images from four digital mobile x-ray units from different vendors. Detail is provided below each radiograph showing the respective retrocardiac and lung regions of each image. There are notable differences in average gray level, equalization, and fine detail contrast, all of which can be modified with image processing adjustment.

in the FOR_PRESENTATION images. The void between static vendor image processing presets and the need for clinical optimization leaves a perpetual opportunity for imaging physicists to engage the clinic at an impactful level. Normalization of the image "look" across systems standardizes radiographic image display and can help to improve diagnostic accuracy, reading efficiency, and reader fatigue [26]. Once satisfactory image processing databases have been established, proper backups and communication with clinical engineers can ensure that the correct machine settings are preserved.

4.3.3.2 Virtual Grids

A notable example of recent development in image processing and analysis has been gridless digital scatter suppression. It is achieved through the use of software-based (Monte Carlo) estimates of the scatter fraction at each pixel for images acquired without a grid. This is desirable for a number of reasons that are summarized in Table 4.4. Vendors with a digital scatter suppression option are often eager to tout the many benefits of these types of technologies and reticent to admit to their limitations. Although digital grids solve the image contrast reduction issues caused by excessive scatter (often matching the contrast improvement fraction of specified grids), vendor claims often neglect to acknowledge other problems such as excess quantum noise. For example, imagine two exams – one is acquired with a grid and the other without. If exposure to the detector is to be maintained, the gridless exam should be acquired with reduced mAs since scatter and primary radiation that would otherwise be stopped by the grid will be allowed to reach the detector. In that scenario, the radiation reaching the detector will have a larger scatter fraction and inferior image quality than the gridded scenario. If both gridded and non-gridded exams are taken at the same detector exposure, the total image signal (and therefore quantum noise) will also be equivalent but the image contrast is not due to excessive scattered radiation which has the effect of reducing subject contrast. To compensate for the loss of contrast, virtual grid software can be applied to selectively

Table 4.4 Benefits and drawbacks of scatter reduction techniques in radiography.

Scatter ManagementTechnique	Pros	Cons
Air Gap	• Simple • No additional hardware	• Greater SID required • Large object magnification • Excess focal spot blur • Small FOV
Grid	• Excellent scatter rejection • Historical precedence • Many options	• Added dose penalty ($T_P < 1$) • Potential for misalignment/misuse • Grid line artifacts
Collimation	• Simple • Reduce excess patient exposure	• Risk of cropping relevant anatomy • Limited effectiveness
Fan-beam (slot scan)	• Excellent scatter rejection • Effectively combines benefits of grids and (extreme) collimation	• Long scan time • Patient motion • Precise detector/source alignment required • Overbeaming often necessary • Dedicated systems only
Digital Scatter Suppression	• Seamless workflow • No misalignment risks • Contrast improvement factor matches actual grid	• Increased noise • Large patient IQ may benefit more from physical grid • Variable performance across vendors

subtract scatter signal from the image. As a result, because the noise remains constant following signal subtraction, the SNR for the gridless exam with digital scatter suppression will suffer a loss in comparison to the gridded exam imaged at equivalent detector dose. To compensate for the loss in SNR, the dose associated with the gridless exam should be increased to deliver a final image with comparable SNR. Otherwise, post processing image noise reduction may be used to compensate for the relative increase in noise at the loss of some resolution [16].

The example of virtual grids is one that embodies the ethos of MP 3.0, as it provides several opportunities for physics to contribute demonstrable clinical value.

1) **Validation of vendor claims** – A few simple calculations can be used to verify what the vendor is claiming while at the same time filling in the gaps to show what the vendor is (in)advertently *not* claiming. For instance, digital scatter suppression is a workflow solution and *not* a dose-saving technology because of the need to increase technique to compensate for excess noise. The imaging physicist should be equipped to prove this point.

2) **Reformulation of technique factors** – It should not be assumed that the same image quality can be achieved simply by replacing physical grids with virtual grids. This implies that some scrutiny of technique factors will be necessary and will likely involve image quality analysis of sample patient images or extrapolation from phantom data.

3) **Adaptation of clinical target EI** – Because excess scatter otherwise stopped by conventional (physical) grids is allowed to reach the detector, target EI values will increase. Also, due to the increased scatter fraction in larger patients relative to smaller patients, the target EI will increase as patient size increases. The physicist should be prepared to justify these claims and educate clinical staff on how to adapt their EI expectations accordingly.

4) **Caveats and precautions** – Bone and metal attenuate radiation much differently than soft tissue at radiographic energies. Therefore, one would expect a virtual grid algorithm to behave differently in image regions containing thick bone and metal (implants). Technologists and radiologists should be advised to scrutinize image quality at bone/metal and tissue interfaces and watch for possible artifacts.

5) **Technological Limitations** – It is not uncommon to encounter scatter fractions near unity in regular clinical practice. The mathematical formulation below shows how grid performance and virtual grid performance in terms of total detector exposure and SNR improvement factor change as functions of scatter fraction. In general, virtual grids are suitable for small patients and low scatter fraction imaging scenarios. But because of the combined constraints from the excess noise associated with virtual grids and detector saturation limits, conventional grids may be a more appropriate recommendation for the largest of patients.

The following are formulations relating common grid parameters primary transmission fraction (T_P), scatter transmission fraction (T_S), total transmission fraction (T_T), selectivity (Σ), scatter fraction (SF), Bucky factor (B), and contrast improvement fraction (C_{IF}) [27]:

$$\Sigma = \frac{T_P}{T_S}$$

$$B = \frac{1}{T_T} = \frac{1}{T_P} \frac{\Sigma}{\Sigma - SF(\Sigma - 1)}$$

$$C_{IF} = \frac{T_P}{T_T} = \frac{\Sigma}{\Sigma - SF(\Sigma - 1)}$$

As mentioned earlier, virtual grids are often used to match C_{IF} of physical grids, and this can be accomplished through selective (scatter) signal subtraction on a pixel-by-pixel basis according to the above formulations. However, according to Poisson statistics, SNR can be estimated in terms of the total number of photons (N) with appropriate modification by SF to yield SNR estimates with and without grid (SNR_0 and SNR_{GRID}, respectively) and SNR improvement factor (SNR_{IF}):

$$SNR_0 = \frac{N(1 - SF)}{\sqrt{N}}$$

$$SNR_{GRID} = \frac{T_P N(1 - SF)}{\sqrt{T_T N}}$$

$$SNR_{IF} = \frac{SNR_{GRID}}{SNR_0} = \frac{T_P}{\sqrt{T_T}} = T_P \sqrt{B}$$

Because a virtual grid stops no photons, the noise associated with the virtual grid image is proportional to $\sqrt{N}$, and the signal of interest is proportional to the number of primary photons $N(1 - SF)$ making the baseline (maximum) SNR associated with the virtual grid image equal to SNR_0. Therefore, as shown in Figure 4.12, the SNR_{IF} associated with the virtual grid image in the best case scenario is unity, and the SNR_{IF} of a typical physical grid is a function of several variables including Σ, T_P, and SF. When $SNR_{IF} > 1$, grid use is recommended, and physical grid performance will exceed that of the

Figure 4.12 Comparison of SNR_{IF} from a hypothetical physical grid ($\Sigma = 7.8$, $T_P = 0.75$) and a virtual grid.

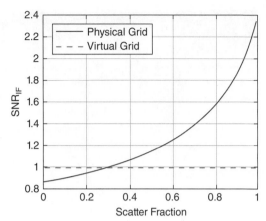

virtual grid in terms of achievable SNR at equivalent technique. To compensate for excess noise, virtual grid images should be obtained with SNR_{IF}^2 times higher exposure than the equivalent physical grid technique to achieve comparable SNR. Note that the techniques for physical grid use are already subject to a recommended increase by Bucky factor B to maintain SNR. As alluded to previously, this can become problematic for high scatter scenarios as the total exposure transmitted through the patient approaches the detector response saturation point resulting in "image burn" artifacts.

4.3.3.3 Rib Suppression

In addition to system- and vendor-specific image processing, third party image processing software can be deployed to provide radiologists with an "enhanced" view of the patient. This software can be implemented several ways, but it usually involves some form of communication with the PACS. One example of third party software performs bone suppression in chest radiographs. This type of software has been shown to improve the identification of lung infiltrates and detection of lung nodules by making lung lesions otherwise obscured by overlying ribs more conspicuous [28, 29]. The challenge for imaging physics is how to analyze the efficacy of this software. Figure 4.13 provides two examples of commercially available bone suppression software performance on clinical images – one optimal and another suboptimal example. Time limitations, complex study designs, radiologist participation, and cost limit the practicality of clinical observer performance studies. Observer models can also be impractical to utilize in the clinical setting. As an alternative, clinical physicists can provide their expertise to scrutinize vendor white papers and collect publications to build an understanding of the software, its purpose, limitations, and how it simplifies, complicates, enhances, or inhibits the existing workflow. While some rudimentary measurements might be performed, it behooves the MP 3.0 physicist to understand how efforts are best spent.

4.3.4 New System Wide Technologies

4.3.4.1 Original Data

In general, compliance with NEMA/MITA XR 30-2016 would mean that physicists have easy access to original data for equitable testing across systems [25]. Despite the efforts of NEMA and the AAPM, universal access to original data (i.e. FOR_PROCESSING images) can still be rather difficult. When testing new systems, information requests often pass through representatives who have little understanding of physics needs and how to satisfy them resulting in testing delays. In the meantime,

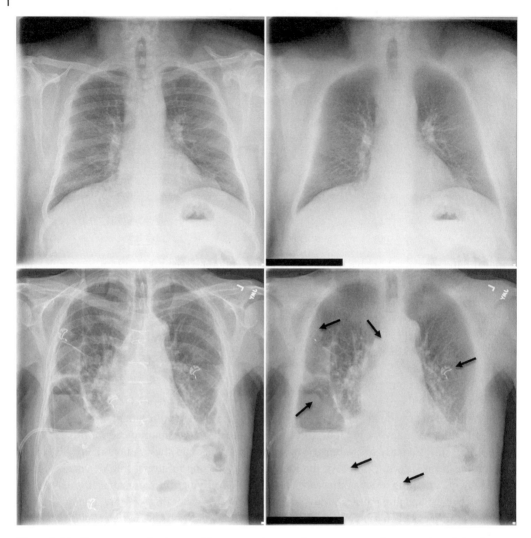

Figure 4.13 Bone suppression images. The top two images demonstrate good suppression of the ribs, vertebrae, and clavicles. The bottom two images provide an example of suboptimal bone suppression performance. The ribs are not completely suppressed in the lower right lung, the spine detail is poorly suppressed below the diaphragm, and various pieces of hardware (EKG leads, tubing, and surgical staples and wires) are subject to varying levels of suppression.

baseline assessments made without access to original data may obfuscate image quality measurements, results, and conclusions. Manufacturers are expected to provide information on original data and its relationship to detector exposure as a part of normal system documentation. Obtaining this system documentation well in advance of testing is recommended. Otherwise, some ad hoc resources (e.g. clinical imaging physics listservs) may be available for troubleshooting purposes.

4.3.4.2 Long Length Imaging

New and sometimes niche technologies can present significant challenges to even the most rudimentary of physics tests. A case study of long-length imaging technologies provides ample evidence to suggest that an MP 1.0 approach is not only insufficient, but potentially misleading when evaluating new imaging technologies. Long-length imaging has two specific applications in radiographic imaging: scoliosis (entire spine) and leg length (entire leg) imaging. There are several commercially available methods for producing images larger than the standard CR or FPD dimensions allow, and a brief overview of each technology, its benefits, and its challenges are presented here for MP 3.0 consideration.

4.3.4.2.1 Slot Scanning Fan beam or slot scanning technology is not new to the radiography landscape. It has been used for decades in niche applications such as panoramic dental imaging and bone mineral densitometry. Although defunct, some dedicated chest imaging systems (Thorascan, Delft Imaging Systems, Veenendaal, Netherlands and Thoravision, Philips Medical Systems, Da Best, Netherlands) [30, 31] have in the past taken advantage of the superior scatter-rejecting properties of the slot scanning geometry to improve the overall quality of lung images. Work in image quality metrology has shown that the clinical performance of slot scanning systems such as these is generally poorly characterized with conventional detector-based metrics such as MTF, NPS, and DQE, the results of which can be misleading [32]. Because the superior image quality attributes of slot scanning systems are achieved through manipulation of the acquisition geometry (as opposed to improvements to the detector), detector-based metrics do not properly characterize the system performance as a whole when clinically deployed. Figure 4.14 shows an example comparison of the contradictory conclusions drawn from DQE and eDQE analysis of a conventional radiographic system and a slot scanning system. By accounting for subject factors such as magnification, primary transmission, and scatter fraction, effective measurements of MTF, NPS and DQE (eMTF, eNPS, and eDQE, respectively) can be derived which are more representative of real-world performance of imaging systems as opposed to measurements of the detector in isolation.

Recently, slot scanning technology has been marketed for some general purpose and long length radiographic imaging applications (EOS Imaging System, EOS imaging, Paris, France). Like its predecessors, the performance of this system is best characterized by replacing conventional MP 1.0 detector-based metrics with their "effective" counterparts. Complicating matters further, factors such as scan speed may be coupled to image quality characteristics like resolution. Figure 4.15

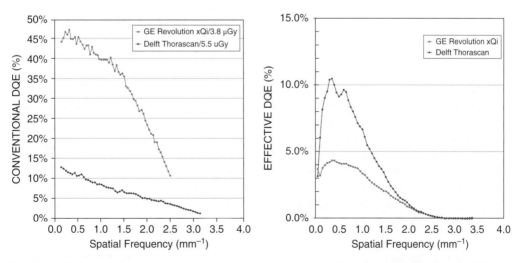

Figure 4.14 Comparison of conventional radiographic and slot scanning systems with DQE and eDQE. Conventional DQE analysis s shows that the conventional radiographic detector is more efficient, however eDQE analysis reveals that the slot scanning system as a whole is superior at rendering the spatial frequencies of most interest. *Source:* Images compliments of A. Mackenzie, K-Care.

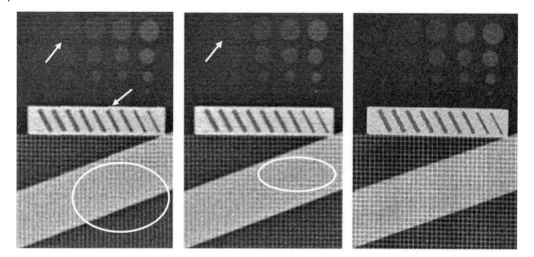

Figure 4.15 Resolution of a slot scanning radiographic system (scanning in the vertical direction) is tempero-spatially and directionally dependent. Red arrows and ovals indicate changes in artifact and resolution performance between fast (left) and slow (center) scan speeds. An image of the same quality assurance phantom with similar filtration, kVp, field of view, and DAP on a conventional FPD system is provided for comparison (right).

shows how resolution of the slot scanning system is not only temporally and spatially dependent but also directionally dependent (as might be expected). Comparison of the resolution performance of the slot scanning device with a conventional FPD radiography system of somewhat comparable native detector pixel pitch (254 and 200 μm, respectively) shows that tube motion and the image formation process are likely contributors to the resolution discrepancies between the imaging systems. Because both resolution and dose are tied to scan speed, care should be taken in protocol design and optimization, and image quality and dose compromises should be carefully communicated to technologists who operate the machinery and must often adapt protocols on a patient-by-patient basis.

Whereas some slot scanning systems (Thorascan and Thoravision) were in the past marketed as dedicated chest imaging systems, a more recent (EOS) slot scanning system has been marketed to also fill the niche of long length imaging of the spine and leg bones. This is a curious move which contradicts the primary image quality benefit of the slot scanning geometry – low-contrast resolution improvement. Figure 4.16 provides an excellent example of how the imaging task should be the ultimate determinant of optimality. In both entire spine and entire leg imaging protocols, bone visualization is the primary task. The bones are inherently high contrast objects against the tissue background, and a device's aptitude for bone visualization is thus best characterized not by the (e) DQE but rather by the (e)MTF. Bone visualization is a contrast-limited task as opposed to low-contrast lesion visualization which is a noise-limited task. The medical physicist should understand this when characterizing imaging system quality as it relates to the imaging application. The metric selected for characterization of system optimality must coincide with the imaging task in order to draw proper conclusions.

4.3.4.2.2 Image Stitching As with slot scanning, some FPD-based long length imaging scans are subject to motion artifact. Several vendors offer long length imaging solutions as add-on packages to conventional digital radiography systems. For upright (wall Bucky) imaging, this generally

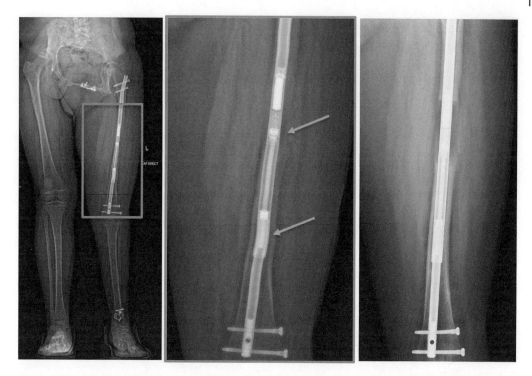

Figure 4.16   Inferior contrast resolution and motion artifact from a slot-scanning long length imaging device compromise the assessment of bone growth and metal hardware (left). The image inset demonstrates poorly visualized bone growth, and the metal implant appears bent as a result of motion artifact (center). This additional conventional radiographic imaging with superior contrast resolution properties and shorter imaging time is required for proper assessment (right).

involves a shoot and translate setup wherein the patient stands in front of a static board while the detector translates and the tube tracks the detector motion.[6] This is then followed by software-based image registration that stitches the separate images together to form a single long view of the anatomy. Perhaps the most obvious vulnerability of such a setup is the possibility of patient motion. Specifically, due to the seconds-long lag between the initial and subsequent images, breath holds may fail and unstable patients may waver. Figure 4.17 shows an example of digital FPD long spine imaging with a failed patient breath hold. The diaphragm is duplicated across the component image junction, and an additional vertebrae has been added into the image, as evidenced by the duplication of ruler markers. The squat appearance of the false vertebral body manifests as a clinically actionable compression fracture. Although this type of problem would likely be difficult to quantify from a physics testing perspective, physics can advise clinicians and administrators to help them understand the likely hardware and software limitations associated with image stitching in addition to variables which may exacerbate the problem such as patient motion, breathing, low exposure, and large patient habitus.

4.3.4.2.3   Long Length CR and Digital FPDs   Perhaps the most obvious solution to circumvent motion-related problems associated with image stitching would be the exposure of a single

---

6 Similar (less common) setups are also available in table Buckys for supine long length imaging.

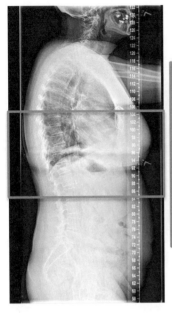
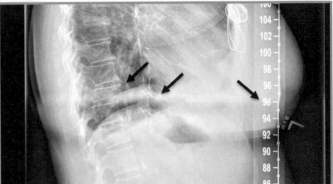

Figure 4.17 Misregistration artifact resulting from automatic FPD image stitching failure (left). Red arrows denote misregistration of the alignment ruler, spine, and diaphragm in the image (right) as a result of a failed patient breath hold. The addition of an extra vertebrae manifests as a clinically actionable compression fracture.

long-form detector. Modern solutions come in several forms: multiple CR screens loaded into a single long-form cassette, multiple individual CR cassettes interleaved in a cassette holder, and a single long-form digital FPD. In all cases, the entire anatomy is acquired in a single exposure that effectively eliminates the risk of misregistration artifact. Some modest stitching artifacts or "structured noise" may still be present at the junction of adjacent plates due simply to the inability of software to seamlessly combine the different images. While it is possible that these imperfections may negatively impact image quality, the physicist should be able to determine a threshold beyond which these types of artifacts impede the physicians' ability to render an accurate diagnosis. In this way, the MP 3.0 task becomes less about simple artifact detection and measurement and more about artifact management.

One issue associated with long length CR and digital FPD imaging is the challenge of appropriate radiation penetration across the entire length of the long view image within the confines of a single exposure. Lateral views of the entire spine are particularly challenging for this reason. The cervical spine, thoracic spine, and lumbosacral spine must all be simultaneously visualized behind the neck, shoulder, lung, abdomen, and pelvis. Exposure must be increased to adequately penetrate the shoulder and pelvis, which can lead to detector over-exposure and saturation in other more radiolucent regions. Figure 4.18 shows an example of entire spine image detector saturation in the neck, lungs, and background. The detector saturation point has been reached due partly to the high technique required to penetrate the thicker portions of the anatomy, and also to the use of a virtual grid. When employing virtual grids (see Section 4.3.3.2), scatter fraction increases significantly at the detector, which can increase the risk of detector saturation, especially for larger patients and poorly collimated studies. Combining knowledge of virtual and physical grid performance, detector target exposure, and recommended technique factors (see Section 4.4.2.1), the MP 3.0 physicist should be able to approximate the detector saturation risk

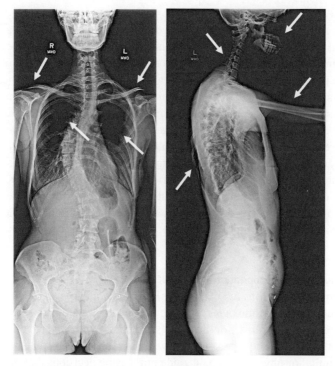

Figure 4.18 AP and LAT scoliosis images exhibiting "image burn" (red arrows) due to detector saturation. In the LAT view, there is also distinctive image underexposure through the shoulder and pelvis. A "virtual grid" was used to produce these images.

of different imaging protocols by taking into account factors such as grid use, patient thickness, scatter fraction, etc.

To help mitigate some problems associated with grossly unequal radiation penetration across long length exams, resurrection of "antiquated" techniques such as the use of wedge filters can help to improve penetration disparities and avoid both detector saturation limits and underexposure of key anatomy. It is also possible that the heel effect is partly responsible for the disparity between penetration of the superior and inferior aspects. Physics acceptance testing of such a device should include a recommendation for optimal SID, anode–cathode axis orientation, and recommendations for the proper detector location commensurate with the limitations of devices such as grids (reference IEC 60627) [33]. These considerations are certainly within the purview of MP 3.0.

4.4 Clinical Integration and Implementation

4.4.1 Training and Communication

Communication is key in the clinical operation of a radiographic unit. As physics reports are produced and presentations delivered, it is important to provide information that is not only succinct and accurate, but easily interpreted by the target audience – oftentimes non-physicists. Providing context and practical rationale for physicist recommendations will help to better convey the important conclusions drawn from physicist efforts.

4.4.1.1 AEC and Patient Alignment

AEC in general radiography is primarily achieved through an array of 1–3 radiosensitive cells coupled to a signal amplifier and controller electronics (Figure 4.1).[7] As the active cells are exposed, voltage accumulates in proportion to the total exposure until a predetermined voltage threshold is reached at which point the exposure is automatically terminated. Of course, these radiosensitive cells are finite in size (about 8 cm diameter) meaning that voltage accumulation is measured as a spatial average across the entire active photocell area. Figure 4.19 shows an example of how the finite size of AEC cells can interfere with the consistent delivery of high image quality. Even partial photocell exposure to the unattenuated beam results in premature AEC termination and suboptimal image quality due to underexposure of the detector. Pediatric patients with smaller body parts and a tendency to wiggle are particularly vulnerable to this type of error (as demonstrated in Figure 4.19). This example shows that, while a well-tuned AEC can afford an increase in the accuracy and precision of radiation delivery, this can only be achieved through sufficient understanding of the hardware and its limitations, adequate technologist education, and proper patient alignment.

4.4.1.2 The Consolidation Appropriations Act of 2016

The Consolidation Appropriations Act of 2016 has been a major driver in the transition from film-screen to CR to fully digital technologies. Because of scheduled Medicare reimbursement reductions for film-screen and CR exams, non-hospital-based clinics will need to convert to digital x-ray technologies lest they risk losing a percentage (eventually all) of their imaging reimbursements. This is an opportunity for physicists to help guide purchasing decisions (see Section 4.4.1.3), but

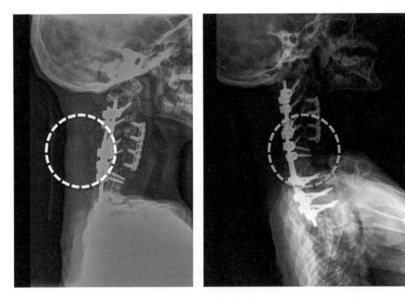

Figure 4.19 Clinical case of AEC cell misalignment of lateral cervical spine in a pediatric patient. The left image (25 × 30 cm cassette) shows poor centering of the neck over the active AEC photocell (red) resulting in dramatic image underexposure. The right image demonstrates the same patient with proper centering over the photocell (green) which corrects the problem.

---

7 AEC in mammography is notably different wherein the digital detector itself performs the AEC functions.

also to train technologists on how to properly adapt their practices and techniques to newer digital equipment – a topic discussed later in Section 4.4.2.

4.4.1.3 Consumer Report

In the modern medical imaging landscape, many equipment options exist to satisfy clinical needs. Vendors compete for business with a variety of offerings, and hospitals and clinics must make their selections within a complex and highly heterogeneous healthcare operation. Healthcare providers are further pressured by increased regulatory scrutiny, limited (financial) resources, and the need to remain competitive and relevant in the healthcare marketplace. As a result, some facilities are faced with making major purchasing decisions with the input and expertise of only a few individuals who may or may not adequately represent the wide range of needs that the equipment must satisfy throughout the clinical operation. First and foremost are the needs of the patient, but the satisfaction of those needs is contingent upon the considerations of those who purchase the equipment (administration), those who operate the equipment (technologists), those who utilize the imaging technologies (radiologists), and those who maintain the equipment (engineers), among others. To avoid sub-optimal use of resources and to provide a quality medical imaging product, it takes a coordinated and concerted effort by the clinical leadership to make the right decision.

The role of clinical physicists in the brokering of medical equipment deals may not be obvious since they often perform annual and acceptance testing of machines only after major purchasing decisions have been made and the equipment installed. In this regard, physicists may represent an "untapped resource." Physicists, with their wealth of knowledge and expertise, pose to greatly improve the quality and confidence of the purchasing process by offering data-driven answers to challenging clinical questions. The AAPM Task Group Report No. 74 states that "The diagnostic medical physicist... possesses a unique vantage point from which to assess the appropriateness of imaging equipment" [17]. Given the needs for unbiased and data-driven decision making in the modern medical imaging landscape, the physicist is uniquely positioned and well-equipped to supervise and supplement these types of efforts.

In an effort to find the right product at the intersection of these considerations, work has been done to provide a template for the objective and comprehensive comparison of medical imaging devices in the form of a "consumer report" style analysis [34]. A sampling of mobile digital radiography units was chosen by the authors to demonstrate the various components of this integrated approach. Although this demonstration focused on mobile digital radiography, the methods presented can be applied to any number of different technologies to aid hospitals and clinics when making purchasing decisions – the Long Length Imaging above serves as an example. The proposed consumer report analysis is conducted under four primary categories: vendor specifications, physicist measurement, technologist survey, and radiologist image review. Note that financial costs of equipment purchase and maintenance were not part of this study, but are inevitable considerations when making equipment purchases and must be weighed in conjunction with desired features, performance, and specific needs of the clinic in question.

4.4.2 Optimization

4.4.2.1 Technique Charts

A working technique chart can be developed with little to no optimization, especially with the large dynamic range of modern digital detectors and the autoranging capabilities of image processing software. However, in the spirit of the ALARA principle, care should be taken to design radiographic techniques that are appropriate per patient per exam. Several publications have outlined methods for developing size-based technique charts for pediatric and adult imaging [35–37]. Size and thickness-based methods for technique chart development have precedence and history in film-based radiography where consistent film exposure was required to achieve an image within the narrow linear range of film densities. This method translates into the digital imaging world as a method to maintain the noise in images. Target exposure of a detector may be determined based on the formulation in Section 4.2.1.2.1 or from manufacturer recommendations. Once a target detector exposure is determined, ongoing quality assurance in terms of technique appropriateness is easily achieved by monitoring clinical EI values. Because of this, it is paramount that EI be properly calibrated, preferably in accordance with IEC standards (see Section 4.2.1.3).

Exposure-based technique charts are merely one way to optimize quality in the digital imaging workflow. Because of the flexibility afforded by digital detectors and software, one could optimize acquisition techniques and geometries to maximize any number of desirable image quality characteristics. For instance, an understanding of imaging tasks and the minimum image quality for their reliable detection may guide technique chart development in a different direction. Technologists have long understood the importance of proper technique and how different patient positions and radiographic views can be used to achieve optimal views of a given diagnostic task. A classic example is the difference between chest (lung) and rib examinations. Both exams cover the thorax but for very different purposes: the former enhances visualization of nodules and infiltrates against the lung background (a noise-limited task) while the latter enhances bony detail (a contrast-limited task). The physicist can contribute to the technologist knowledge base through targeted optimization on the basis of task object visualization. If patient dose is held constant, the ideal technique for low-contrast conspicuity would be optimized through (e)DQE maximization while bone imaging would depend on optimization of the x-ray spectrum to maximize bone-tissue contrast resolution via (e)MTF maximization. Through careful integration of technologist and physicist expertise, the efforts of both parties may be more meaningful toward optimization of the imaging workflow.

4.4.2.2 Image Processing

Image processing is perhaps one of the most underappreciated yet most significant links in the imaging chain. Even the most finely tuned imaging system with appropriate imaging technique factors and geometries can render adequate images unusable if image processing is not adequately optimized. Image processing assessment may be as simple as a cursory review of the image processing database when new equipment is installed or software upgraded. It is not uncommon to see the link between image acquisition protocols and the image processing database break during service, and image quality may suffer if the correct processing is not linked to its respective imaging protocol. A more thorough approach to image processing assessment would be the regular check of image processing parameter settings to ensure consistency with manufacturer or institution standards. Ideally, an objective image quality-based approach to image processing assessment is merited to truly optimize this parameter space. Therefore, as image quality specialists, it is crucial that physicist support of radiography include some assessment of image processing.

Image processing can be managed in a number of ways. It is an attractive prospect to use phantoms for image quality optimization as they eliminate a number of variables associated with patient imaging. However, even anthropomorphic phantoms may not adequately simulate the fineness of detail and other nuances necessary for translating phantom-based results to full time clinical use. Furthermore, the prospect of phantom-based optimization is an expensive one as image processing tends to be highly protocol-specific thus requiring a multitude of anatomy-specific phantoms. Therefore, image processing optimization on a small set of representative patient images is merited

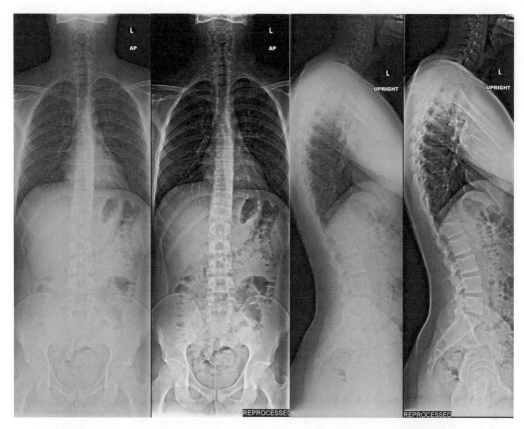

Figure 4.20 Protocol-specific image processing optimization in entire spine imaging. Default image processing settings were appropriate for bone (extremity) imaging – not scoliosis imaging. Adjustment of the default image processing settings was necessary to enhance the spine detail and account for the large changes in image intensity along the length of the body through equalization.

during imaging system acceptance and maintenance. Figure 4.20 demonstrates how the default image processing parameter set was inadequate for entire spine imaging on a new system install. In this example, the relative contrast of the thoracic and lumbar vertebral bodies was maximized while the intensity difference between the two was minimized to ensure adequate visualization of the spine within a single window/level setting. A more subjective limitation was set on optimization to ensure the image did not look "overly processed" or "artificial," which can negatively impact reader confidence.

Even different views of the same anatomy may require view-specific image processing adaptation. Chest image quality is notoriously difficult to manage, and Figure 4.22 demonstrates how image processing optimized for a PA chest view does not necessarily produce the same optimality of image quality in the lateral view. Differences in patient thickness, radiolucency, and anatomical arrangement and overlap of the lung region in the lateral view all contribute to an intensity histogram which deviates from that of the PA view. This in turn can influence the results of automatic image processing and window-leveling yielding an image of undesirable quality.

It is sometimes the case that clinics with multiple radiographic units will have a variety of vendors or machine models represented. This can present a challenge to maintaining image quality consistency across the fleet. Figure 4.22 demonstrates how image processing can be optimized

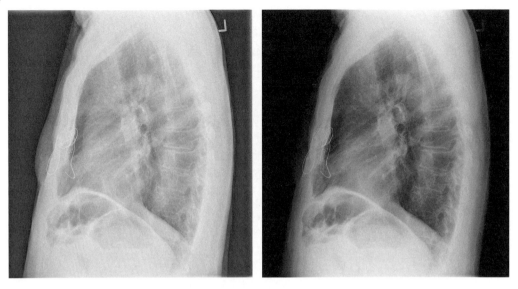

Figure 4.21 Lateral chest images. The first image was produced after the default lateral chest image processing settings were erroneously set to the PA chest settings. Correction of the default lateral chest image processing protocol produced more favorable image quality.

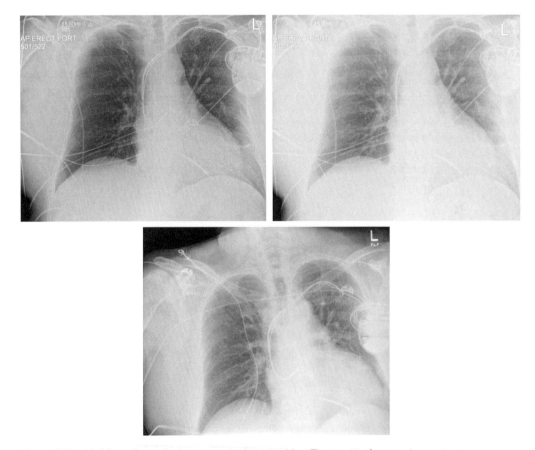

Figure 4.22 Mobile radiography image processing matching. The top two images demonstrate modification of the image processing "look" from one vendor's default settings before (left) and after (right) matching the "look" from a second vendor (bottom) using the code from Patient-Based Image Quality.

(matched) to a preferred "look" in order to maintain consistency in clinical care. The top and bottom mobile AP chest radiographs of the same patient were acquired on different days of an inpatient stay with two different vendor devices. In this case, any day-to-day discrepancies in the images should be due to changes in the patient or disease state and not the result of changes in acquisition geometry, patient positioning, image processing, or device differences. Using the code described in Section 4.2.2.2, image processing settings of one vendor were adjusted to match the image quality delivered by another vendor consistent with the image quality preferences of inter-preting radiologists reading at the facility. In the movement from digital image post-processing toward adaptive processing, knowledge of clinical imaging tasks will help the MP 3.0 physicist to optimize image processing in an intelligent manner such that the diagnostic quality of each image is truly optimized to each anatomical site, view, and the diagnostic task at hand.

4.4.3 Automated Analysis and Data Management

Automated data analysis and management in radiography is a simple way to improve the objectiv-ity and consistency of clinical testing results without devoting excess time to data collection and analytics. To exemplify how automation can add value to the clinical operation, this section will be divided into three specific spheres of MP 3.0 practice.

4.4.3.1 Prospective Performance Assessment

Prospective performance assessment generally refers to the MP 1.0 canon of tests. These tests are a means by which physics can infer the quality of system performance through assessments made outside of the normal clinical workflow. These repeated assessments performed (annually) on radi-ographic systems can benefit greatly from automation. Something as simple as maintaining a template for system testing can greatly accelerate the pace at which analysis is performed by stand-ardizing data entry forms and programming basic calculations. It can also free time for additional, more sophisticated analysis. Some physicists have even proposed the establishment of a "structured physics report" in the spirit of "structured dose reports" as part of the digital imaging and commu-nications in medicine (DICOM) family of formatted files [38]. While proposals have thus far been CT-centric, the same concept can be applied to any imaging modality, radiography included.

Automation of image and data analysis is another easy way to enhance the objectivity and con-sistency of physics test results. For example, some software-based solutions for baseline detector performance characterization include source code for detector response curve, MTF, NPS, and DQE analyses [39]. Other software packages include automatic CR and digital imaging analysis routines for defective pixel, uniformity, dark field, and lag analysis, among others [40, 41]. Still, some users may elect to write their own programs to analyze quality assurance and QC data to suit their own specific needs and testing preferences.

A third means by which prospective performance assessment can be enhanced relates to vendor-based QC. Many vendors offer hardware or software tools for imaging equipment quality assur-ance that can be run on a regular basis to monitor system performance. In general, the results of these tests remain on the imaging system where they were performed, and action is only taken if values exceed static manufacturer-defined QC bounds. Additional value can be extracted from these assessments by collecting, automatically analyzing, and compiling the results from the entire imaging fleet into a user-friendly format. Once collected, trend analysis can be performed on QC data to catch anomalous patterns or drifting values that point to developing problems. Ideally, the identification of developing problems would be acted upon before negatively impacting patient care and perhaps even before QC values exceed manufacturer thresholds. If data are available from multiple systems, the performance of like systems can be compared to uncover any actionable discrepancies between machines across the imaging fleet.

4.4.3.2 Prospective Protocol Definition

QC by way of prospective protocol definition is a way to assure and control quality through the prescription of imaging protocols. Historically, this has been synonymous with the definition of acquisition technique factors (see Section 4.4.2.1), but following the digital renaissance in radiography, this has come to include the management of image processing presets as well (see Section 4.4.2.2). Physics oversight and management within this domain can be difficult. Several parties may need to access and modify acquisition protocols, processing presets, and machine databases including physicists, technologists, and field service engineers. This is but one reason why ongoing physics support of radiography must not stop at annual QA. Rather, physics support should be integrated such that all significant modifications to either the equipment or database is followed by physics assessment so that proper QC checks of acquisition and processing databases can be performed prior to continued patient imaging. Physics may elect to orchestrate, delegate, or automate the maintenance of database master copies so that any modifications can be cross-checked and validated by relevant parties or programs. Establishment of a centralized server may be justified to aid in this effort.

4.4.3.3 Retrospective Quality Assessment

Retrospective quality assessment refers to the quantification of characteristics related to imaging outcomes for the purposes of ongoing QC. This includes but is not limited to analysis of patient dose and image quality but also includes considerations like image reject and repeat analysis. Interrogation of the imaging deliverable is necessary to better inform the clinical practice, especially with regard to how imaging can be better utilized and how imaging prescriptions (i.e. acquisition technique factors and processing) can be optimized to enhance patient care.

While individual patient dose monitoring is generally not formally mandated by either regulatory or accrediting bodies for radiography, it is merited for the purposes of optimizing the consistency and quality of clinical images. Dose monitoring quantities and caveats are discussed at length in Section 4.2.3. To obtain these data, many modern systems are capable of sending radiation dose structured report (RDSR) data that can be automatically delivered to and collected on PACS or a dedicated dose monitoring server. Otherwise, much radiometry data can be easily obtained from DICOM image header data that can also be automatically delivered from the imaging system to an alternate dose monitoring server or harvested from the PACS itself using query-retrieve operations. Automation of dose monitoring data retrieval, extraction, and analysis is key to the success of any dose monitoring system, and several commercial solutions are available for purchase to ease the burdens associated with the development and integration of such a program.

Automation of dose monitoring, while laudable, is scarcely adequate to assure image quality optimality. A multitude of clinical variables can impact the delivery of high quality images – even those images that are adequately exposed. A complete MP 3.0 approach to retrospective quality assessment recognizes the need to monitor dose quantities in conjunction with image quality-related metrics. EI monitoring is a reasonable and easily accessible starting point. As discussed above in EI is an image quality index correlated with detector exposure and the resultant image noise and can be used as a metric of dose appropriateness, especially when compared to target EI values *vis-à-vis* DI. However, one cannot infer the myriad of other image quality attributes that constitute a quality diagnostic image from EI alone. For this additional information, some form of explicit assessment of image quality attributes directly from the patient images would be required.

If access to DICOM image data is available, software such as that proposed in Section 4.2.2.2 may be automated and used to quantify relevant parameters on a patient-by-patient basis. Population means may then be computed from individual scores as a function of any number of variables including station name and technologist ID to uncover clinical trends.

Lastly, a comprehensive image reject tracking program is an important and valuable contribution to technologist workflow analysis. The World Health Organization suggests that reject rates less than 5% are optimal and rates higher than 10% are unacceptable [42]. However, AAPM Task Group 151 suggests that abnormally low reject rates may indicate issues with reject tracking compliance or manipulation by users as opposed to actual low rates of rejection [43]. While a reasonably low and achievable reject rate should be targeted, it is of greater importance to understand the reasons for image reject so that unacceptable rates can be remedied. This requires reject data to be tracked and stratified by factors such as anatomy, view, technologist, and reason for reject among other variables. In multi-vendor and multi-model imaging facilities, standardization of reject reports is another important step to enable fleet-wide analysis. Automatic sending of reject reports from individual systems to a centralized server helps to maintain the continuity of reject data tracking. For those systems without an auto-send feature, technologists may be called upon to push reports for (automatic) analysis.

4.4.4 Meaningful QC

As stewards of dose and arbiters of quality, physicists have a great role to play in radiography management. The call to leadership will require physicists to be judicious with their efforts, keeping in mind the limits of resource, time, and capital. Three themes prevail throughout this chapter – efficacious quantification, clinical integration, and variance reduction. These guiding principles form the basis for meaningful QC in radiography.

Efficacious quantification does not need to be elaborate and sophisticated. In fact, simple automation of routine measurements or processes can be far more beneficial in terms of time savings than the development of a complicated and nuanced metrology that may have only incremental (and perhaps even abstruse) clinical benefit.[8] In this way, some training in informatics, computer programming, and databasing may be of greater benefit to the MP 3.0 radiography physicist than time spent developing more complex and esoteric metrology. The sheer abundance of radiographic equipment necessitates this level of efficient assessment in the interest of good time management.

Whereas physics assessment can only be pared down and optimized so much, the acute timing of said assessment can save additional time and resource elsewhere. In the spirit of clinical integration, physics may elect to synchronize testing with preventative maintenance performed by clinical engineers. In doing so, any deficiencies identified by physics can be more quickly and efficiently addressed. Even "minor" repairs and adjustments that take little time to address can become costly if extra hours must be devoted to travel, scheduling, and machine down time. Ultimately, schedule synchronization can allow more physics input to have real clinical impact by allowing quick integration of recommended changes without undue burden to other clinical partners.

A strong clinical effect can be made through quantification and communication at the administrative level as well. Practical indicators of clinical efficiency and proficiency known as key performance indicators (KPIs) can provide a quick and easy conduit for communication with nonclinical personnel at the administrative, vendor, and regulatory levels. Relatively simple measurements

---

8 https://xkcd.com/1205.

mined from information sources available to physicists can provide much needed input to influence the clinical trajectory and practice. Metrics such as images or exams per system per month can provide critical input toward optimizing resource and personnel allocation within and between clinics. Such a data-driven approach can be used to easily justify equipment purchases. Reject rate can be an indicator of technologist proficiency and the need for ongoing training through continuing medical education which physicists can provide. EI/DI mean and variance sorted by anatomical region and view can highlight inconsistencies in patient care from one system to another. Paired with estimates of patient dose and objective measures of patient-based image quality, this KPI can identify systems in need of a technology upgrade. By partnering with administrators, physics insight can help to shape the standard of clinical care as the right technology is selected to suit the particular needs of the clinic served.

As radiography has grown and matured as a modality, a shift to newer digital technologies has eliminated some problems and introduced others. In place of film and processor chemical control, technologists contend with spotty wireless network connectivity in mobile radiography. Instead of film processor temperature and silver recovery, the clinic is now subject to the health and longevity of wireless detector batteries. Whereas screen-film contact and screen resolution testing has gone by the wayside, wireless detector drops and damage pervade. More apropos QC of these newly relevant problems is an opportunity for engineering, physics, and technologist integration. Physics may consider adding wireless transmission signal strength to their canon of tests. Engineers may be asked to regularly log maximum battery capacity and number of total charge cycles for monitoring long-term battery health to predict impending battery failures. Technologists may be asked to implement a login credential system for radiography equipment to track operators and hold them accountable for machine use allowing better monitoring and tracking of costly detector drops. Physicist oversight and recommendations within these practices can bring much value to the clinical workflow as novel sources of variance come to dominate the radiography landscape.

Moving forward with a focus on regulatory oversight, it would be ideal to transition the modality from exposure-centric regulatory practice toward one of image quality optimality and consistency. While a focus on patient exposure does have image quality consequences, there remain many other (perhaps even more impactful) sources of quality variability left untested – namely an outright lack of explicit image quality regulation, a lack of balance between patient exposure and the need to achieve exam- and patient-specific EI (detector exposure) targets, and image processing inconsistency. Absolute thresholds for dose delivered to a standard patient (i.e. DRLs) can help to push clinics in the direction of adopting more radiosensitive digital equipment and avoid chronic overexposure. On the other hand, image quality standards can help to ensure optimality of implementation and use of equipment and software in an effort to prevent chronic *underexposure* and underutilization of image quality enhancement tools such as image processing. A robust informatics infrastructure, integration of physics QC with PACS, and a "big data" approach to QC can provide additional resource to better handle image quality variability and justify exam- and patient-specific exposures in addition to more apt identification of operational outliers in the pursuit of diagnostic quality radiographs.

Ultimately, as a member of the clinical care team, the radiography physicist must *confidently* deliver recommendations, especially in a modality with few regulatory requirements on which to rely. The MP 3.0 physicist should always be thinking about what can and should be done to affect a positive clinical change beyond simply maintaining regulatory compliance. In this way, the physicist can claim a stake in the department as a true arbiter of quality and safety. But even the most ambitious physicist must temper expectations of what can be reasonably accomplished across a large radiography enterprise. Physics testing time is costly both to the physics enterprise and to the healthcare provider. Imaging units may at times need to be taken out of service to accommodate physics testing and recommendations that impact revenue generation. What remains to be done is the advancement of a deliberate and effective policy change in the direction of image quality performance in the wake of a digital renaissance in radiography. It is therefore essential that physics look critically at which tests result in meaningful clinical change so that precious time is not wasted on remedial exercises. In doing so, radiography physicists will position themselves within the imaging enterprise as essential support staff and less so as mere regulatory compliance officers.

References

1 Gallagher, A., Dowling, A., Faulkner, R. et al. (2014). Quality Assurance Testing in the 21st Century – Are We Still in the Dark Ages?, Radiological Society of North America 2014 Scientific Assembly and Annual Meeting.

2 Dobbins, J.T., Samei, E., Chotas, H.G. et al. (2003). Chest radiography: optimization of X-ray spectrum for Cesium iodide–Amorphous silicon flat-panel detector. *Radiology* 226: 221–230.

3 Huda, W. (2005). The current concept of speed should not be used to describe digital imaging systems. *Radiology* 234: 345–346.

4 Haus, G. and Jaskulski, S.M. (1997). *The Basics of Film Processing in Medical Imaging*. Medical Physics Publishing.

5 Internation Organization for Standardization (2004). 9236-1:2004 Photography – Sensitometry of Screen/Film Systems for Medical Radiography – Part 1: Determination of Sensitometric Curve Shape, Speed and Average Gradient. pp. 20.

6 Shepard, S.J., Wang, J., Flynn, M. et al. (2009). An exposure indicator for digital radiography: AAPM Task Group 116 (executive summary). *Medical Physics* 36((7): 2898–2914.

7 International Electrotechnical Commission (2008). Medical electrical equipment - Exposure index of digital X-ray imaging systems - Part 1: Definitions and requirements for general radiography, *Vol. Publication 62494-1*, (IEC, Geneva.

8 Eastman Kodak Company (2005). ADJUSTMENTS AND REPLACEMENTS for the Kodak DirectView CR 825/850 SYSTEMS, edited by Eastman Kodak Company (Rochester, NY), pp. 160.

9 Brateman, L.F. and Heintz, P.H. (2015). Meaningful data or just measurements? Differences between ionization chamber and solid-state detectors. *J. Am. Coll. Radiol.* 12: 951–953.

10 International Electrotechnical Commission (2014). Medical electrical equipment - Characteristics of digital x-ray imaging devices - Part 1–1: Determination of the detective quantum efficiency: Detectors used in radiographic imaging, *Vol. Report No.: 62220-1-1*, (IEC, Geneva), pp. 37.

11 International Electrotechnical Commission (2005). Medical diagnostic X-ray equipment - Radiation conditions for use in the determination of characteristics, *Vol. Publication 61267-2*, (IEC, Geneva).

12 Conway, J., Duff, J.E., Fewell, T.R. et al. (1990). A patient-equivalent attenuation phantom for estimating patient exposures from automatic exposure controlled x-ray examinations of the abdomen and lumbo–sacral spine. *Med. Phys.* 17: 448–453.

13 Baydush, H., Ghem, W.C., and Floyd, C.E. (2000). Anthropomorphic versus geometric chest phantoms: a comparison of scatter properties. *Med. Phys.* 27: 894–897.

14 Chotas, H.G., Floyd, C.E., Johnson, G.A., and Ravin, C.E. (1997). Quality control phantom for digital chest radiography. *Radiology* 202: 111–116.

15 Samei, N.T., Ranger, A., MacKenzie, I.D. et al. (2009). Effective DQE (eDQE) and speed of digital radiographic systems: an experimental methodology. *Med. Phys.* 36: 3806–3817.

16 Wells, J.R. and Dobbins, J.T. III (2013). Frequency response and distortion properties of nonlinear image processing algorithms and the importance of imaging context. *Med. Phys.* 40: 091906.

17 American Association of Physicists in Medicine (2002). *Quality Control in Diagnostic Radiology*, vol. 74. Madison: Medical Physics Publishing.

18 Jones, K., Heintz, P., Geiser, W. et al. (2015). Ongoing quality control in digital radiography: report of AAPM imaging physics committee task group 151. *Med. Phys.* 42: 6658–6670.

19 Lin, Y., Luo, H., Dobbins, J.T. III et al. (2012). An image-based technique to assess the perceptual quality of clinical chest radiographs. *Med. Phys.* 39: 7019–7031.

20 Samei, Y.L., Choudhury, K.R., and Page McAdams, H. (2014). Automated characterization of perceptual quality of clinical chest radiographs: validation and calibration to observer preference. *Med. Phys.* 41: 111918.

21 Vañó, E., Miller, D., Martin, C. et al. (2017). ICRP Publication 135: Diagnostic Reference Levels in Medical Imaging, Ann. ICRP.

22 Kofler, J.M., Jordan, D.W., and Orton, C.G. (2014). Exposure tracking for x-ray imaging is a bad idea. *Med. Phys.* 41 (1): 010601.

23 Wall, B., Haylock, R., Jansen, J. et al. (2011). *Radiation risks from medical x-ray examinations as a function of the age and sex of the patient.* (Centre for Radiation, Chemical and Environmental Hazards, Health Protection Agency).

24 Littleton, J.T. (1970). A phantom method to evaluate the clinical effectiveness of a tomographic device. *Am. J. Roentgenol.* 108: 847–856.

25 N. E. M. Association (2016). Quality Control Tools for Digital Projection Radiography, *Vol. XR 30-2016*, (NEMA, Rosslyn, VA).

26 Krupinski, E.A., Williams, M.B., Andriole, K. et al. (2007). Digital radiography image quality: image processing and display. *J. Am. Coll. Radiol.* 4: 389–400.

27 Aichinger, H., Dieker, J., Joite-Barfuß, S., and Säbel, M. (2012). *Radiation Exposure and Image Quality in X-Ray Diagnostic Radiology*, 2e. Berlin, Germany: Springer.

28 Freedman, M.T., Lo, S.-C.B., Seibel, J.C., and Bromley, C.M. (2011). Lung nodules: improved detection with software that suppresses the rib and clavicle on chest radiographs. *Radiology* 260: 265–273.

29 Li, F., Engelmann, R., Pesce, L. et al. (2012). Improved detection of focal pneumonia by chest radiography with bone suppression imaging. *Eur. Radiol.* 22: 2729–2735.

30 Samei, E., Saunders, R.S. Jr., Lo, J.Y. et al. (2004). Fundamental imaging characteristics of a slot-scan digital chest radiographic system. *Med. Phys.* 31: 2687–2698.

31 Chotas, H.G., Floyd, J.C.E., and Ravin, C.E. (1995). Technical evaluation of a digital chest radiography system that uses a selenium detector. *Radiology* 195: 264–270.

32 Samei, E., Ranger, N.T., MacKenzie, A. et al. (2008). Detector or system? Extending the concept of detective quantum efficiency to characterize the performance of digital radiographic imaging systems. *Radiology* 249: 926–937.

33 International Electrotechnical Commission (2013).Diagnostic X-ray imaging equipment: characteristics of general purpose and mammographic antiscatter grids, *Vol. Publication 60627-3*, (IEC, Geneva).

34 Wells, J., Christensen, J., and Samei, E. (2015). TH-AB-201-12: a consumer report for mobile digital radiography: a holistic comparative evaluation across four systems. *Med. Phys.* 42: 3720–3720.

35 Wells, J.R., Mann, S.D., and Samei, E. (2017). We-AB-601-02: advanced methods for the development of system-specific and size-specific radiographic technique charts across the radiology enterprise. *Med. Phys.* 44: 3195–3196.

36 Shah, C., Jones, A.K., and Willis, C.E. (2008). Consequences of modern anthropometric dimensions for radiographic techniques and patient radiation exposures. *Med. Phys.* 35: 3616–3625.

37 Sánchez, A.A., Reiser, I., Baxter, T. et al. (2017). Portable abdomen radiography: moving to thickness-based protocols. *Pediatr. Radiol.* 48 (2): 210–215.

38 Boone, J.M., Mahesh, M., Gingold, E.L., and Seibert, J.A. (2016). A call for the structured physicist report. *J. Am. Coll. Radiol.* 13: 307–309.

39 Samei, E., Ikejimba, L.C., Harrawood, B.P. et al. (2018). Report of AAPM Task Group 162: software for planar image quality metrology. *Med. Phys.* 45: e32–e39.

40 Desai, N. and Valentino, D.J. (2011). A software tool for quality assurance of computed/digital radiography (CR/DR) systems, 7961, 79614E-79614E-79611.

41 Donini, B., Rivetti, S., Lanconelli, N., and Bertolini, M. (2014). Free software for performing physical analysis of systems for digital radiography and mammography. *Med. Phys.* 41.

42 Lloyd, P.J. (2001). *Quality Assurance Workbook for Radiographers and Radiological Technologists*. World Health Organization.

43 Dunn, M.A. and Rogers, A.T. (1998). X-ray film reject analysis as a quality indicator. *Radiography* 4: 29–31.

Part II

Mammography

5

Clinical Mammography Physics: Perspective

Douglas E. Pfeiffer

Boulder Community Health, Boulder, CO, USA

5.1 Historical Perspective

Mammographic imaging has undergone significant development over the last century [1]. Beginning with simple radiography of mastectomy specimens, *in vivo* breast imaging was started in 1930 by Dr. Warren Stafford at the Rochester Memorial Hospital, using fine-grain, double-emulsion film produced by Kodak paired with dual, fine-grain Patterson screens. Interpretation and diagnosis continued to improve throughout the 1930s and 1940s. Technical developments also took place during this period, along with pathological correlation, although there was still no wide-spread acceptance of the technique.

During this period, mammography was performed using standard radiographic equipment and technical parameters similar to 60 kV, 150 mAs. Around 1950, Raul Leborgne reported the prevalence of microcalcifications and recognized that compression of breast tissue was important for improved image quality. He began using technical parameters of approximately 20–30 kV and 5 mAs per cm compressed breast tissue [2]. Interest in mammography continued to grow as imaging methodologies improved. During this developmental period, much of the work was done by surgeons and radiologists [3–5].

In 1960, the application of xerographic imaging to mammography was published [6], which represented the introduction of imaging systems specifically designed for mammography. In 1965, the CGR company introduced the Senographe unit, which was the first system designed to be dedicated to breast imaging (Figure 5.1). This device incorporated a molybdenum target and a 0.7 mm nominal size focal spot. Many manufacturers entered the market and a wide variety of units designed on the physics of this unit were marketed.

The next decades witnessed the further development of mammographic systems. Improvements touched essentially all aspects of the imaging chain: focal spots, automatic exposure controls, grids, generators, film-screen imaging systems, and film processors. The improvement in image quality and the associated improvements in sensitivity and specificity, the American Cancer Society (ACS) began promoting mammography as a screening tool for asymptomatic women [7]. It formed an ACS Mammography Physics Committee to work with the American College of Radiology Breast Task Force, which was developing new guidelines. Both groups were comprised of radiologists and medical physicists.

Clinical Imaging Physics: Current and Emerging Practice, First Edition. Edited by Ehsan Samei and Douglas E. Pfeiffer.
© 2020 John Wiley & Sons, Inc. Published 2020 by John Wiley & Sons, Inc.

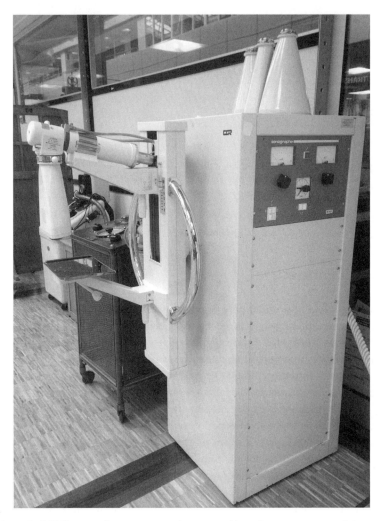

Figure 5.1 An early CGR Senographe mammography system. Note the cones on top of the system for collimating the x-ray beam. *Source:* Răzvan Iordache, PhD, GE Healthcare.

In 2000, digital mammography was introduced with the General Electric 2000D. Digital systems have improved and gained wide acceptance, with digital mammography holding over 95% of the installed base in the US at this time. At least 33 models from 11 manufacturers are currently available (Figures 5.2 and 5.3).

During this time, the quality control (QC) of mammographic systems also underwent dramatic development. Through the mid-1980s, little special attention was paid to mammographic QC, treating mammographic units much the same as other diagnostic imaging equipment. Over time, however, the technical demands of mammography were recognized to demand greater QC, particularly as the need for contrast and detail pushed the limits of the image receptor technology.

In 1986, the National Council on Radiation Protection published *Mammography – A User's Guide* [8], a consensus document of concerned organizations that provided QC recommendations. This was updated about two decades later, with Report No. 149, *A Guide to Mammography and Other Breast Imaging Procedures* [9].

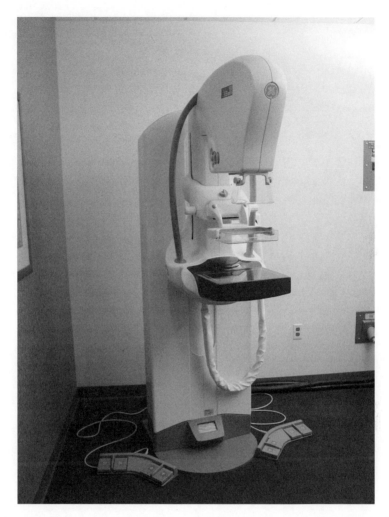

Figure 5.2 A modern digital mammography system. Note that the detector is thicker than in the old CGR system in Figure 5.1, making getting into the axilla challenging for technologists.

Conducted in 1985 and published in 1987, a study of dedicated mammography machines by the Nationwide Evaluation of X-Ray Trends (NEXT) demonstrated wide variations in image quality and dose [10]. Further, in 1998 report on the technical quality of 32 mammography services in regional screening programs found inadequacies in a number of them [11].

The ACS/ACR (American College of Radiology) committee was to choose devices and methods for image quality and dosimetry, and to establish minimum QC standards. In response, the committee promoted the use of a phantom very similar to what is currently accepted as the ACR Accreditation Phantom, and included a thermoluminescent dosimetry (TLD) strip for it.

In parallel, the American Association of Physicists in Medicine (AAPM) developed and published Report No. 29, *Equipment Requirements and Quality Control in Mammography*, in 1990 [12].

In 1987, the ACR Breast Task Force developed the Mammography Accreditation Program (MAP), a voluntary accreditation program with standards for personnel qualifications, equipment performance, clinical image quality, phantom image quality, and dose [13]. Within four years, approximately 25% of nearly 10 000 mammography facilities had achieved accreditation. The peer review

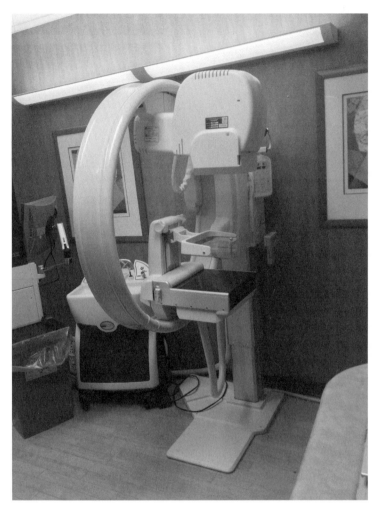

Figure 5.3 A system incorporating unusual annular geometry. This system allows for positioning the patient from the front, through the annulus, rather than only from behind or beside.

process aimed not only at passing judgment on facilities, but also had a large educational component, focusing on improving the overall quality of breast imaging. If a facility did not pass accreditation, the College and the experts within the program provided recommendations and feedback as to how the facility could achieve appropriate quality.

As part of this effort, the ACR later published the detailed *Mammography Quality Control Manual* [14]. The manual has sections for the radiologist, technologist, and medical physicist, each of whom has an important function in establishing and maintaining a quality mammography program. For the technologist and medical physicist, the manual defines specific QC tests, providing full procedures for each test. These tests have remained at the heart of mammographic QC since their publication.

At the time that the ACR was establishing the MAP, several states passed legislation mandating that facilities meet certain quality standards for mammography, and also that State Radiation Control personnel carry out inspections to enforce those standards. Extending these state regulations, in 1990 the US Congress authorized Medicare coverage of mammography, and required facilities to register with the Health Care Finance Administration (HCFA) and to maintain quality standards like those of the ACR MAP. At this point, many facilities in the United States had to comply with a patchwork of federal, state and voluntary standards and programs, while others underwent little oversight at all. The issue gained national attention, and imaging professionals and politicians recognized that there was a need for uniform quality requirements for all screening and diagnostic facilities across the country.

In 1992, the United States enacted the federal Mammography Quality Standards Act [15]. This legislation required accreditation for most mammographic facilities in the US, and it directed the US Food and Drug Administration (FDA) to promulgate federal regulations to implement the fundamentals of the MAP. It also gave the FDA authority to enforce these regulations. The FDA first published its interim rules that went into effect in February of 1994; they required all mammography facilities to become accredited by October of 1994, and also set standards for accrediting bodies. The regulations effectively codified the ACR Mammography QC Manual. The final regulations, published in the Federal Register [16] came into effect in April 1999. These set the standards for personnel qualifications, equipment function, phantom image quality and dose. In 1998 Congress enhanced the effectiveness of the Mammography Quality Standardization Act (MQSA) by promulgating the Mammography Quality Standards Reauthorization Act (MQSRA), because of which the FDA issued a stricter set of regulations that became effective in October 2002.

While the MQSA and MAP programs in the US have received most attention, other international societies have also made substantial efforts in developing and promoting quality assurance in mammography. Most notably, the European Commission established the European Protocol for the QC of the Technical Aspects of Mammography Screening starting in 1993 [17].

In 2005, the International Atomic Energy Agency published a "state of the practice" survey of five eastern European countries [18]. This study involved a series of tests performed on units throughout the five countries to establish the existing status of image quality and dose status of their facilities. Following this initial testing, QC and improvement measures were implemented, along with training for the staff. The tests were repeated, and the report concludes that, "considerable reductions in dose were achieved at low cost while keeping the image quality at the highest level compatible with diagnostic requirement." Not only is establishment of a QC program vital to good mammography, but appropriate training for personnel in performing QC tests is also mandatory.

The IAEA has published two documents for QC in mammography though their Human Health Series. Publication No. 2, *Quality Assurance Programme for Screen Film Mammography* [19], and Publication No. 17, *Quality Assurance Programme for Digital Mammography* [20] are complementary documents for these two breast imaging implementations.

In the US, experience gained through the program and advances in equipment technology, especially digital mammography, pushed the FDA to publish a number of guidance documents and regulatory interpretations. FDA also developed the MQSA Policy Guidance Help System [21], which incorporated these documents and interpretations and serves as a vehicle for keeping pace with necessary changes. However, it was impossible to make QC for digital systems fit into the MQSA paradigm, so the FDA opted to require each manufacturer to develop its own QC manual. Facilities were required to follow the requirements of these manuals.

The problem with this approach was that each manual was significantly different from the others, and even different models from the same manufacturer could have different requirements. Additionally, each workstation, display, and printer could also have its own manual. This led to the situation that a physicist covering a large number of facilities could be required to be familiar with literally hundreds of QC manuals.

Recognizing the difficulty, the ACR stepped in and formed the Subcommittee on QA in Mammography, with the charge of developing a digital mammography QC manual along with a

QC phantom more appropriate to digital mammography. The draft of this manual has been submitted to FDA for approval as an alternative standard at the time of this writing.

5.2   Current and Upcoming Technologies

As was stated earlier, more than 95% of the installed base of mammography systems are now digital. These systems are grossly divided into two types: computed radiography (CR) and flat panel. The details of these systems have been described elsewhere [22–24].

CR systems replace film-screen cassettes with CR cassettes containing photostimulable phosphor (PSP) screens. While a standard screen-film mammography unit is used with CR, it is necessary to recalibrate the unit for the different exposure requirements of CR. After exposure, these screens are processed in the CR reader. The reader scans the plates with a typically red laser, causing the latent images to be released as typically blue light. This light is collected and converted to digital signals as the laser is scanned across the plate and the plate is translated though the beam path. Compared to standard CT systems, mammographic CR systems have a reduced pixel size (typically 50 µm); increased detective quantum efficiency (DQE) via thicker screens, double-sided readout, and smaller grain size; and mammography-specific image processing. The DQE of CR systems typically peak between 50 and 60%.

Flat panel systems do away with cassettes entirely. Several detector types are available. Cesium iodide (CsI) detector systems incorporate CsI having a needle-like structure coupled to an amorphous silicon (aSi) array. X-rays are absorbed by the CsI, which subsequently emits light that is detected by the aSi. The needle structure improves spatial resolution by limiting the spread of the light within the scintillator. With a pixel size of 100 µm, CsI systems have a DQE up to about 70%. Other flat panel systems use a amorphous selenium (aSe) plate coupled to a TFT active matrix array for x-ray detection. In these systems, x-rays stopped by the aSe plate create charge-hole pairs. The charges are transported to the pixel electrodes, from which the image is created. These systems have typically a 70–85 µm pixel size and a maximum DQE of about 75%. One aSe detector incorporates dual aSe layers and a 50 µm pixel size with a maximum DQE greater than 80%.

One unique device is a slot scanning system that uses a silicon detector connected to a photon counter. A narrow band of x-rays is swept across the breast while the detector array is swept below the breast (Figure 5.4). The detector array is composed of 3 mm deep silicon detectors (Figure 5.5) having approximately 95% x-ray absorption at mammographic energies. These count individual photons that are digitized upon detection. Energy discrimination allows for noise suppression by setting energy thresholds. The detection rate is at least 5×10^6 x-rays per sec per pixel. The system has a 50 µm pixel size and a peak DQE of about 63% in the detector array direction and about 61% in the scan direction. Unlike other detectors, the DQE for this system is largely independent of dose.

Improved detectors and increased computing power have led to further advances in digital mammography, including digital breast tomosynthesis (DBT) and contrast-enhanced spectral mammography (CESM). Without question, further advances will continue to improve the screening and diagnostic value of mammographic imaging.

Each of these presents new challenges for medical physics testing. Slot scanning devices such as photon counting systems have different failure modes than conventional digital mammography systems, and many of the test methods typically employed are not amenable to the different geometry of these systems.

CESM uses a significantly different beam quality than is typically used. Advanced image processing is central to the modality. Current test protocols do not address these aspects.

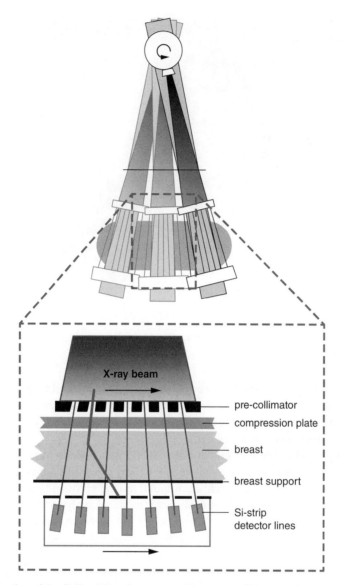

Figure 5.4 Illustration of the Philips Microdose system. The sweep of the x-ray beam paired with a sweeping detector array is demonstrated. The unit incorporates pre-patient collimators as well as post-patient collimation. *Source:* Philips Medical systems.

DBT is widely accepted clinically, and the ACR Digital Mammography QC Manual has established a unified testing paradigm for these units. It is an alternative to the manufacturer QC manuals.

5.3 The Movement from 1.0 to 3.0

Since the inception of the ACR accreditation program, testing and QC of mammography systems has been largely dictated by the ACR Mammography QC Manual. With the advent of digital mammography, MQSA mandated that all testing be done according to manufacturer QC manuals.

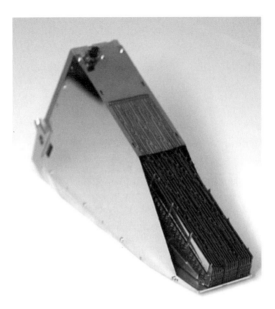

Figure 5.5 The Philips Microdose photon counting detector, with multi-slit configuration. *Source:* Philips Medical systems.

While these manuals describe generally thorough evaluations of the imaging systems, it is not clear that common equipment failure modes are emphasized. It is essential that regular QC focuses on those aspects that have the highest clinical impact. Further, the focus must be on capturing failures before they become clinically evident.

Due to the design and stability of modern equipment, many of the traditional measurements made by medical physicists have been rendered moot. X-ray generators are now self-regulated and extremely stable, meaning that tube potential, output reproducibility, and beam quality essentially will not drift except for catastrophic failure. Many of the visual analyses of image quality, such as the accreditation phantom and line-pair patterns, are not sensitive measures of image quality. While radiation dose remains a focus, it is possible that dose has been over-emphasized, and that rebalancing dose and image quality might be in order.

Medical physics support in mammography has been almost solely relegated to the equipment. Comparatively little time is spent on use or optimization of the equipment or the images. This has been left to the manufacturers. The limitation of this situation is that manufacturers must standardize their settings for mass approval, and optimization for local preferences is rarely achieved. Marketing pressures may necessitate emphasizing low radiation dose at the possible expense of sensitivity or specificity.

A shift to clinically driven measures of image quality, such as the detectability index d' or dose-image quality figures of merit [25] need to become more prominent in the developing practice of clinical medical physics. Such metrics will allow medical physicists to assist with local optimization (Table 5.1).

This type of involvement necessitates improved communication and interaction with the facility. It has been the case that physicists may see only the technologist, or even no-one from the facility, during a visit. While this may be efficient for the current paradigm, it is not a sustainable model. Medical physicists must transition to a more truly consultative role, being

Table 5.1 Comparison of medical physics 1.0 and 3.0 paradigms.

Mammography	1.0	3.0
Focus of MP's attention	Equipment	Patient
Image quality evaluation	Visual, subjective	Mathematical, quantitative
MP "tools of the trade" for image quality evaluation	Line pairs, simulated fibers, specks, and masses	Modulation transfer function (MTF), noise power spectrum (NPS), DQE, signal to noise ratio (SNR) uniformity, noise component analysis
Ongoing QC	Individual subjective evaluation of image quality, manufacturer-specified tests	Automated, remote of advanced image quality metrics
Patient dosimetry	Average glandular dose	Average glandular dose
Radiation risk estimation		
Commonly used imaging technologies	CR, digital radiography (DR)	DR and advanced apps (tomosynthesis, DE, etc.)
X-ray source technology	Rotating anode tube	Rotating anode tube

available for questions and advice, working closely with the facility on a more than annual basis, which is the current typical practice.

It is likely that changes to regulations will be a slow process. It will be necessary to implement the consultative, clinically-driven model of Medical Physics 3.0 largely in parallel with regulatory compliance. During this transition period, it will be important to demonstrate to the regulatory authorities that the new approach will yield better mammography at reasonable radiation dose, and will therefore achieve improved patient care.

References

1 Gold, R.H., Bassett, L.W., and Widoff, B.E. (1990). Highlights from the history of mammography. *Radiographics* 10 (6): 1111–1131.
2 Leborgne, R. (1951). Diagnosis of tumors of the breast by simple roentgenography. *AJR* 65: 1–11.
3 Salomon, A. (1913). Beiträge zur pathologie und klinik der mammakarzinome. *Arch. Klin. Chir.* 101: 573–668.
4 Warren, S.L. (1930). Roentgenologic study of the breast. *AJR* 24: 113–124.
5 Egan, R. (1964). *Mammography*, 3–16. Chicago: Thomas.
6 Gould, H.R., Ruzicka, F.F. Jr., Sanchez-Ubeda, R., and Perez, J. (1960). Xeroradiography of the breast. *AJR* 84: 220–223.
7 McLelland, R., Hendrick, E., Zinninger, M., and Wilcox, P. (September 1991). The American college of radiology mammography accreditation program. *AJR* 157: 473–479.
8 National Council on Radiation Protection and Measurements. Mammography – A User's Guide, NCRP Report No. 85 (National Council on Radiation Protection and Measurements, Bethesda, Maryland).
9 National Council on Radiation Protection and Measurements. A Guide to mammography and Other Breast Imaging Procedures, NCRP Report No. 149 (National Council on Radiation Protection and Measurements, Bethesda, Maryland).

10 Reuter, F.G. (1986). Preliminary Report – NEXT-85. National Conference on Radiation Control. Proceedings of the 18th Annual Conference of Radiation Control Program Directors (CRCPD Publication 86-2), pp. 111–120.

11 Galkin, B.M., Feig, S.A., and Muir, H.D. (1988). The technical quality of mammography in centers participating in a regional breast cancer awareness program. *Radiographics* 8: 133–145.

12 American Association of Physicists in Medicine Equipment Requirements and Quality Control in Mammography, AAPM Report No. 29 (American Institute of Physics, New York, New York).

13 Destouet, J.M., Bassett, L.W., Yaffe, M.J. et al. (2005). The ACR's mammography accreditation program: ten years of experience since MQSA. *J. Am. Coll. Radiol.* 2 (7): 585–594.

14 Hendrick, R.E., Bassett, L., Botsco, M.A. et al. (1999). *Mammography Quality Control Manual*. Reston (VA): American College of Radiology.

15 Mammography Quality Standards Act of 1992. Public Law 102-539. As amended by the Mammography Quality Standards Reauthorization Act of 1998, Pub. L. No. 105-248, Title 42, Subchapter II, Part F, Subpart 3, § 354 (42 USC 263b), certification of mammography facilities.

16 Quality Mammography Standards Final Rule, Federal Register, October 28, 1997; 62(208): 55 852-55 994.

17 European Commission (1999). The European Protocol for the Quality Control of the Physical and Technical Aspects of Mammography Screening. In: European Guidelines for Quality Assurance in Mammography Screening, Office for Official Publications of the European Communities, Luxembourg. CEC Report EUR 14821, 1st ed, 1993; 3rd ed.

18 International Atomic Energy Agency (2005). Optimization of the radiological protection of patients: Image quality and dose in mammography (coordinated research in Europe). Results of the Coordinated Research Project on Optimization of Protection in Mammography in some eastern European States. Austria, May.

19 International Atomic Energy Agency (2009). Human Health Series Publication No. 2, Quality Assurance Programme for Screen Film Mammography. Vienna.

20 International Atomic Energy Agency (2011). Human Health Series Publication No. 2, Quality Assurance Programme for Digital Mammography. Vienna.

21 CDRH, FDA (2014). MQSA Policy Guidance Help System. http://www.fda.gov/radiation-emittingproducts/mammographyqualitystandardsactandprogram/guidance/policyguidancehelpsystem/default.htm. Last updated 9/9/2014.

22 Pisano, E.D., Yaffe, M.J., and Kuzmiak, C.M. (2004). *Digital Mammography*, 15–26. Philadelphia, PA: Lippincott, Williams, and Wilkins.

23 Noel, A. and Thibault, F. (2004). Digital detectors for mammography: the technical challenges. *Eur. Radiol.* 14: 1990–1998.

24 Yaffe, M.J. and Rowlands, J.A. (1997). X-ray detectors for digital radiography. *Phys. Med. Biol.* 42: 1–39.

25 Bloomquist, A.K. et al. (2014). A task-based quality control metric for digital mammography. *Phys. Med. Biol.* 59: 6621.

6

Clinical Mammography Physics: State of Practice

Melissa Martin[1] and Eric Berns[2]

[1] *Therapy Physics, Inc., Signal Hill, CA, USA*
[2] *Radiological Sciences, University of Colorado, Aurora, CO, USA*

6.1   Introduction

As was detailed in Chapter 5, mammographic imaging has undergone tremendous development and change over the last 40 years [1–6]. Testing paradigms have struggled to keep pace with those changes.

As mammography equipment developed and improved over the decades, so did quality assurance standards and legislation. In the mid-80s, several studies suggested that large variations from site to site were still present in patient dose, image quality, and film processor performance [7–9]. During this time, the American Cancer Society (ACS) was beginning its National Breast Cancer Awareness Screening Programs and was concerned about advising women over the age of 40 to have screening mammograms without some level of confidence that mammography was being performed at a reasonably low dose and reasonably high image quality. It was at this point that the ACS approached the American College of Radiology about testing and designating mammography sites as meeting ACR-established quality standards. As a result, in October 1986, the ACR Mammography Accreditation Program was initiated. The goals of the accreditation program were to establish quality standards for mammography, compare performance from site to site, and encourage high quality mammography.

In the fall of 1990, the ACR published quality control manuals for radiologists, technologists, and medical physicists recommending a full quality control program at every mammography site [10]. These manuals provided procedures for quality control tests, frequencies, and recommended action limits. ACR Mammography Quality Control Manuals were revised and updated in 1992, 1994, and 1999 [11–13]. The mammography quality control manual provides a cookbook for quality control test procedures and provides forms for recordkeeping.

Congress passed the Mammography Quality Standards Act (MQSA) on October 27, 1992 to establish quality standards for mammography. Interim Rules were then published on December 21, 1993 [14]. MQSA required by law that all sites providing mammography meet the requirements listed in the Interim Rules by October 1, 1994. The Interim Rules mandated that all sites perform quality control testing as prescribed by the ACR Mammography QC Manuals (1992 or 1994 versions) [14]. On October 28, 1997, the Food and Drug Administration published the Final MQSA

Regulations in the Federal Register; they became effective on April 28, 1999 [15]. This effectively codified the 1999 ACR QC manual.

This paradigm worked well for film-screen units for many years. The advent of full-field digital mammography [16] led to some confusion. Much of the testing mandated under MQSA did not apply to digital units. In response, Food and Drug Adminiustration (FDA) required manufacturers of full-field digital mammography (FFDM) units to develop quality control (QC) manuals specific to their systems; facilities were required to follow the appropriate manual for their system. In facilities with several different manufacturers, each system required different testing protocols. For associated systems, such as interpretation workstations or printers, facilities were required to follow the most restrictive testing requirements for that device. With the vast number of models of mammography systems and allied devices, it became challenging to be sure that the appropriate testing was being performed.

In response to this, the ACR began developing a Digital Mammography QC Manual. The intent of this manual was to provide a standardized testing paradigm applicable to all existing systems.

Full-field digital mammography units now compose over 95% of the clinical units in the field. Quality control requirements still come from the FDA MQSA guidelines that, for digital units, require a facility to follow the Manufacturer Quality Control programs specific to the unit. In February of 2016 the FDA approved the ACR request for an alternative standard that allows facilities to use the new ACR Digital Mammography Quality Control Manual in place of a Manufacturer's QC program. This manual has been published and updated for digital breast tomosynthesis (DBT) units.

6.2   System Performance

System performance in the clinical setting is typically approached by performing the testing required under the MQSA regulations. These tests include the use of external test equipment and production of test and phantom images. These tests are very well defined in the tests, test procedures, and action limits that must be met. Previous generation screen-film units use the tests that are detailed in the ACR Mammography Accreditation Manual [17]. Newer generation digital mammography systems use their respective manufacturer quality control manual that describes the tests, procedures, and action limits. With the FDA acceptance of the ACR Digital Quality Control Manual as an alternative standard, facilities could start using this in 2017 as the basis for their testing.

6.2.1   Intrinsic Performance

There are several important intrinsic tests relevant to digital mammography. In particular specifications on x-ray tube, detector type and size, and the most importance in system performance.

6.2.1.1   kVp Measurement

In mammography, tube potential, or kVp, is easily measured by an external kVp meter or kVp divider. The kVp measurement was introduced, and required, in the original FDA MQSA regulations in 1997. This requirement called for systems to be within $\pm5\%$ of the indicated kVp, to be measured at the lowest clinical kVp, the most common kVp, and the highest available clinical kVp. Additionally, at the most commonly used kVp, the coefficient of variation or reproducibility of the kVp shall be equal to or less than 0.02. This measurement is to be measured at acceptance (Mammography Equipment Evaluation, abbreviated to MEE) and annual testing per MQSA requirements.

With modern systems however, kVp performance is rarely found to fail. Most manufacturer QC manuals follow the MQSA requirements for annual testing, but the ACR Digital QC Manual only requires kVp measurements be made at MEE.

6.2.1.2 Radiation Output and Half Value Layer

Two characteristics, in addition to the kVp, determine the radiation dose to the patient. These are the radiation output of the unit and the half value layer (HVL), which is a measure of the quality of the x-ray beam.

Radiation output is defined as the air kerma rate in $mGy\ s^{-1}$ when operating at 28 kVp for a Mo/Mo target/filter combination at 4.5 cm above the breast support surface. The original set two minimum values of a radiation output rate, depending upon when the system was manufactured: greater than $4.5\ mGy\ s^{-1}$, or $513\ mR\ s^{-1}$, in units manufactured prior to October 28, 2002; and $7.0\ mGy\ s^{-1}$, or $800\ mR\ s^{-1}$ in units manufactured after October 28, 2002. The measurement is to be averaged over a 3.0 s time period.

The radiation output was originally intended to make sure mammography x-ray units could produce enough exposure to create an image within a short enough time so that patient motion did not become an issue. With modern digital mammography systems, the radiation output measurement rarely fails the requirement but is still important in terms of radiation dose and patient motion reduction. In the 1999 ACR QC manual the measurement was required annually. Starting with the 2016 ACR Digital Mammography QC Manual it is only required at MEE.

Beam quality, as measured by the HVL, is important in mammography as the measured value directly effects patient dose and patient image contrast. HVL values are traditionally measured using an ion chamber and making exposure measurements with no additional filtration in the beam and then with varying thicknesses of aluminum to calculate the HVL in millimeters of aluminum. Modern solid state detectors can determine the HVL directly from a single exposure.

If using an ion chamber and aluminum sheets, and making several different measurements, the HVL can be calculated using the equation given in the ACR manual. The FDA MQSA requirements for beam quality performance are listed in Table 6.1.

6.2.1.3 Collimation

A collimator is used to allow only the x-rays exiting the x-ray tube to impinge on the image receptor and nowhere else. In the case of mammography, there are typically two sizes the x-ray field collimated to, 18×24 cm and 24×30 cm, or the Imperial unit equivalents of $8''\times10''$ and $10''\times12''$. Since the advent of digital mammography, manufacturers have chosen a fixed detector size close to 24×30 cm but deviate slightly to accommodate their own design requirements. The field is collimated down to the smaller size depending upon the compression paddle being used.

X-ray beam collimation has three performance requirements. The first requirement is that the x-ray field and light field shall not be misaligned by more than 2% of the SID (source-to-image

Table 6.1 X-ray tube voltage (kilovolt peak) and minimum HVL.

Designed Operating Potential (kV)	Measured Operating Voltage (kV)	Minimum HVL (millimeters of aluminum)
Below 50	20	0.20
	25	0.25
	30	0.30

distance). This means that when a user looks at the light field during patient positioning, they should be able to trust that the light field closely defines the actual x-ray field.

The second is that all systems shall allow the entire chest-wall edge of the x-ray field to extend to the chest wall edge of the image receptor and provide the means to assure the x-ray field does not extend beyond any edge of the image receptor by more than 2% of the SID. This requirement ensures the x-rays will be reasonable close to the image receptor in all directions, but especially the chest wall where the patient is aligned.

The third requirement is that the chest-wall edge of the compression paddle shall not extend beyond the chest's wall edge of the image receptor by more than 1% of the SID. This requirement assures the compression paddle is in alignment with the image receptor and no significant patient tissue is lost outside the image.

To measure collimation, one can use coins or other markers to delineate the light field and use film or other exposure recording devices to measure the deviations between the light, x-ray, paddle, and image receptor. The precise step-by-step methodology of this test can be found in the ACR Digital Mammography QC Manual.

The significance of this test is twofold. First to make sure the entire image receptor is receiving the x-ray data need to create the image. The second is to prevent unnecessary patient exposure to radiation. Years of experience have indicated that this component is not prone to failure, and so testing collimation is required only at MEE under the ACR DM QC Manual. It is required as an annual test under all manufacturer mammography QC manuals and for digital breast tomography systems.

6.3 Qualimetry

Image quality performance in mammography typically utilizes two kinds of measurements. The first is evaluation of the limiting spatial resolution of a system. The second is overall image quality assessment using a phantom. In mammography, the primary phantom is defined and mandated by the FDA MQSA regulations, used as part of the ACR Mammography Accreditation Program since its inception.

6.3.1 Resolution

Limiting spatial resolution in mammography is mostly dependent on the detector element size (pixel) inherent in the detector itself, though other factors influence it, such as laser light scatter in the case of computed radiography. The pixel size is determined by the manufacturer and manufacturing process and also relates to the type of digital detector. Typical pixel sizes in mammography range from 50 to 100 μm. There are many ways to measure limiting spatial resolution. The screen-film method typically used a line-pair test phantom imaged and visually scored using a reticle. The line-pair phantom included line-pairs both parallel and perpendicular to the anode–cathode axis of the x-ray film.

Minimum requirements for a screen-film mammography system in contact mode is 11 line-pairs per mm for line-pair bars perpendicular to the anode–cathode axis and 13 line-pairs/ per mm for line-pair bars parallel to the anode–cathode axis. Digital mammography manufacturer's all took modified approaches to measuring spatial resolution, with many making a single measurement of a line-pair phantom at a 45° angle on top of a 4 cm acrylic block and visually scoring the line-pair phantom on a workstation. Or, if film was available, line-pair measurements could be made and scored on film. Typically, manufacturers chose action limits that were closely related to the pixel size of their respective detectors.

Another approach used by some manufacturers is to determine the value of the modulation transfer function at specific line-pair frequencies. This method, while more time consuming than a visual determination, removes the objective nature of a visual measurement.

6.3.2 Image Quality

Image quality in mammography is measured using an FDA MQSA approved phantom (Figure 6.1). The phantom is imaged under clinical conditions and scored using a viewbox or monitor and under clinical lighting conditions. The ACR Screen-Film (SFM) phantom is a 4.5 cm thick acrylic block with a wax insert with test objects embedded to simulate clinical morphology. The ACR Digital Mammography (FFDM) Phantom was developed to meet all of the FDA MQSA mandated image quality requirements (test objects visibility and radiation dose measurement) but enlarged to cover the majority of the larger digital detector sizes (Figure 6.2).

Figure 6.3 is an image of the SFM phantom. The SFM phantom consists of six fibers, five speck groups, and five masses all going from larger to smaller sizes arranged in a square wax insert. A small acrylic disk is provided for measuring the contrast in a screen-film image. Figure 6.4 is an image of the FFDM phantom in a rectangular shape with the test objects arranged in a linear fashion with the top row consisting of six fibers, the next row of six speck groups, and the third of six masses. Additionally, there is a 1 mm deep, 20 mm diameter hole milled into the center of the phantom to measure contrast-to-noise (CNR). Figure 6.5 compares the FFDM phantom test object configuration to the SFM phantom test object configuration.

Table 6.2 lists the total number of test objects in each phantom comparing the SFM to FFDM phantom. The ACR SFM Phantom has a total possible score of six fibers, five speck groups, and five masses. The ACR FFDM Phantom has a total possible score of six fibers, six speck groups, and six masses.

Figure 6.1 Original Mammography Screen-Film Phantom.

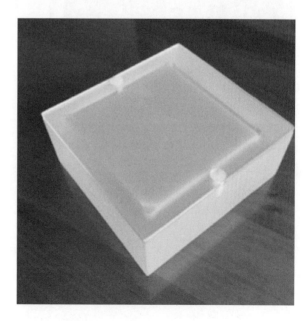

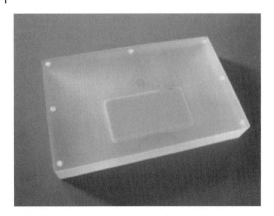

Figure 6.2   ACR Digital Mammography Phantom.

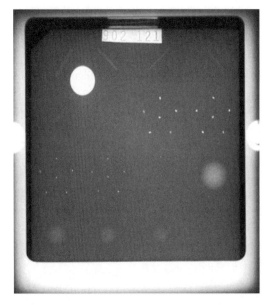

Figure 6.3   Image of Original Mammography Screen-Film Phantom. The large white circle is a 4 mm acrylic disc glued to the top of the phantom to provide an optical density contrast measurement.

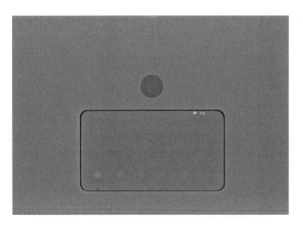

Figure 6.4   Image of ACR Digital Mammography Phantom.

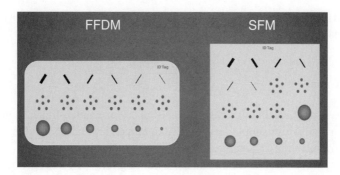

Figure 6.5 Test object comparisons of Original Mammography Screen-Film Phantom and ACR Digital Mammography Phantom.

Table 6.2 Total number of test objects in the Original Mammography Screen-Film Phantom and ACR Digital Mammography Phantom.

	ACR Mammography Phantom Total Number of Test Objects	ACR Digital Mammography Total Number of Test Objects
Fiber Score	6	6
Speck Group Score	5	6
Mass Score	5	6

Table 6.3 Minimum passing phantom scores for the Original Mammography Screen-Film Phantom and ACR Digital Mammography Phantom.

	ACR Mammography Phantom Minimum Passing Scores	ACR Digital Mammography Minimum Passing Scores
Fiber Score	4.0	2.0
Speck Group Score	3.0	3.0
Mass Score	2.0	2.0

To score the phantom after imaging, the observer counts how many test objects of each type can be visualized. Once the observer cannot visualize any further test objects of that type, the scoring is stopped. For the SFM phantom a minimum of four fibers, three speck groups, and three masses must be visualized. For the FFDM phantom a minimum of two fibers, three speck groups, and two masses must be visualized. Table 6.3 lists the minimum passing scores for both the SFM and FFDM phantoms.

For digital mammography, in addition to the test object visual evaluation, a CNR measurement is performed. This can only be done using the new FFDM phantom and using the quantitative software on the digital unit itself or on a workstation with region-of-interest (ROI) tools. The CNR value is defined as the mean cavity signal minus the mean background signal divided by the standard deviation of the background:

$$CNR = \frac{signal_{cavity} - signal_{background}}{SD_{background}}$$

All digital units should be able to produce a CNR of 2.0 or greater. In addition to a fixed CNR measured value, a digital unit should be able to maintain an annual CNR value of at least 85% or greater of the previous year's CNR value.

Signal-to-noise (SNR) is also measured and has a limiting value of 40.0 or greater. SNR is defined as the mean background signal minus the DC offset (if any from a given manufacturer) divided by the standard deviation of the background:

$$CNR = \frac{signal_{cavity} - DC\,offset}{SD_{background}}$$

6.3.3 Artifacts

Artifacts in digital mammography arise from different areas of the imaging chain. In the new ACR Digital Mammography QC Manual, evaluation for artifacts can now result in a documented failure of the QC Test. Most artifacts arise from the condition or performance of the detector. Contamination of the calibration files or deterioration of the detector itself is the most common cause of failure. X-ray tube and filter failures are the second most common reason for failures. Grid, bucky, and paddle components are the third most likely causes of artifacts. Unknown electronic noise, thermal contributions, and other miscellaneous reasons can also cause artifacts. For mobile mammography vans, electronics noise, physical vibrations, and power conditioners can often be the cause of artifacts.

When evaluating for artifacts it is often more helpful to see what an artifact-free image is rather than trying to detail the almost infinite causes of an artifact. Artifact testing typically involves imaging a "flat-field" image, usually using a uniform block of acrylic 2–4 cm thick and covering the entire detector. After imaging, the flat-field image is displayed on a monitor and evaluated for any clinically significant artifacts that may impede clinical interpretation. Figure 6.6 shows an "artifact free" flat-field image and has a very clean, uniform, appearance. Figure 6.7 shows an "artifact free" SFM phantom image. When evaluating for artifacts, it is recommended to adjust the window width and level to various settings to help emphasize any artifacts that are present. When doing this it is important to make decisions based on reasonable WW and WL settings, as too narrow a width can overemphasize artifacts that are not of clinical relevance, while a WW that is too wide can mask clinically important artifacts. Figures 6.8–6.13 are examples of typical artifacts in digital mammography. Artifacts continue to be the most significant performance issue in mammography.

6.3.4 Mammography Display Evaluation

Mammography displays (monitors) are typically divided into an acquisition workstation (AW), which is the monitor attached to the x-ray acquisition device that the technologist uses. The radiologist workstation (RW) is typically of much higher resolution and higher brightness than the AW. The RW typically has more sophisticated manufacturer built-in quality control hardware and software which allows much more detailed evaluation.

Figure 6.6 Example of an artifact-free flat-field image.

Figure 6.7 Example of a good SFM Phantom image.

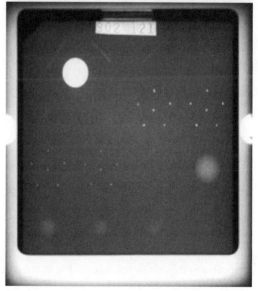

Monitor evaluation typically includes visual evaluation of a test pattern, such as the AAPM TG18-QC test pattern (Figure 6.14), physical inspection of the monitor and screen, luminance checks, and DICOM Gray-Scale Display Function (GSDF) tests. In mammography, tests are required by either the digital unit manufacturer, the monitor manufacturer, or the ACR depending on the QC Manual used by the facility. Unlike other modalities, monitor evaluations for both technologist and radiologist are required by MQSA. This requirement leads to the complexity of QC records being maintained

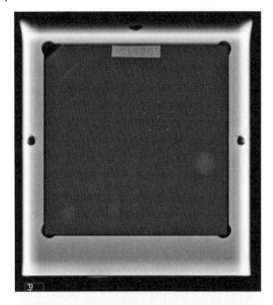

Figure 6.8 SFM Phantom with non-uniform vertical banding. This is typically due to corrupt calibration files.

Figure 6.9 Flat-field phantom exhibiting bright white pixel artifacts. This was due to a failing detector.

when images are being interpreted at off-site facilities. The ACR Digital Mammography QC Manual is the first manual to directly address the evolution of off-site reading and quality control.

6.3.5 Radiometry

6.3.5.1 Average Glandular Dose and Patient Dosimetry

Evaluation of radiation dose to the patient in mammography uses average glandular dose (AGD) from a single cranial-caudal view to a single breast as its metric. There have been a variety of ways to measure and calculate this over the years. Most recently, Dance et al. [18], presented a method that has been adopted by the majority of digital mammography vendors and also the ACR Digital Mammography QC Manual [17]. This method uses the following equation:

$$D = \text{kgcs}$$

Where,

D = average glandular dose (mGy)

K = entrance exposure (mR)

g = g-factor for breast simulated with acrylic or BR-12
c = c-factor for breast simulated with acrylic or BR-12
s = s-factor for clinically used x-ray spectra

Figure 6.10 SFM Phantom with non-uniform vertical banding. This is typically due to corrupt calibration files.

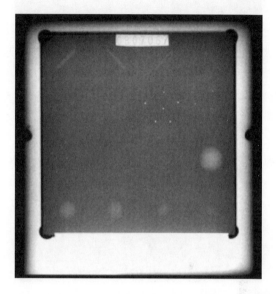

Figure 6.11 Magnified corner of a SFM Phantom with hexagonal mesh pattern. This is typically due to in improperly functioning grid from a manufacturer who uses the cross hatch grid.

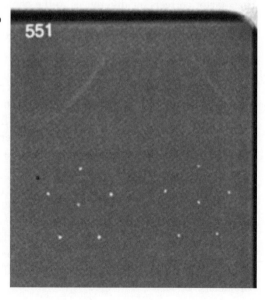

Figure 6.12 Magnified corner of a SFM Phantom with linear, vertical line pattern. This is typically due to in improperly functioning grid from a manufacturer who uses the linear grid design.

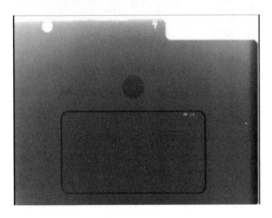

Figure 6.13 Flat-field phantom imaged on a screen-film system. A multitude of artifacts can be seen that are typical of screen-film. These include dust, roller marks, non-uniformities, and screen defects.

The factor K is the exposure in the absence of backscatter at the entrance surface of the breast. The g-factor corresponds to the glandularity of 50% and derived from values calculated from the Dance paper. The c-factor corrects for any difference in breast composition from 50% glandularity. The s-factor corrects for differences to the choice of x-ray spectrum. The Dance paper presents methods for calculating the g- and c-factors that all depend on the beam energy, HVL, and breast thickness. The ACR Digital Mammography QC Manual contains tables for the g-, c-, and s-factors for the FFDM phantom thickness and additional breast thicknesses for both acrylic and BR-12 phantom material.

The radiation dose limit mandated by the FDA MQSA regulations is 3.0 mGy for a single cranio-caudal view. In practice, systems use variations of exposure mode that can range from fully automatic exposure control (AEC) where the target-filter, kVp, and mAs are selected to optimize the image quality and dose, to an auto-time AEC where the target-filter and kVp are fixed by the operator, all the way to a fully manual mode where the operator selects all the technical factors to make an exposure.

When an automatic mode is selected, units may pre-select the target-filter and kVp on compressed breast thickness, then make a short pre-exposure to determine the exposure time required along with the target-filter combination, if these have not been predetermined, then make the exposure. The exposure time will depend on breast thickness and breast composition or density. Unlike screen-film mammography that determines x-ray exposure required to reach a certain optical density on film, digital imaging requires a certain amount of signal reaching the detector to determine final exposure parameters.

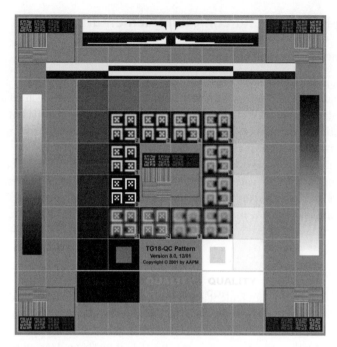

Figure 6.14 The AAPM TG18-QC test pattern.

In mammography, AEC is almost always employed. All current manufacturers seek to ensure AEC performance tracks across different breast thicknesses including magnification modes. Typically, phantoms simulating breast thicknesses of 2, 4, 6, and 8 cm in contact mode and 4 cm magnification modes are used to measure signal or SNR ratio and ensure they are all within an acceptable range. However, with more modern and current digital mammography units emerging, manufacturers are continuing to optimize their equipment resulting in the ability to maintain image quality and reduce patient doses at higher breast thicknesses. As a result, the ACR has introduced a new approach to track AEC consistency across the same breast thicknesses instead of making all breast thickness seek the same performance. This will allow manufacturers to move forward in the future to continue to optimize patient exposure for all breast sizes instead of trying to match signal to breast sizes.

An additional feature of mammography units worth mentioning is that most digital mammography units have one or two target materials and two or three filter materials to choose from. The unit or operator has the ability to select the target–filter combination, which directly effects the patient dose and exposure time. Certain target–filter combinations have harder beams that reduce patient dose and exposure time, but slightly decrease patient contrast.

Radiation doses in mammography have dropped substantially since the advent of digital mammography, especially for larger breast sizes. This is a result of a more controlled feedback loop from exposure to image receptor in digital units and the machines doing more of the selecting of techniques for clinical imaging. With newer target–filter combinations and improved detector technology, along with improved image processing algorithms, patient radiation dose in mammography will continue to go down while image quality will be maintained or improved.

6.4 Testing Paradigm and Clinical Implementation

6.4.1 Acceptance Testing and Commissioning

Acceptance testing and commissioning is required by the FDA in the MQSA regulations. After installation, a major service event, a certified part replacement, or other specified activity, and prior to imaging patients, a digital mammography unit must be tested by a qualified medical physicist.

Acceptance testing in mammography is also known as a MEE, which is a term used by the FDA in the MQSA regulations. As a minimum, a physicist must perform all required tests outlined in the quality control manual appropriate to the system. It is up to the physicist if they would like to expand their testing to acquire measurements using different acquisition modes, different magnification modes, or different target-filter settings beyond that required by the QC manual. Most quality control manuals cover the majority of system components and often times expanded measurements are not necessary.

6.4.2 Quality Control

Current there are two ways to implement a quality control program for a clinical digital mammography system. A facility may either adopt the manufacturers quality control program, or, implement the ACR Digital Quality Control Manual. An alternative standard, approved by the FDA, can be used in place of another quality control program after it has been deemed to provide mammographic quality substantially the same as the original MQSA standard.

The ACR Digital Mammography Quality Control program was approved as an alternative standard in February 2016. It contains radiologist, technologist, and medical physicist sections. The technologist and physicist sections have specific quality control test procedures, frequencies, action limits, and forms (Table 6.4).

Table 6.4 ACR Digital Mammography quality control tests.

Test	Minimum Frequency	Corrective Action Timeframe
Technologist Tests		
1) ACR DM Phantom Image Quality	Weekly	Before clinical use
2) Computed Radiography (CR) Cassette Erasure (if applicable)	Weekly	Before clinical use
3) Compression Thickness Indicator	Monthly	Within 30 days
4) Visual Checklist	Monthly	Critical items: before clinical use; less critical items: within 30 days
5) Acquisition Workstation (AW) Monitor QC	Monthly	Within 30 days; before clinical use for severe defects
6) Radiologist Workstation (RW) Monitor QC	Monthly	Within 30 days; before clinical use for severe defects
7) Film Printer QC (if applicable)	Monthly	Before clinical use
8) Viewbox Cleanliness (if applicable)	Monthly	Before clinical use
9) Facility QC Review	Quarterly	Not applicable
10) Compression Force	Semiannual	Before clinical use

Table 6.4 (Continued)

Test	Minimum Frequency	Corrective Action Timeframe
11) Manufacturer Detector Calibration (if applicable)	Mfr. Recommendation	Before clinical use
Optional – Repeat Analysis	As Needed	Within 30 days after analysis
Optional – System QC for Radiologist	As Needed	Within 30 days; before clinical use for severe artifacts
Optional – Radiologist Image Quality Feedback	As Needed	Not applicable
Medical Physicist Tests		
12) Mammography Equipment Evaluation (MEE) – MQSA Requirements	MEE	Before clinical use
13) ACR DM Phantom Image Quality	MEE and Annual	Before clinical use
14) Spatial Resolution	MEE and Annual	Within 30 days
15) Automatic Exposure Control System Performance	MEE and Annual	Within 30 days
16) Average Glandular Dose	MEE and Annual	Before clinical use
17) Unit Checklist	MEE and Annual	Critical items: before clinical use; less critical items: within 30 days
18) Computed Radiography (if applicable)	MEE and Annual	Before clinical use
19) Acquisition Workstation (AW) Monitor QC	MEE and Annual	Within 30 days; before clinical use for severe defects
20) Radiologist Workstation (RW) Monitor QC	MEE and Annual	Within 30 days; before clinical use for severe defects
21) Film Printer QC (if applicable)	MEE and Annual	Before clinical use
22) Evaluation of Site's Technologist QC Program	Annual	Within 30 days
23) Evaluation of Display Device Technologist QC Program	Annual	Within 30 days
MEE or Troubleshooting – Beam Quality (Half-Value Layer) Assessment	MEE or Troubleshooting	Before clinical use
MEE or Troubleshooting – kVp Accuracy and Reproducibility	MEE or Troubleshooting	MEE: before clinical use; troubleshooting: w/in 30 days
MEE or Troubleshooting – Collimation Assessment	MEE or Troubleshooting	MEE: before clinical use; troubleshooting: w/in 30 days
Troubleshooting – Ghost Image Evaluation	Troubleshooting	Before clinical use
Troubleshooting – Viewbox Luminance	Troubleshooting	NA

The ACR Quality Control manual has incorporated many new methods, tests, and, most importantly, the new ACR Digital Mammography Phantom. Tests are now relevant to modern equipment, modern mammography facilities, while still addressing MQSA requirements, and have been standardized across all manufacturers and models. As stated earlier, the new phantom contains more challenging test objects and a larger uniform field for artifact evaluation. While under the old paradigm the test object score could be reduced for artifacts but not fail solely due to artifacts, with the new phantom a system may fail strictly due to objectionable artifacts.

Display monitors also get special attention for quality control procedures. Image quality, luminance output, and luminance uniformity all get a single approach along with ways to track and document multiple review workstations across an imaging network. Repeat analysis has been moved to a troubleshooting and is no longer required. Beam quality, kVp, and collimation are now MEE tests only and are no longer an annual requirement. The AEC test for the physicist now tracks consistency for each breast thickness instead of combining performance for all thicknesses. SNR and CNR tests that were often technologist tests are now only in physicist testing. And, finally, a formal technologist quarterly QC review test was added to ensure that the lead interpreting radiologist, technologists, and facility manager (if any) all review the previous quarter's quality control records.

6.4.3   Accreditation and Compliance-Related Matters

To perform mammography legally in the United States, a facility has to be accredited by an FDA-approved accrediting body. The American College of Radiology, and the states of Texas, Iowa, and Arkansas are the only four approved bodies. The accrediting states have borrowed heavily from the accreditation process the ACR uses.

The accreditation process has an applying facility demonstrating that they meet the FDA MQSA requirements to perform mammography. This is a complex process and beyond the scope of this chapter to detail, but in general facilities have to document that personnel meet initial and ongoing educational and clinical requirements, equipment meets minimum standards, quality control programs are in place, and image quality and radiation doses are adequate. Both clinical and phantom images are submitted to the accrediting body for approval before accreditation can be granted. Accreditation certificates are typically on three cycles.

6.4.4   Training

The FDA requires that eight hours of training, specific to the modality, be obtained by each new user (technologist, radiologist, or medical physicist) before independent use or testing can be performed. This is very different from other imaging modalities. Users can get this training by attending conferences, training from the manufacturer, or training from another trained trainer. A user must obtain documentation of the training and have these records available to the MQSA inspector.

6.5   Mammography 1.5 – The Shifting Landscape

Mammography has always been an extremely dynamic imaging modality with many technical and equipment advances over the years. Within the last decade full-field digital mammography has almost fully replaced screen-film mammography, significantly lowering patient radiation dose and significantly improving image quality. DBT and Contrast-Enhanced Mammography (CEM) have matured with their technology, with DBT at approximately a 30% market share across the US. Breast cancer screening continues to make headlines with continued controversy regarding the right frequency to screen and at what age to start. All of this attention continues to reinforce the importance of mammography and it will continue to evolve.

In addition to equipment advancement, the less visible component of the future of mammography is the growth of the networking and transmitting of digital images and digital information. This will have a tremendous impact on the facility, medical physicist, and the regulators as images are interpreted more and more at locations that are separate from the unit of origin. Mammography, like other commodities, will continue to work toward an economy of scale to continue to allow breast imaging facilities to provide the best possible health care.

6.6 Conclusion

The vast majority of testing performed in mammography is prescribed in published documents from either the unit manufacturer or the ACR. This is due to the heavily regulated nature of mammography compared to other modalities. Additionally, mammography facilities are required by the FDA to undergo annual inspections by not only the medical physicist but also an MQSA inspector that may or may not be associated with the State. These inspections have raised the level of awareness and interest by technologists, physicians and facility managers well beyond the recognition of other modalities making mammography unique within the imaging community.

References

1 Gros, C.M. (1967). Methodologie: symposium Sur Le Sein. *Journal de Radiologie, d'Électrologie, et de Médecine Nucléaire* 48: 638–655.
2 Price, J.L. and Butler, P.D. (1970). The reduction of radiation and exposure time in mammography. *The British Journal of Radiology* 43: 251–255.
3 Ostrum, B.J., Becker, W., and Israd, H.J. (1973). Low-dose mammography. *Radiology* 109: 323–326.
4 Weiss, J.P. and Wayrynen, R.E. (1976). Imaging system for low-dose mammography. *Journal of Applied Photographic Engineering* 2: 7–10.
5 Buchanan, R.A., Finkelstein, S.I., and Wickersheim, K.A. (1976). X-ray exposure reduction using rare earth Oxysulfide intensifying screens. *Radiology* 118: 183–188.
6 Haus, A.G. (1990). Technologic improvements in screen-film mammography. *Radiology* 174: 628–637.
7 Conway, B.J., McCrohan, J.L., Reuter, F.G., and Suleiman, O.H. (1990). Mammography in the 80s. *Radiology* 177: 335–339.
8 Reuter, F.G. Preliminary Report: NEXT-85. In: National Conference on Radiation Control: Proceedings of the 18th Annual Conference of Radiation Control Program Directors. CRCPD Publication 86–2. Charlseton, W. Va: CRCPD 1986; 111–120.
9 Galkin, B.M., Feig, S.A., and Muir, H.D. (1988). The technical quality of mammography in centers participating in a regional breast cancer awareness program. *Radiographics* 8: 133–145.
10 McLelland, R., Gray, J.E., McCrohan, J. et al. (1990). *ACR Mammography Quality Control Manuals*. Reston, VA: American College of Radiology.
11 American College of Radiology (1992). *Mammography Quality Control*. Reston, VA: American College of Radiology.
12 American College of Radiology (1994). *Mammography Quality Control Manual* Revised Edition. Reston, VA: American College of Radiology.
13 American College of Radiology (1999). *Mammography Quality Control Manual*. Reston, VA: American College of Radiology.

14 Mammography Facilities-Requirements for Accrediting Bodies and Quality Standards and Certification Requirements; Part VII. Interim Rules, 21 CFR Part 900. Federal Register. 1993

15 Quality Mammography Stands; Final Rule. Part II. 21 CFR Part 16 and 900. Federal Register. 1997

16 Lewin, J.M., Hendrick, R.E., D'Orsi, C.J. et al. (2001). Comparison of full-field digital mammography with screen-film mammography for cancer detection: results of 4,945 paired examinations. *Radiology* 218: 873–880.

17 Berns, E.A., Baker, J.A., Barke, L.D. et al. (2016). *ACR Digital Mammography Quality Control Manual*. Reston, VA: American College of Radiology.

18 Dance, D.R., Skinner, C.L., Young, K.C. et al. (2000). Additional factors for the estimation of mean glandular breast dose using the UK mammography dosimetry protocol. *Physics in Medicine and Biology* 45: 3225–3240.

7

Clinical Mammography Physics: Emerging Practice

Andrew Karellas and Srinivasan Vedantham

Department of Medical Imaging, College of Medicine, University of Arizona, Tucson, AZ, USA

7.1 Philosophy and Significance

7.1.1 Background

Mammography started as a diagnostic imaging modality and it was practiced largely in women who were symptomatic of a breast abnormality. Therefore, breast cancers were detected at a much later stage than in today's screening practice of asymptomatic women. Many anatomic features such as microcalcifications, subtle masses and spiculations were difficult to visualize with early mammography which used harder x-ray beams at a higher tube potential compared to the typical 24–39 kVp used today and with special beam filtration. Early image receptors were film without intensifying screens and operated at high radiation dose. Soon after, important developments in high-resolution screen technology and dedicated x-ray generator and tube led to screen–film mammography and eventually to digital mammography. There has been a long history of research and development before the technology evolved to the "gold standard" of using an x-ray tube with a molybdenum, rhodium or tungsten x-ray target, with about 1 mm of beryllium window and very thin filtration – 0.03 mm of molybdenum for a Mo target, 0.05 mm of Rh for Mo, Rh or W targets, or 0.07 mm of Al or 0.05 mm of Ag for a W target. The tube voltage was restricted mostly between 24 and 35 kV and the antiscatter moving grid became a permanent feature in all equipment with the exception of slot-scan systems. The geometry of projection was refined providing standard and magnification views using equipment that was designed exclusively for mammography. From the year 2000 onwards, digital mammography became commercially available, and this was a major turning point in breast imaging.

7.1.2 The Development of Digital Mammography

The potential of digital mammography was envisioned on the basis of physical principles and computations, which predicted that this technology would increase tissue contrast and it would enable improved detection of tumors in dense fibroglandular tissue. This early foresight has generated significant rewards because today's digital mammography has been shown to be superior in detecting cancers in the dense breast [1]. Currently, the sensitivity of digital mammography is similar to

Clinical Imaging Physics: Current and Emerging Practice, First Edition. Edited by Ehsan Samei and Douglas E. Pfeiffer.
© 2020 John Wiley & Sons, Inc. Published 2020 by John Wiley & Sons, Inc.

screen-film mammography for women with predominantly adipose breasts [1]. The advantages of digital mammography in terms of throughput efficiency along with digital storage and communication are unquestionably superior to the old analog technology for both screening and diagnostic use. In its early days of research and development, there was considerable uncertainty about the potential of digital mammography to even meet the minimum requirements for mammography in terms of spatial resolution. One of the main concerns was the smallest attainable x-ray detector element (pixel) size for imaging microcalcifications. Even though spatial resolution remains inferior to that of a screen-film system, microcalcification visibility is acceptable and digital mammography is now a universally accepted, robust technology.

Today medical physicists are confronted with a large number of approaches to mammography using different x-ray detectors and image acquisition techniques. Mammography systems, which were very much alike using similar hardware platforms in the screen-film versions, have evolved to be dramatically different in their digital reincarnation. For example, most manufacturers use amorphous selenium as the primary detector [2], while one uses amorphous silicon with scintillator [3]. Another variant has used a slot-scan configuration for the x-ray beam with a photon-counting silicon strip detector [4].

7.2 Compliance Assurance, the Medical Physicist's Current Role

The Mammography Quality Standards Act (MQSA), which was enacted by the US Congress, has greatly enhanced the role and responsibilities of the medical physicist in mammography. The regulations from US Food and Drug Administration (FDA) mandate an extensive list of measurements that must be performed on an annual basis and for follow-up testing after a component or function fails to meet certain criteria. This evaluation was well standardized with screen-film mammography and a single guidance document, the Mammography Quality Control Manual [5] by the American College of Radiology was applicable to virtually all mammography equipment. With the advent of digital mammography, many of these well-established quality assurance standards and procedures had to be reinterpreted or modified so that they would meet the requirements of MQSA, FDA regulations and ACR accreditation.

As digital mammography equipment exhibited vastly different characteristics, accrediting and regulatory agencies required physics surveys to follow the manufacturer's recommendations for the most part of the compliance and performance evaluation rather than a generic approach previously provided by the American College of Radiology (ACR) Mammography Quality Control Manual [5]. Although the lack of uniformity in testing procedures among different mammography systems contributes to time inefficiency, medical physicists have adapted to this process.

Several of the tests performed in the annual physics evaluation are clearly very important in terms of patient safety and image quality. For example, the measurement of the radiation dose under clinically relevant conditions is meaningful but this is also a test that rarely fails in modern equipment. At times the dose may be higher than needed, or lower than the level required for good image quality, but the record of modern mammography equipment consistently meeting regulatory requirements in terms of radiation dose is considered very good. However, current methodology for radiation dosimetry relies on dose measurements using a "standard" phantom which was intended to represent the average breast thickness and composition. Although this approach is reasonable as a reference point, the medical physicist may be required to provide more insight on the Average Glandular Dose (AGD) for an individual patient. This issue is discussed later in this chapter.

Since digital mammography systems have a wider range of linear response with incident air KERMA (exposure) compared to screen-film systems, there was a concern regarding radiation "dose creep" with digital mammography [6]. However, the radiation dose from digital mammography is lower than screen-film systems as evidenced from the results of the American College of Radiology Imaging Network-Digital Mammography Imaging Screening Trial (ACRIN-DMIST) study [7, 8]. Image quality is critically important and this can vary substantially between different equipment and over time. Image artifacts due to detector defects or inadequate calibration must be identified, reported in the periodic survey and remediated. Radiologists and technologists may observe image artifacts between annual surveys and it is critical that they contact the medical physicist and engineering for timely remediation of the problem.

Certain performance characteristics may not be as critical for good-quality mammography and patient safety, whereas other characteristics are of high importance for ensuring patient safety and high-quality mammography. Nevertheless, it is important to ensure that the system is in compliance with applicable requirements. For example, if the x-ray field extends 2 mm outside of the detector beyond the regulatory limit on the distal part of the x-ray field (breast nipple side) the impact to safety and image quality is practically of no significance but it must be brought to compliance. By comparison, the same magnitude of deviation at the chest wall is cause for timely correction because of the obvious effect of irradiating excess tissue at the chest wall, which will not be included in the image. It may also be argued that other tests like kV accuracy may not be critically important because drifts beyond approximately 1–2 kV are not too common and in digital mammography a small drift in kV may not have a substantial effect on image quality. However, a slight change in kV may affect the response and function of the automatic exposure control with possible over or under compensation in the exposure time. Therefore, the evaluation of kV accuracy is currently considered important until proven otherwise.

7.3 Operational Resource, the Medical Physicist's Expanded Role and Frequency of Medical Physics Services

Limiting the participation of medical physics to an annual visit to the facility with little if any meaningful communication between annual surveys can lead to overlooked deficiencies and these deficiencies may linger until the date of the next annual survey. Assuring safety and compliance is an important responsibility of the medical physicist in mammography. However, this practice can easily degenerate into an annual routine where only major and obvious problems are identified and remediated and the prevailing objective is to simply comply with the regulation. Under such a plan it is possible, and actually very likely, that the medical physicist has minimal to no communication with a responsible individual in a particular facility until the next annual medical physics survey. During that time, subtle changes in image quality may or may not be noticed by the technologists or the radiologists and suboptimal imaging for a prolonged period of time is possible. Depending on the facility, the medical physicist may receive occasional calls with questions about equipment performance or about regulatory compliance, and engineering service may be called without concurrent notification to the medical physicist. In many cases, follow-up by the medical physicist is not needed but certain types of engineering services require follow-up evaluation by the medical physicist. Replacement of the x-ray tube or detector is an obvious example where the medical physicist is always called upon to ensure optimal performance of the system. However, removal of the x-ray imager to test if it works on a nearby unit and replacing it back on its original system may not be recorded as an action that needs notification to the medical physicist. While this may seem innocuous, as the x-ray imager had been replaced onto the original system, there are potential sources for suboptimal image quality and patient safety. For example, if appropriate recalibration is not performed upon reinstalling the x-ray imager onto the original system this could lead to suboptimal image quality. Also, upon reinstalling the x-ray imager to the system, the congruence between the x-ray field and the imager may not be the same as prior to removal. This may adversely affect patient safety, for example, by unnecessary irradiation of the chest that does not contribute to the image.

Recommendations: An electronic recording and notification system must be implemented for entry of all actions taken by engineering service. Such actions include periodic calibrations, electronic or mechanical adjustments, replacement of major components, and removing and reinstalling of major components. Service recording systems are already in use, but the notification aspect for efficient tracking and communication between engineering, the technologist, and the medical physicist is not adequately practiced. Implementing and auditing the implementation is intended to identify and reduce the number of events where follow-up by the medical physicist was needed but was not performed.

Regulatory compliance is essential but regulations alone cannot guarantee optimal results. These regulations are intended to provide minimum performance/acceptance criteria but superior quality mammography is achievable by identifying optimal criteria above and beyond the minimum performance/acceptance levels. The determination for annual versus some other time period for routine tests and surveys is based on a combination of data on failure rates and convenience. Regardless, for mammographic and other radiographic equipment we could use more reliability data to better define routine testing intervals. The proposed recommendation of implementing an electronic recording and notification system can be of value in better defining the testing intervals.

The medical physicist must also act as an operational resource providing input on the ongoing issues relating to quality and safety in mammography. This means that the medical physicist must play a continuous role rather than sporadic involvement with the issues that relate to how equipment and equipment performance affect patient care and radiation safety. The following are currently areas that the medical physicist can pay more attention to as an operational resource and are ordered from screening to post-diagnosis patient care:

- quantitative assessment of breast density
- guidance on implementing appropriate breast cancer-risk related models to ensure quality of breast cancer screening procedure
- collection of technique data (kV, mAs, filter, breast thickness)
- collection of dose related data (air KERMA at skin entrance, HVL, AGD)
- use of CAD
- focus on diagnostic mammography (magnification and spot views)
- verifying the targeting accuracy of stereotactic biopsy equipment
- verifying the size and distance measurements reported on review workstations is concordant with truth
- Assistance in determining outcome measures from mammography.

7.4 Metrics and Analytics

The routine annual physics survey of digital mammography equipment is important for safety and compliance but there is other important information that is not captured by this survey. For example, in a given population of screening or diagnostic mammography the medical physicist may not be aware of the following:

- information on actual kV, mAs and exposure time
- information on breast compression and thickness
- information on breast glandularity
- percent of screening versus diagnostic procedures
- prior mammography history for a given patient
- radiation dose differences between screening and diagnostic mammography

Some of the aforementioned information is recorded on the DICOM image headers. Statistics on the exposure parameters such as kV and exposure time can be very important in identifying problems in the function of the x-ray generator and tube. A particular system may behave normally during the annual survey but during the interval between successive annual surveys its performance may be erratic causing problems with image quality. Currently, we have no clear information on how a mammography system performs over an extended period in actual clinical use. Extreme values in kV or exposure time can be useful to identify operational problems as well as studying the influence of breast density and thicknesses encountered in a particular practice on these exposure parameters. This information may be useful in the proper calibration of the automatic exposure control, which can be based on realistic variations in breast thickness and composition rather than on homogenous phantoms. Analysis of the trends in breast compression force and compressed breast thickness could help in identifying equipment related issues as well as operator related factors such as adequacy of breast compression. This feedback to the operator could improve the quality of mammography practice and patient safety. Currently, there are several methods, techniques, and software implementations that provide for a quantitative estimate of breast density or glandularity [9–16]. While these quantitative estimates of breast density are mostly intended for risk estimation [17] and to identify patients who may be best served with a supplemental screening procedure, these data may be useful for optimizing the automatic exposure control mechanism.

The differences between screening and diagnostic mammography is often overlooked, especially when reporting dose in mammography. For example, in an inquiry on dose to the breast from mammography without additional details, the assumption may be made that the inquiry is about screening mammography. In contrast to screening mammography where two standard views viz., craniocaudal (CC) and mediolateral oblique (MLO) are acquired, the AGD in diagnostic mammography can be much higher than in screening [18–20]. The higher dose is the result of multiple views that include spot compression and magnification views depending on the patient-specific clinical need. There is little information in the literature on dose trends in diagnostic mammography [19] but medical physicists may be surprised to find out that at large number of views may be acquired for some diagnostic mammography procedures.

Increasingly, patients demand more detailed information about the radiation dose from x-ray procedures and this trend is likely to continue. In future, this information will be based on patient specific data rather than a literature value. Providing a textbook value may be instructive in a general inquiry, but increasingly this will not be considered responsible in an inquiry from a patient or a physician for an actual mammography procedure. The AGD for a single mammographic view can be calculated as shown in Figure 7.1. For multiple mammograms of the same breast, the AGD

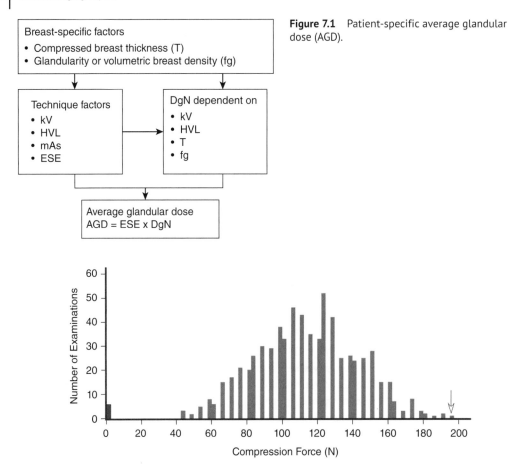

Figure 7.1 Patient-specific average glandular dose (AGD).

Figure 7.2 Variation of the breast compression force to the right breast in a routine digital mammography screening practice over a continuous 30 day period. The arrow shows the highest value recorded for one view during this period.

can be cumulated [21]. Access to prior mammography history for a given patient could enable estimation of patient specific cumulative dose over time.

The investigation of trends in radiation dose, breast compression force, and other parameters must extend beyond the "average" or "typical" values. Reliance on such general trends may lead to lack of understanding of the magnitude of potential problems. The following are just two examples of observations as shown in Figures 7.2 and 7.3. These figures show the recent trend in compression force and AGD respectively within a continuous 30 day period in a mammography screening examinations. Digital breast tomosynthesis (DBT) was not included in these observations. These examples do not represent a comprehensive and systematic statistical survey but they can be instructive about the type of variations that are expected in digital mammography systems in clinical practice.

Figure 7.2 shows the readout of the variation in the applied compression force in this sample of examinations. While this is not an unusual distribution, the extreme high and low breast compression values are of interest and improvements may be possible. At the very least, medical physicists must pay attention to the accuracy of the compression force and measuring mechanism for proper

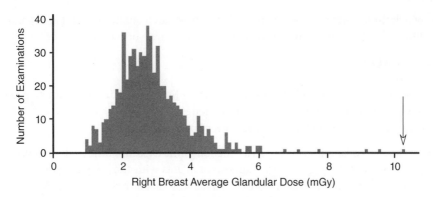

Figure 7.3 Variation of the right breast average glandular dose (AGD) in a routine digital mammography screening practice over a continuous 30 day period. The arrow indicates the highest cumulated dose from all views for the right breast (sometimes more than the standard two views).

operation. Medical physicists must become more involved in the collection, analysis and interpretation of physical data such as breast compression force and investigate the root cause of values that exceed a certain range above or below the mean value.

Figure 7.3 shows the variation of the right breast AGD in a digital mammography screening practice over a continuous 30 day period. The arrow indicates the highest cumulated dose from all views for the right breast. Sometimes more than the typical two views may be required because of breast size or repeat views. In most cases the reason for the outliers at the high dose end of the distribution is high breast thickness and density. The AGD for a high density breast with 80 mm compressed thickness for example can exceed two or three times higher the AGD for an "average" breast. A persistent trend of high AGD may warrant a more in-depth evaluation of the automatic exposure control mechanism and in particular on the kV and filtration selected for large and dense breasts.

The aforementioned examples in Figures 7.2 and 7.3 represent a very limited view of trends in just two parameters in digital mammography. A closer examination of other trends like kV and filtration in conjunction with breast thickness and composition may reveal deficiencies in acquisition techniques that may need attention. Medical physicists are encouraged to become more engaged, not only with the testing of equipment in isolation, but also with the equipment as used in patients. Until recently, image acquisition techniques were not easily accessible by the medical physicist and this may have been especially challenging for some consulting medical physicists. The advent of commercially available radiation dose monitoring software is now facilitating access to image acquisition and dose related parameters and this presents a great opportunity for all diagnostic medical physicists to gain more insight into image acquisition trends before and after the annual survey. In the case of outlier values as demonstrated in Figures 7.2 and 7.3, a more in-depth analysis can be performed to identify the root causes of certain trends and find solutions for improved image quality at reduced discomfort and radiation dose to patients.

7.4.1 Intrinsic Performance

Mammography physics surveys include of a comprehensive list of tests. Even with this thorough evaluation, the medical physicist rarely has access to the more esoteric aspects of x-ray generation, which may have profound effects on image performance. In addition, the intrinsic performance of the system can be more thoroughly characterized using well-established physics-based quantitative metrics, which unfortunately have been used only in research studies [22, 23] and not as part of routine clinical practice. The following are a few tests that are worth consideration:

- radiation waveform
- x-ray spectrum
- spatial resolution characterization using pre-sampled Modulation Transfer Function (MTF)
- spatial resolution under various magnification modes
- system noise characterization using Noise Power Spectrum (NPS)

The recording of the radiation output as a function of the exposure time (radiation waveform) is a well-known test that is performed to diagnose problems with the x-ray generator or the x-ray tube. Modern x-ray systems are expected to be stable in terms of radiation and kV waveform but there is a paucity of data to support this assumption. A non-invasive device to continually monitor the radiation output could be of benefit.

Currently, the limiting spatial resolution is determined either by visual analysis of a test bar pattern or by quantitative analysis of the bar pattern at manufacturer-specified spatial frequencies. Determination of the pre-sampled MTF [24] provides the advantage of a nearly continuous measure of system response as a function of spatial frequency. This may help identify spatial resolution degradation over time at spatial frequencies that may not be captured with bar pattern-based analyses. There is currently a paucity of data to indicate if measurement of pre-sampled MTF over time could identify degradation of spatial resolution of the imaging system earlier than the current standard using bar patterns. Magnification views play an important role during diagnostic mammography particularly for evaluating suspicious microcalcifications. It is important to quantify the spatial resolution characteristics of a system under various magnification modes. Given the asymmetric focal spot size, characterizing the pre-sampled MTF along the two orthogonal directions, in particular for magnification views, rather than using a bar pattern will be of value.

Currently, image noise is quantified using standard deviation of the background region in a phantom with targets or using homogenous material. While this is a valid measure, it does not provide spatial frequency dependence of the noise. NPS estimated using well-established techniques could provide a near-continuous measure of imaging system noise as a function of spatial frequency. In particular such NPS analysis inclusive of structured noise component could also identify periodic noise patterns that could not be readily recognized during visual analysis of image artifacts due to flat-field correction.

7.4.2 Qualimetry

Quantitative characterization of the imaging system in terms of the pre-sampling MTF, which provides a measure of spatial resolution, and the NPS at a given detector entrance exposure, which provides a measure of image noise, facilitates computation of the Noise Equivalent Quanta (NEQ) at that exposure. The NEQ provides the square of the signal-to-noise ratio transfer characteristics of the system as a function of spatial frequency. The NEQ, when combined with a description of an imaging task in terms of spatial frequency, such as detection of a lesion of a give shape, size, and composition, provides the International Commission of Radiological Units (ICRU) recommended detectability index, d' [25]. Determining the NEQ with the NPS measure inclusive of structured noise component provides a better understanding of the qualitative and quantitative effect of periodic image artifacts on overall system performance. The NEQ, when used to determine the detectability index, can be further generalized to include the x-ray scatter contribution to the image and the background breast structure, commonly referred to as anatomical noise [26]. This unifying metric can be of profound value in task-specific evaluation and optimization of mammography systems.

Another approach to determine the combined effects of radiation dose, and consequently the image noise and spatial resolution, is to assess the threshold contrast-detail characteristics of the system. One potential phantom for such evaluation is the CDMAM phantom [27]. For this specific phantom, automated analysis software has been developed, providing a time-efficient test that could even be used on a more frequent basis to characterize and identify temporal changes in mammography system performance. One limitation of this approach is that it does not include the anatomic noise arising from normal breast structures, which has been shown to be a major factor in limiting detection of lesions, particularly soft tissue abnormalities [26].

7.4.3 Radiometry

The measured air KERMA at skin entrance and AGD based on a phantom acquisition can be of value in determining the consistency and assessing temporal changes in the tested system. However, they are of limited use in determining the actual dose to the patient. For a more accurate assessment of the patient dose the medical physicist must have the actual exposure parameters used to acquire that patient's images. The system generates a value for AGD that is included in the DICOM Radiation Dose Structure Report (RDSR), but its accuracy may have to be verified by the medical physicist – especially important with magnification views. Ideally the medical physicist should have access to advanced simulation programs that can compute the AGD based on the input of the important parameters of exposure geometry and approximate tissue composition. Further, with the availability of quantitative tools for estimating breast density, which is likely to be become more widespread, utilizing this patient/breast-specific density could further refine the dose estimate.

7.5 Testing Implication of New Technologies

7.5.1 Hardware

7.5.1.1 Digital Mammography

As noted earlier in this chapter, the hardware in mammography has advanced significantly in terms of technology and approach compared to the technology of just a few years ago. The most common technologies used today are:

- flat panel detector using direct conversion amorphous selenium detector
- flat panel detector using indirect detector amorphous silicon detector
- slot-scan approach using silicon detector.

The establishment of a uniform set of specifications for digital mammography across various systems is challenging because each system has unique characteristics. For example, the spatial resolution as shown by the MTF or by the visual and more subjective test pattern imaging can vary widely for systems from different manufacturers [4]. Digital mammography systems employing hexagonal pixels [28] have been introduced in clinical practice. Hexagonal pixel arrays provide the advantage of increased sampling density. However, these raw images have to be resampled to square pixels to ensure display without distortion. While the pre-sampled MTF and NPS can be readily estimated after resampling, ideally it would be preferable to determine these physical metrics prior to resampling. This would allow the effect of resampling on image quality to be understood. We do not know if detectors with hexagonal pixels will be translated for other x-ray imaging equipment, but the medical physicist must understand the fundamental principles and issues that may arise in the evaluation of image quality.

7.5.1.2 Digital Mammography with Tomosynthesis

The addition of DBT as a feature of digital mammography adds to the complexity of these systems. Systems acquire tomographic views by taking a number of projections along an arc ranging from $\pm7.5°$ to $\pm25°$ depending on the particular system [29]. In such combined DBT and mammography systems, the x-ray detector may be operated in a different mode, such as employing pixel binning; hence, the spatial resolution is likely to be different between the DBT and mammography modes. Additionally, factors such as oblique x-ray incidence on the detector and tube motion during acquisition will also contribute to degradation of spatial resolution. Importantly, the spatial resolution in planes parallel to the breast support (x–y planes) and along the axis orthogonal to the breast support (z-axis) will be substantially different due to the limited-angle acquisition during DBT. The z-axis resolution, or, alternatively, the slice sensitivity profile, will also vary between systems because of the differences in angular sampling. The variability in specifications and performance has made it difficult for accrediting organizations such as the American College of Radiology and regulatory Agencies such as the US FDA to enforce strict minimum standards on specifications. In recent years, these agencies are willing to adopt certain performance standards as specified by the manufacturers of mammography and DBT equipment. This practice has been well accepted and it has been reasonably successful. However, whether this approach provides for maintaining the highest image quality consistent with the aim of effective screening and diagnostic use needs further investigation. Currently, the AAPM has a task group to provide guidelines and recommendations for quality control of DBT systems. The American College of Radiology has completed a quality control manual for DBT. In addition to the aforementioned variability between systems based on their design characteristics, the same system may provide for multiple modes of operation in terms of angular range of tube motion and pixel size either by binning or resampling that are targeted towards either screening or diagnostic use.

7.5.2 Software: The Medical physicist's Role

Currently, there are at least two US FDA approved image analysis software packages to estimate breast density. One approach to validate the accuracy of the breast density estimation software is to develop a set of 3D physical breast phantoms with known breast densities that replicate the structures observed in a normal breast [30]. The availability of 3D printers makes it feasible to pursue such an approach. An alternate approach is to have a collection of mammograms from patients for whom the breast density has been determined either from MRI or dedicated breast CT. It is relevant to note that the software used for estimating breast density requires the DICOM "for processing" images and not the DICOM "for presentation" images, which are subjected to additional image processing such as for visualizing the skin line near the periphery of the breast. These tasks, however, are generally beyond the scope of the clinical medical physicist.

While the major focus of mammography quality control is targeted toward screening, mammography also plays an important role for diagnosis and post-diagnosis evaluation, such as in the determination of the size of tumor to determine appropriate treatment. For example, for pathology-verified tumors with no nodal involvement, tumor size and location, and breast size are important factors in determining whether the patient would be suitable for breast conserving surgery or would need to undergo mastectomy. Hence, it is important that the accuracy of the measurement scale provided with the image display software either as part of the review workstation or picture archiving and communication system is quantified. At present, while quality control procedures do address the displayed image quality and the performance of the image display, little attention is paid to determining the accuracy of size, area, and distance measurement scale provided with the review workstations. When review workstations are installed or upgraded, it is important to verify that the quantitative image evaluation tools are accurate.

For systems capable of DBT, the implications of the reconstruction algorithms on the image quality need to be understood. Most DBT systems use either a variant of filtered back-projection (FBP), iterative reconstruction methods, or a combination thereof. For systems using FBP, the choice of filter kernel could have a profound impact on reconstructed image quality similar to CT systems. For iterative reconstruction methods, the factors included in the forward model, the objective function, the regularization function, the number of iterations as well as the implementation of the algorithm could all contribute the reconstructed image quality. In future it is quite likely that the reconstruction algorithms are tuned to a specific imaging task. For example, it may be possible that we may use one setting each for screening, diagnostic evaluation of soft tissue abnormalities and diagnostic evaluation of microcalcifications. This is likely to pose additional challenges in quality control of such systems. In such cases, the importance of task-based evaluation would be even more profound. When modifications are made to the image reconstruction software, it is essential to perform a thorough quality control testing, preferably from a set of clinical images with anatomical structure to understand its implications in clinical use.

7.5.3 Image Processing

Two-dimensional digital mammograms synthesized from DBT using image processing algorithms, primarily to reduce the additional dose to patient from an acquired digital mammogram, pose an additional challenge in terms of quality control testing. At present, published data suggest that, according to phantom-based measures and quality control tests, the synthesized digital mammograms need further refinement to match the image quality of an acquired digital mammogram [31]. Clinical studies indicate progressive improvement with the algorithms used for generating the synthesized mammogram [29, 32–34]. Hence, it is quite likely that the software used to generate the synthesized digital mammogram will continue to be refined. When modifications are made to the algorithm/software it is essential to evaluate the implications of these changes. Further, it is essential to ensure that synthesized 2D mammograms provided by a system meet the radiologists' needs for diagnostic image quality.

7.5.4 System-Wide Technologies

It is important for the medical physicist to recognize that mammography and DBT, while playing a critical role in breast cancer imaging, are only part of the continuum of breast-related care. This care ranges from risk-assessment models to identify patients suitable for adjunctive imaging with more sensitive but often more expensive and restrictive imaging modalities in terms of eligibility for such imaging, to genetic testing to identify patients for prophylactic intervention or increased surveillance, to CT imaging for radiation therapy treatment planning. In the future there is likely to be a large growth in system-wide technologies that integrate these multiple modalities in terms of the interpretation and study results to multimodality image registration. Medical physicists can play a constructive role in critically evaluating these approaches and determining optimal solutions to ensure the overall health and safety of the patient beyond quality control of mammography alone.

7.6 Clinical Integration and Implementation

7.6.1 Training

In order for the medical physicist to implement these new paradigms into clinical practice, the most essential requirement is continually updating one's skill set and undergoing training in all aspects pertaining to system-wide technologies relevant to breast-related care. It is important that the medical physicist is in the forefront of understanding the various imaging technologies in terms of the physics, operational characteristics, and clinical benefits. Combining this knowledge with a good understanding of the system-wide technologies would be of great benefit in developing the implementation plan. It is also critical that the plan for implementation is clearly outlined and communicated to the leadership at the clinical practice. Engaging all stakeholders early in the planning stages would facilitate a cohesive plan that is less likely to encounter technical and logistical challenges.

7.6.2 Optimization

It is important that the medical physicist develop an approach for optimizing the image acquisition protocol based on clinical tasks. At present, automatic selection of technique factors including target (if selectable), filter, kVp, and mAs is mostly performed by an AEC mechanism without consideration for the clinical imaging task. For example, during diagnostic evaluation where there is *a priori* knowledge as to whether the radiologist is concerned with an area of soft tissue, or if the evaluation is for microcalcifications. Ideally the image acquisition protocol needs to be tailored for that clinical task. This is likely to be particularly important for diagnostic evaluation with DBT, where selection of angular range, detector pixel size, and reconstruction method may be possible. This implies that the medical physicist should be well versed in the physics and implementation aspects of task-specific evaluation methods. In order for the medical physicist to implement such optimization of protocols, it is essential to understand the workflow. In the diagnostic imaging example above, it is essential that the images are made available to the radiologist in a reasonable timeframe to determine the next course of action, as the patient is waiting for the radiologists recommendation. An image reconstruction method that could take several hours would be unsuitable for such implementation. On the other hand, considering that screening mammograms are often batch-read at most institutions, an increased time between acquisition and availability of the images for interpretation by the radiologist would be of lesser concern.

7.6.3 Automated Analysis and Data Management

One potential phantom and automated analysis that can provide a framework for a future was designed and used for quality control during the ACRIN-DMIST study [7]. This phantom enabled simultaneous visual analysis targets simulating microcalcification clusters as well as automated analysis of pre-sampled MTF. Another phantom and automated analysis tool is the CDMAM [27], mentioned previously, which allows determination of threshold contrast-detail characteristics of the mammography system. Considering that determination of the system response function, pre-sampled MTF, NPS, and scatter-to-primary ratio would enable determination of the generalized NEQ for task-specific evaluation, a phantom could be potentially designed to facilitate automated analysis. The imaging tasks needed to perform such an analysis can be provided as part of the automated analysis tool. Such a metric would be clinically meaningful in assessing task-based performance of the system. The International Atomic Energy Agency currently has a working group in place developing just such a phantom and software tool.

Tracking image acquisition technique factors and image analysis may facilitate quantitative breast density estimates, lifetime risk from established risk-assessment models, and clinical outcome measures for each patient. Analyzing these data would enable patient-specific dose estimates based on the individual's breast density, identifying patients who are likely to benefit from supplemental imaging, identifying resource utilization in terms of the appropriateness of the modality(ies) used, refining the risk models to incorporate breast density estimates based on outcome measures, identifying any aberration in a specific system in a clinical practice with multiple mammography systems, and identifying if appropriate compression is used during image acquisition.

7.6.4 Meaningful QC

In order for the new paradigm to be effective and clinically relevant, the quality control procedures need to be timely, expedient, minimally intrusive, and optimally, automated, while providing the sensitivity needs to alert for changes that could impact image quality and to address the clinical challenges. The medical physicist should be integrated with the clinical practice so that they can monitor for any change in the metrics between periodic surveys that might adversely affect image quality or patient safety. Any such event that triggers an engineering service should be tracked, the remediation documented and communicated through an automated process, followed by verification by the medical physicist. In addition, the medical physicist, with their physics and quantitative skills, should have access to outcome measures so that they are able to provide constructive recommendations to improve the overall system-wide performance of breast imaging practice. It is important for medical physicists to serve the role of enabling quality practice rather than limiting themselves to auditing mammography equipment.

7.7 Summary

In summary, the future of mammographic quality control is likely to include more quantitative metrics that are aimed at evaluating the system for specific clinical tasks. Some of the tests performed as part of quality assurance today would remain, mainly for adherence to regulatory or accreditation requirements. Additionally, there will be a tremendous growth in informatics and analytics based on the collected data. This could potentially be integrated with real-time notification to engineering service and medical physicists so that possible issues with equipment performance can be identified early and remedied promptly. This requires that the medical physicist be continuously engaged within the clinical practice, rather than just for annual surveys and ad hoc verification after a major service. In order for medical physicist to keep abreast of these impending changes, it is important to seek continued training.

7.8 Acknowledgments

The data used in Figures 7.2 and 7.3 were obtained as part of quality improvement process, while employed at the University of Massachusetts Medical School. Some of the knowledge gained were from National Cancer Institute (NCI) of the National Institutes of Health (NIH) grants R21CA134128, R01CA195512 and R01CA199044. The contents are solely the responsibility of the authors and do not necessarily reflect the official views of the NCI or the NIH.

References

1 Pisano, E.D., Gatsonis, C., Hendrick, E. et al. (2005). Diagnostic performance of digital versus film mammography for breast-cancer screening. *N. Engl. J. Med.* 353 (17): 1773–1783.

2 Zhao, W., Ji, W.G., Debrie, A., and Rowlands, J.A. (2003). Imaging performance of amorphous selenium based flat-panel detectors for digital mammography: characterization of a small area prototype detector. *Med. Phys.* 30 (2): 254–263.

3 Vedantham, S., Karellas, A., Suryanarayanan, S. et al. (2000). Full breast digital mammography with an amorphous silicon-based flat panel detector: physical characteristics of a clinical prototype. *Med. Phys.* 27 (3): 558–567.

4 Monnin, P., Gutierrez, D., Bulling, S. et al. (2007). A comparison of the performance of digital mammography systems. *Med. Phys.* 34 (3): 906–914.

5 ACR (1999). *Mammography Quality Control Manual*. Reston, VA: American College of Radiology (ACR).

6 Seibert, J.A. (2004). Mammography "dose creep": causes and solutions. *Acad. Radiol.* 11 (5): 487–488.

7 Bloomquist, A.K., Yaffe, M.J., Pisano, E.D. et al. (2006). Quality control for digital mammography in the ACRIN DMIST trial: part I. *Med. Phys.* 33 (3): 719–736.

8 Hendrick, R.E., Pisano, E.D., Averbukh, A. et al. (2010). Comparison of acquisition parameters and breast dose in digital mammography and screen-film mammography in the American College of Radiology Imaging Network digital mammographic imaging screening trial. *AJR Am. J. Roentgenol.* 194 (2): 362–369.

9 Malkov, S., Wang, J., Kerlikowske, K. et al. (2009). Single x-ray absorptiometry method for the quantitative mammographic measure of fibroglandular tissue volume. *Med. Phys.* 36 (12): 5525–5536.

10 Yaffe, M.J., Boone, J.M., Packard, N. et al. (2009). The myth of the 50-50 breast. *Med. Phys.* 36 (12): 5437–5443.

11 Vedantham, S., Shi, L., Karellas, A. et al. (2011). Semi-automated segmentation and classification of digital breast tomosynthesis reconstructed images. *Conf. Proc. IEEE Eng. Med. Biol. Soc.*: 6188–6191.

12 Vedantham, S., Shi, L., Karellas, A., and O'Connell, A.M. (2012). Dedicated breast CT: fibroglandular volume measurements in a diagnostic population. *Med. Phys.* 39 (12): 7317–7328.

13 Tagliafico, A., Tagliafico, G., Astengo, D. et al. (2013). Comparative estimation of percentage breast tissue density for digital mammography, digital breast tomosynthesis, and magnetic resonance imaging. *Breast Cancer Res. Treat.* 138 (1): 311–317.

14 Alonzo-Proulx, O., Mawdsley, G.E., Patrie, J.T. et al. (2015). Reliability of automated breast density measurements. *Radiology* 275 (2): 366–376.

15 Vedantham, S., Shi, L., Michaelsen, K.E. et al. (2015). Digital breast tomosynthesis guided near infrared spectroscopy: volumetric estimates of fibroglandular fraction and breast density from tomosynthesis reconstructions. *Biomed. Phys. Eng. Exp.* 1 (4): 045202.

16 Puliti, D., Zappa, M., Giorgi Rossi, P. et al. (2018). DENSITY Working Group. Volumetric breast density and risk of advanced cancers after a negative screening episode: a cohort study. *Breast Cancer Res.* 20 (1): 95. doi: 10.1186/s13058-018-1025-8.

17 McCormack, V.A. and dos Santos Silva, I. (2006). Breast density and parenchymal patterns as markers of breast cancer risk: a meta-analysis. *Cancer Epidemiol. Biomark. Prev.* 15 (6): 1159–1169.

18 Liu, B., Goodsitt, M., and Chan, H.P. (1995). Normalized average glandular dose in magnification mammography. *Radiology* 197 (1): 27–32.

19 Vedantham, S., Shi, L., Karellas, A. et al. (2013). Personalized estimates of radiation dose from dedicated breast CT in a diagnostic population and comparison with diagnostic mammography. *Phys. Med. Biol.* 58 (22): 7921–7936.

20 Law, J. (2005). Breast dose from magnification films in mammography. *Br. J. Radiol.* 78 (933): 816–820.

21 Hendrick, R.E. (2010). Radiation doses and cancer risks from breast imaging studies. *Radiology* 257 (1): 246–253.

22 Vedantham, S., Karellas, A., Suryanarayanan, S. et al. (2000). Mammographic imaging with a small format CCD-based digital cassette: physical characteristics of a clinical system. *Med. Phys.* 27 (8): 1832–1840.

23 Suryanarayanan, S., Karellas, A., and Vedantham, S. (2004). Physical characteristics of a full-field digital mammography system. *Nucl. Instrum. Methods Phy. Res. Sect. A* 533 (3): 560–570.

24 Samei, E., Buhr, E., Granfors, P. et al. (2005). Comparison of edge analysis techniques for the determination of the MTF of digital radiographic systems. *Phys. Med. Biol.* 50 (15): 3613–3625.

25 . ICRU (1996). Medical Imaging – The Assessment of Image Quality, Report No. 54, (International Commission on Radiation Units and Measurements, Bethesda, MD).

26 Burgess, A.E., Jacobson, F.L., and Judy, P.F. (2001). Human observer detection experiments with mammograms and power-law noise. *Med. Phys.* 28 (4): 419–437.

27 Suryanarayanan, S., Karellas, A., Vedantham, S. et al. (2002). Flat-panel digital mammography system: contrast-detail comparison between screen-film radiographs and hard-copy images. *Radiology* 225 (3): 801–807.

28 Okada, Y., Sato, K., Ito, T. et al. (2013), Proc. SPIE 8668). A newly developed a-Se mammography flat panel detector with high-sensitivity and low image artifact. In: *Medical Imaging 2013: Physics of Medical Imaging* (eds. R.M. Nishikawa, B.R. Whiting and C. Hoeschen), 86685V. Orlando, FL: SPIE.

29 Vedantham, S., Karellas, A., Vijayaraghavan, G.R., and Kopans, D.B. (2015). Digital breast tomosynthesis: state-of-the-art. *Radiology* 277 (3): 663–684.

30 Kiarashi, N., Nolte, A.C., Sturgeon, G.M. et al. (2015). Development of realistic physical breast phantoms matched to virtual breast phantoms based on human subject data. *Med. Phys.* 42 (7): 4116–4126.

31 Nelson, J., Wells, J., and Samei, E. (2015). Intrinsic image quality comparison of synthesized 2-D and FFDM images. *Med. Phys.* 42 (6): 3611–3612.

32 Spangler, M.L., Zuley, M.L., Sumkin, J.H. et al. (2011). Detection and classification of calcifications on digital breast tomosynthesis and 2D digital mammography: a comparison. *AJR Am. J. Roentgenol.* 196 (2): 320–324.

33 Zuley, M.L., Guo, B., Catullo, V.J. et al. (2014). Comparison of two-dimensional synthesized mammograms versus original digital mammograms alone and in combination with tomosynthesis images. *Radiology* 271 (3): 664–671.

34 Skaane, P., Bandos, A.I., Eben, E.B. et al. (2014). Two-view digital breast tomosynthesis screening with synthetically reconstructed projection images: comparison with digital breast tomosynthesis with full-field digital mammographic images. *Radiology* 271 (3): 655–663.

Part III

Fluoroscopy

8

Clinical Fluoroscopy Physics: Perspective

Ehsan Samei

Departments of Radiology, Medical Physics, Physics, Biomedical Engineering, and Electrical and Computer Engineering, Duke University Medical Center, Durham, NC, USA

Fluoroscopy was adapted for medical use as early as radiography, and as such has claimed clinical physics support since the early years. It is the modality in which clinical physicists have demonstrated the most rigorous estimation of dose and visual image quality. It is also the modality that is the bedrock of image-guided interventional procedures, providing physicists models of practice that are unique. These attributes set the role of physicists in fluoroscopy apart compared to that in other medical imaging modalities. This provides unique opportunities for improved care through physics expertise. Many such opportunities are detailed in the Chapters 9 and 10.

Casting the opportunities for clinical physics in fluoroscopy in terms of a transition from a Medical Physics 1.0 mindset to a Medical Physics 3.0 is summarized in Table 8.1. Many of these are reflected in the following two chapters. In this brief perspective, we highlight a few that can inform the expanding role of physicists in this area.

8.1 Changing Technologies

Fluoroscopy, similar to mammography and radiography, has experienced and is currently experiencing a change from analogue to digital detectors. The analogue Image Intensifier (II) detectors are being replaced by newer flat panel systems. This has notable implications for physics. Flat-panel detectors have unique noise characteristics, in that noise tends to be a more significant issue at low doses than was exhibited in II systems. Further, the systems with flat panel detectors do not exhibit the same resolution change as a function of field of view that is well-known for II systems. Finally, digital signals from flat-panel detectors provide opportunities for temporal filtering as well as other post-processing functions that can affect image quality. These attributes should be incorporated in the physics-based evaluation and optimization of fluoroscopic systems and procedures.

8.2 Quantitative Metrics

Image quality can be more readily assessed, optimized, and tracked if quantified. The transition to digital technology enables more convenient quantitation of image quality. However, that has not yet been realized even as the fluoroscopy technology has been transitioning to digital; while

Clinical Imaging Physics: Current and Emerging Practice, First Edition. Edited by Ehsan Samei and Douglas E. Pfeiffer.
© 2020 John Wiley & Sons, Inc. Published 2020 by John Wiley & Sons, Inc.

Table 8.1 Comparison of Medical Physics 1.0 and emerging 3.0 paradigm in fluoroscopy physics.

Fluoroscopy	1.0	3.0
Focus of MP's attention	Equipment, focused on individual systems and isolated performance	Patient, focused on consistency of care across practice
Image quality evaluation	Visual and subjective, in and through phantoms	Quantitative, in and through phantoms and patient cases
Evaluation condition	Standardized techniques	Techniques most closely reflecting clinical use and variation across cases
MP "tools of the trade" for image quality evaluation	Visibility of dots/holes, line pairs, wire meshes	MTF, NPS, detectability, quantitative characterization of temporal performance
Patient dosimetry	Dose area product (DAP), Air KERMA, fluoro time, skin exposure	Standard dosimetry, organ dose, risk index
Image processing	Often ignored	Incorporated in quantitative evaluation and optimization
System evaluation	Focused on x-ray source and detector alone	Focused on the system as a whole including the anti-scatter technologies
Applications	Focused on 2D applications	Expansion to 2.5–3D applications
Protocols	*Ad hoc*	Systematic analysis of dose and image quality patterns informing refinements of the interventional procedures

physicists actively evaluate the quality of clinical images visually, robust quantitation has been lacking. There is an opportunity to extend the measurements of the modulation transfer function (MTF), noise power spectrum (NPS), and detectability to fluoroscopy, in both spatial and temporal domain. This is particularly valuable as newer clinical applications extend imaging capability of the newer systems to 2.5D and 3D, in both static and temporal renditions. This enables comparison of task-based performance across different operating modes. Figure 8.1 demonstrates a measured temporal MTF through a moving edge enabling temporal characterization of the system performance in dynamic mode.

Being adaptive to patient size, fluoroscopy units use variations in mA and kV to achieve a consistent signal from the detector. This creates variable imaging conditions that a physics evaluation should ideally sample. Thus, a quantitative evaluation of system performance should represent a sampling of conditions under which the system is used so that the results can inform setting up and using the system in an optimized fashion. Such evaluation methods and procedures are essential to maximize the use of the imaging technology.

Dose-wise, while the entrance skin exposure is a relevant and established metric, the metric does not fully represent the radiation burden, particularly when comparing differing modes of the system use (e.g. 2D versus 3D) and comparing those to other modalities (e.g. computed tomography (CT)). Dose metrics need to capture the multi-organ radiation burden and quantification of effective dose and risk indices as denoted Chapter 13. Using unified metrics of both task-based image quality and patient dose across modalities is essential to ascertain the comparative utility of different imaging techniques for maximum benefit of the patient.

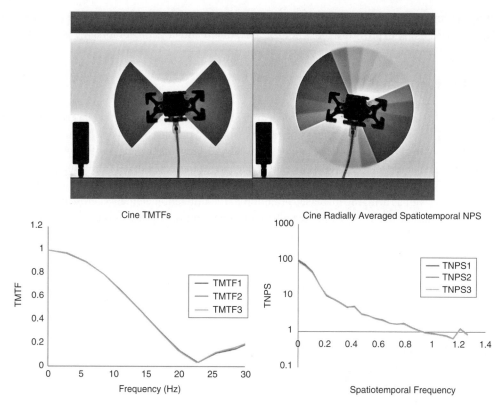

Figure 8.1 Temporal MTF and NPS of a fluoroscopy system measured under multiple acquisition conditions and an image of a moving edge phantom (top) used to capture the performance [1].

8.3 Emerging Applications

Digital technology has enabled a multiplicity of clinical applications for fluoroscopic systems. They include 2.5–3D acquisition modes including cone-beam imaging for a variety of applications: multi-dimensional subtraction angiography, dental, and maxi-facial imaging, extremities imaging, neurological imaging, and interventional imaging in the surgery suites. Each of these applications targets particular indications that should inform the methods that a physicist should use to best capture the performance of the system, and then subsequently use the results to guide the optimal use of the imaging system. This is a growing area for a seasoned physicist to actively engage and aid in the design and details of new applications.

8.4 Performance Monitoring

Performance monitoring is yet another emerging technology across imaging including fluoroscopy. Initially motivated by patient safety, accreditation bodies now require monitoring of entrance skin dose in fluoroscopic procedures. New offerings include automated assessment of skin dose across variable exposure conditions of a given procedure so the peak skin dose can be more reliably assessed. Clinical physics should own and inform the use of these systems to ensure their accuracy and impactful use. Further, as envisioned across other modalities, monitoring can be expanded to patient image quality to provide a more holistic assessment and targeting of imaging performance.

8.5 Interventional Physics

Fluoroscopy is largely an interventional procedure. The use of this imaging is markedly different from diagnostic use of imaging where images are produced and used at two separate stages. The intractability of the clinician with the system creates conditions that can be positively informed by physics knowledge and engagement. Areas of involvement include hands-on training on the safe and effective use of the equipment (in consideration of time, shielding, and distance that are well established) as well as bringing increased attention to the utilization elements across patient sizes, protocol optimization (e.g. DRLs per size), use optimization (e.g. grid, automatic exposure rate control (AERC)), "user" optimization considering the differing habits of different operators, and retrospective analysis of performance from monitoring data and catalyzing corrective actions for improved consistency of quality and safety.

Modern clinical fluoroscopy physics requires active clinical participation of the physicist in designing precise performance metrics, task-specific optimization, integrated, patient-centric optimization, and retrospective audits toward operational quality. The examples discussed above are only a sample of the opportunities where clinical physics can take a more active and engaged presence in the clinical use of modern fluoroscopy systems. Expanded and additional opportunities are highlighted in Chapters 9 and 10.

Reference

1 Russ, M., Mann, S., Richards, T., and Samei, E. (2019). Quantitative evaluation of clinical fluoroscopy systems: reproducibility of temporal modulation transfer function and temporal noise power spectrum measurements using a rotating edge phantom. *Medical Physics* 46 (6): E528–E529.

9

Clinical Fluoroscopy Physics: State of Practice

Beth A. Schueler[1] and Keith J. Strauss[2]

[1] *Department of Radiology, Mayo Clinic Rochester, Rochester, MN, USA*
[2] *Department of Radiology and Medical Imaging, Children's Hospital Medical Center, Cincinnati, OH, USA*

9.1   Introduction

The current state of practice in medical physics support of fluoroscopy systems includes quality control tests to verify equipment performance and ensure patient and staff safety. Fluoroscopy is used for specific clinical imaging tasks that are quite varied, from viewing a radiographic contrast agent in the gastrointestinal tract or circulatory system to guiding the positioning of interventional devices for therapeutic techniques. Consequently, patient and staff radiation exposure ranges from minimal levels to levels high enough to cause radiation tissue reactions. Medical physics support of fluoroscopic equipment should ensure the production of images with appropriate quality at a radiation dose appropriate for the specified task. This is accomplished through qualitative image quality evaluation of phantoms and test objects, radiation dose measurement, and other system component performance tests.

Guidelines to assist the medical physicist in developing a comprehensive quality control program and detailed test procedures have been developed by various professional societies, including the American Association of Physicists in Medicine (AAPM), the National Council on Radiation Protection and Measurements (NCRP) and the Institute of Physics and Engineering in Medicine (IPEM). Several of these documents applicable to fluoroscopy equipment are listed below:

AAPM 1990 Summer School Proceedings: Specification, Acceptance Testing, and Quality Control of Diagnostic X-Ray Imaging Equipment [1]: The proceedings from this course include multiple chapters describing QC tests for fluoroscopy equipment. Testing instructions, diagrams, sample data forms and minimum performance levels are provided for image intensifier (II) fluoroscopy systems [2–4].

AAPM Report No. 70 Cardiac Catheterization Equipment Performance [5]: A comprehensive set of quality control test procedures for cardiac angiography systems is included in this report. In addition to image quality and radiation exposure measurements, collimation, beam quality, generator and automatic exposure rate control (AERC) function tests are described.

IPEM Report 91 Recommended Standard for the Routine Performance Testing of Diagnostic X-ray Imaging Systems [6]: A recommended list of tests is provided with specified frequencies and

Clinical Imaging Physics: Current and Emerging Practice, First Edition. Edited by Ehsan Samei and Douglas E. Pfeiffer.
© 2020 John Wiley & Sons, Inc. Published 2020 by John Wiley & Sons, Inc.

both remedial and suspension performance levels. Image quality tests are based on the Leeds test objects (Leeds Test Objects Ltd, Boroughbridge, North Yorkshire).

NCRP Report No. 168 Radiation Dose Management for Fluoroscopically Guided Interventional Medical Procedures [7]: This report includes an extensive discussion of features available on modern fluoroscopy equipment, along with recommendations for equipment specifications for various types of interventional procedures.

AAPM Report No. 125 Functionality and Operation of Fluoroscopic Automatic Brightness Control/ Automatic Dose Rate Control Logic in Modern Cardiovascular and Interventional Angiography Systems [8]: Testing procedures for evaluation of AERC operation are provided, in addition to sample data from multiple manufacturers/models.

European Commission Radiation Protection No. 162 Criteria for Acceptability of Medical Radiological Equipment used in Diagnostic Radiology, Nuclear Medicine and Radiotherapy [9]: This report provides control limits for acceptable performance of imaging systems.

9.2 System Performance

9.2.1 Intrinsic Performance

9.2.1.1 Mechanical Evaluation Survey

This evaluation is an assessment of various mechanical functions of the system and presence of safety equipment. Inspection items include cumulative fluoroscopy time display and functional five-minute warning, high-level-control activation alerts, operational safety interlocks and x-ray indicator lights, minimum source to skin distance, radiation protection shields available and functional and operational crash guards.

9.2.1.2 Half-value Layer

For measurement of x-ray beam half-value layer (HVL), a fixed high voltage should be selected by locking the technique after driving the AERC with sufficient attenuators to the desired high voltage, if this function is present. Manual selection of a set high voltage may also be possible, though possibly only in the service mode. At 80 kVp, the HVL should be at least 2.9 mm aluminum (Al) [10] for units manufactured on or after June 10, 2006. For systems that include variable added spectral filtration, it is important to measure the HVL in a mode that has the minimum level of filtration. The addition of 0.2 mm copper filtration will generally increase the HVL by 2–3 mm Al.

9.2.1.3 High Voltage Measurement

Verification of the generator calibration is generally limited to non-invasive measurement of high voltage. This is easily measured by most modern solid state radiation detector devices. Accuracy should meet or exceed manufacturer's specifications or regulatory limits (typically ±5%). It should be noted that modern high frequency x-ray generators are very stable and rarely fail high voltage accuracy control limits.

9.2.1.4 Collimation

X-ray beam collimation accuracy should be evaluated for all available primary fields of view (FOVs). For systems with variable x-ray source to image receptor distance (SID), the tracking of the collimators with SID should be assessed by measuring collimation accuracy at both the minimum and maximum SID. Ideally, x-ray beam collimator blades are adjusted so that they are just visible within the fluoroscopic image so that collimation accuracy can be visually verified. If not visible, a computed radiography cassette, radiochromic film, or the like, with radio-opaque rulers can be positioned at the entrance to the image receptor to determine the location of the x-ray field at all four edges (top, bottom, right, and left) as compared to the visible markings in the fluoroscopic image. Federal regulations specify that neither the length nor width of the x-ray field in the plane of the detector shall exceed the visible area by >3% of the SID and the sum of the length and width excess shall be <4% of the SID.

9.2.1.5 Display Monitors

Image displays in the procedure room and control room should have appropriate brightness and contrast for acceptable performance. Each monitor should be evaluated by display of video test patterns, if available. The SMPTE pattern is a common test pattern that allows for assessment of low and high contrast performance. Modern monitors often come equipped with the more advanced TG18-QC test pattern [11].

9.2.2 Qualimetry

The assessment of fluoroscopic image quality includes evaluation of spatial resolution, contrast sensitivity, and noise. Since availability of image manipulation tools (such as region of interest, mean pixel, and standard deviation) is limited in fluoroscopic systems and access to unprocessed images is generally not possible, image quality assessment is typically restricted to qualitative evaluation of images acquired with various test objects. Specific image quality tests include high contrast resolution (HRC), low contrast resolution (LRC), and assessment of image uniformity, distortion, and artifacts.

9.2.2.1 High Contrast Resolution

A number of different factors influence spatial resolution in a fluoroscopic imaging system. For image intensifier-based (II) video systems, these include the resolution of the video camera, the focus of the II itself, and focus of the optical coupling between the II output and video camera. Image sharpness due to these three components may degrade suddenly or deteriorate slowly over time. For flat panel detector (FPD) systems, light spread and scatter in the scintillator, pixel size, and pixel binning will affect HRC. Though the physical properties of the FPD and pixel size are stable over time, changes in system software may alter the degree of pixel binning or spatial averaging that occurs during image processing, resulting in variations in image blur [12]. Other factors that are independent of the detector type include focal spot size and geometric magnification, image processing settings, and matrix size of the display monitor.

High contrast resolution can be measured by imaging a line pair test object, which contains lead bar patterns with frequencies ranging from 0.5 to 5 line pairs mm^{-1}. A mesh large enough to cover the entire detector is also useful for II-video fluoroscopy systems to evaluate uniformity of focus across the entire imaging area. Alternatively, smaller test objects can be located at various positions in the image. Example test objects are shown in Figure 9.1. To assess spatial resolution of the image receptor, the line pair test object should be placed directly on the entrance surface of the detector, with the grid removed if possible. The line pairs are typically placed at an angle of 45° with respect to the pixel matrix to minimize aliasing artifacts that arise from discrete pixel sampling of the parallel lines of the bar pattern. A small amount of additional attenuator is typically needed to stabilize the x-ray technique. The limiting spatial resolution in each FOV should be recorded in both fluoroscopy and acquisition modes. Figure 9.2 shows typical HRC results measured at the detector for several different fluoroscopy systems. In a 20–25 cm FOV, limiting resolution of 1.8–2.0 lp mm^{-1} is expected for II-video systems [5] and 3–4 lp mm^{-1} for FPD systems.

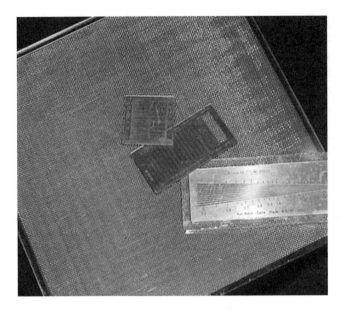

Figure 9.1 Photograph of high contrast spatial resolution test objects.

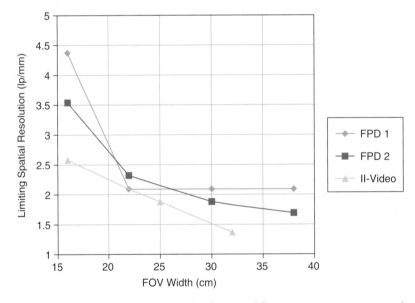

Figure 9.2 Graph of high contrast spatial resolution for several fluoroscopy systems measured at the image receptor.

Reductions in resolution of more than 20% from baseline should be investigated and service adjustment made if necessary. For II-video systems, vibrations or impacts to the image receptor can cause movement of the optical coupling lenses, resulting in a defocused image. Degradation in focus on the outer edges of an II may also occur over time.

To evaluate full system spatial resolution, the line pair test object should be placed on the table-top or at isocenter for C-arms to more accurately reflect the spatial resolution that will be seen clinically. In this configuration, the limiting spatial resolution will partially depend on the focal spot size which may differ for fluoroscopy and acquisition modes.

9.2.2.2 Low Contrast Resolution

Low contrast resolution or discrimination is affected by both contrast and noise characteristics of an imaging system. Factors influencing image contrast include x-ray beam energy, scatter, detector contrast (veiling glare, video contrast) and display contrast (image processing, viewing conditions). Factors influencing image noise include quantum mottle, electronic noise and fixed pattern noise. For FPD systems, fixed pattern noise is eliminated by gain and offset correction maps.

There have been a number of different test tools developed that evaluate LRC [2, 3, 13–15]. An example is shown in Figures 9.3 and 9.4 [16]. Some test tools incorporate a measurement of spatial resolution by including small objects or mesh patterns. Test methods vary depending on the test object selected, but generally the object is imaged at a clinical geometric magnification with attenuating material equivalent to an average patient. The number of objects in the image that are just visible to the operator are counted to determine an evaluation score.

To minimize operator detection variability, viewing conditions should be standardized with dimmed overhead lights, minimal reflections on the display monitor and a standard viewing distance. Also, since x-ray beam energy has such a large effect on image contrast, LRC test results will depend strongly on the high voltage that the AERC system drives to. Therefore, it is helpful to set the high voltage to a specific value, if the system allows this. Alternatively, the percent contrast as a function of indicated high voltage has been published [13]. Expected values for contrast levels are <2% during acquisition and <2.5% during fluoroscopy [5].

9.2.2.3 Image Uniformity, Distortion and Artifacts

The design of an II inherently results in geometric distortion and grayscale non-uniformity [17]. The projection of electrons originating at a curved input surface to a flat output phosphor results in falloff in signal intensity (vignetting) and pincushion distortion. External magnetic fields rotate and shift electron paths within the II to cause S distortion (see Figure 9.5). For FPDs, geometric distortion does not occur and grayscale non-uniformity is minimized with dark noise and gain

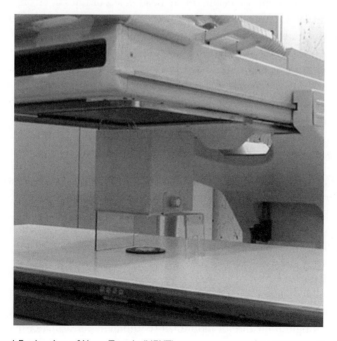

Figure 9.3 National Evaluation of X-ray Trends (NEXT) survey program fluoroscopic phantom.

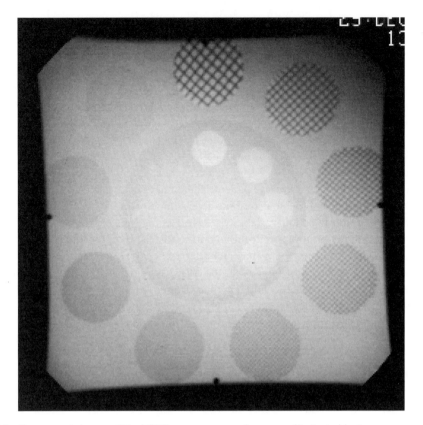

Figure 9.4 Fluoroscopic image of the NEXT survey program image quality test object.

calibrations maps. Artifacts can still occur, due to dead pixels or lines or errors in gain calibration. For both types of image receptors, artifacts may result from damage to grids and filters or contrast material or other contamination along the x-ray beam path.

Image distortion can be evaluated by imaging a test object with a square grid pattern. Image non-uniformity and artifacts can be assessed from uniform field images viewed with a narrow window. The cause of non-uniformity and artifacts should be determined and removed if possible. Minor artifacts that are deemed insignificant should be followed over time to track changes in system performance.

9.2.3   Radiometry

Determination of radiation dose levels in fluoroscopy systems is needed to assess patient and staff safety, select appropriate equipment configurations, monitor system stability, and ensure regulatory compliance. Dose quality control monitoring includes four different tests: entrance detector air kerma (EDAK), maximum patient entrance skin air kerma (ESAK) rate, internal dose monitoring system validation, and typical patient ESAK.

9.2.3.1   Entrance Detector Air Kerma (EDAK)

The quantum flux rate incident upon the detector is a critical parameter determining both image quality and radiation dose. As a result, measurement of EDAK is a useful tool for ensuring appropriate equipment configuration and for monitoring equipment performance over time.

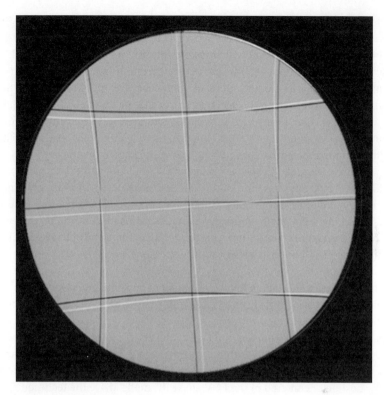

Figure 9.5   Photograph of II distortion image.

Equipment required for EDAK measurement includes a dosimeter and attenuating phantom. Since the absorption of photons in the II or FPD scintillator layer varies with photon energy, it is important to maintain a consistent x-ray beam energy by standardizing the attenuating phantom material and high voltage selection. Aluminum is typical as an attenuator, but copper (Cu) or acrylic may also be used. Due to differences in beam hardening, an acrylic attenuator will result in an EDAK value that is about 30% higher than either Al or Cu, which produce similar results [18]. The attenuating phantom should be configured to allow for adjustment in thickness so that the AERC system will drive the technique to 80 kVp (±5 kVp) for both fluoroscopy and acquisition modes. A total Al thickness of 5–10 cm with increments of 0.5 cm or Cu thickness of 3–5 mm with increments to 0.5 mm is suggested.

To minimize the effect of scattered radiation on the EDAK value, the attenuating phantom should be placed as close as possible to the x-ray tube, the image receptor adjusted to maximum SID and the dosimeter placed midway between the attenuator and detector face. The dosimeter reading should then be corrected for the inverse square distance to the detector input surface. Alternatively, for a solid-state dosimeter with a lead backing, the dosimeter can be placed directly on the detector input surface. If possible, air kerma rate measurements should be made with the grid removed. If the grid cannot be easily removed, a correction factor for grid attenuation must be applied to determine the air kerma rate at the detector input surface. This factor (typically between 1.4 and 1.6) can be determined from a one-time set of measurements with and without the grid in place.

The EDAK should be repeated for all FOVs and all fluoroscopy and acquisition modes. For IIs, the EDAK will generally be inversely proportional to the FOV area. For FPDs, the change in EDAK with FOV will vary depending on the system. The manufacturer-recommended setting may keep EDAK constant for each FOV or adjust the EDAK to be inversely proportional to the FOV diameter.

In addition, for an FOV mode where pixel binning is being implemented, a lower EDAK can be adopted due to the decrease in noise resulting from pixel signal averaging. The EDAK-FOV relationship for FPDs may also be adjusted when system software revisions are installed.

For an II system without added spectral beam filtration in the FOV mode closest to 23 cm diameter, acceptable fluoroscopy EDAK rate values are in the range of 300–1300 nGy s^{-1} [8]. With additional filtration, fluoroscopy EDAK rates will typically be at least two times higher [5]. FPD systems generally require two to four times higher rates as compared to II systems [8]. For acquisition modes, acceptable EDAK values are 450–900 nGy/frame for digital acquisition, 4500–9000 nGy/frame for digital subtraction angiography and 90–130 nGy/frame for digital cardiac [19]. For acquisition, FPD systems can be set to EDAK levels that are slightly lower than II systems.

A control limit of $\pm 20\%$ from baseline values is recommended. For II-video systems, the brightness gain of an II will decrease over time as the input phosphor material ages and the vacuum degrades. As a result, the EDAK will increase to compensate for the lost brightness level. When the increase reaches the suggested control limit, service adjustment of the optical coupling aperture is needed to restore the EDAK to the baseline value.

9.2.3.2 Maximum Fluoroscopy Patient Entrance Skin Air Kerma Rate (MESAK)

Federal regulations limit the MESAK to 88 mGy min^{-1} in regular AERC-mode fluoroscopy and 176 mGy min^{-1} if a high-level control mode is activated [20]. The location for measurement of MESAK is specified to be 30 cm from the input surface of the detector assembly for a C-arm system or 1 cm above the tabletop for an undertable x-ray tube system. The measurement should be made without backscatter or attenuation from any table or pads that can be removed from the x-ray beam. With the dosimeter centered in the FOV, in AERC mode, drive the technique parameters to their maximum values by placing a lead attenuator over the detector – 3 mm lead thickness should be sufficient. If the system is equipped with a software mode that terminates exposure when excessive attenuation is present, it may be necessary to instead use a Cu attenuator and add additional thickness until the maximum technique parameters are reached. If the system includes a manual mode, the measurement should be repeated with the highest selectable technique parameters.

It should be noted that some units operate with MESAK that is lower than the regulatory maximum value. This may be due to limitations of the x-ray tube or generator or as a patient dose reduction feature.

9.2.3.3 Internal Dose Monitoring System Validation

For equipment sold in the United States after June 2006, the FDA requires display of air kerma at the reference point ($K_{a,r}$) within sight of the primary operator [20]. The $K_{a,r}$ value is specified at a defined reference point on the central axis of the x-ray beam that approximates the location of the patient's entrance skin surface. For C-arms, the reference point is located 15 cm from the isocenter of rotation toward the x-ray tube. Note that the reference point location differs from the MESAK measurement point 30 cm from the image receptor assembly. However, for other types of equipment configurations, the reference point is the same as the measurement point specified for the MESAK. In addition to $K_{a,r}$, many units display air kerma area product (KAP), which is a requirement for IEC-compliant equipment [21, 22].

The most common method manufacturers employ to measure patient dose is to mount a parallel-plate transparent ionization chamber at the x-ray tube collimator. Since the dose decreases proportionally to the square of the distance from the focal spot and the area of the irradiated field increases proportionally in the same way, KAP is the same value at any distance from the focal spot. The $K_{a,r}$ is typically calculated by dividing the measured KAP value by the irradiated field size, which is derived from the collimator positions. Alternatively, $K_{a,r}$ can be estimated from actual technique factors and a look-up table of measured radiation output values. For either measurement method, verification of the accuracy of the system dose display is needed to ensure accurate patient dose assessment.

For internal dose monitoring system validation, the system dose readout value is compared to an external dosimeter in a scatter-free configuration. Recommended measurement methods are described in AAPM Report 190 [23]. Using an attenuator of 8 mm Cu to cover the detector, compare the system dose readout to the external dosimeter result for both fluoroscopy and a typical acquisition mode series. To validate accuracy of the KAP value, replace the dosimeter with a field size test plate with radio-opaque distance markings to measure the FOV size.

The FDA and IEC specify that the $K_{a,r}$ shall not deviate from actual values by more than 35% for values greater than 100 mGy [20, 22]. For KAP accuracy, the IEC specifies a control limit of $\pm 35\%$ for >2.5 Gy cm^2 [22]. The correction factor (equal to the external dose value divided by the displayed system value) should be determined to allow for accurate patient dose estimation.

9.2.3.4 Typical Patient ESAK

Measurement of ESAK for a typical patient attenuator allows for estimation of patient dose, comparison between different systems and comparison with available benchmark values. Even if two systems have the same EDAK setting, ESAK can vary greatly due to differences in beam filtration, high voltage selection, geometry and table/pad attenuation. When measuring ESAK, the set up should mimic a clinical equipment configuration, including the SID, table height (if adjustable) and typical grid use. A phantom consisting of varying thickness of acrylic or Al is recommended. For the patient equivalent of a child, small adult, and large adult, 10, 20, and 30 cm acrylic or 2.5, 5, and 7.5 cm Al are appropriate. Air kerma values displayed by the internal system dose display should be corrected using the correction factor determined in the previous test. A backscatter factor should also be applied if comparison to other measurements or benchmark values acquired with backscatter is desired. A table of backscatter factors for varying irradiated field size and beam energy can be found in ICRU Report 74 [24]. Typical backscatter factors range from 1.4 to 1.6. Alternatively, a dosimeter can be placed close to the entrance surface of the attenuator. This value will include backscatter if the dosimeter does not incorporate a lead back.

ESAK measurements should be repeated for all FOVs and all fluoroscopy and acquisition modes. Laskey et al. [25] provides benchmark data from 41 cardiac fluoroscopy systems. Dose measurements are for the 15–18 cm FOV, with backscatter included. For a 20 cm acrylic phantom, median ESAK was 26 mGy min^{-1} (interquartile range 12 mGy min^{-1}). For a 30 cm phantom, median ESAK was 110 mGy min^{-1} (interquartile range 42 mGy min^{-1}). In order to assess the function of the AERC algorithm, it is helpful to make measurements with smaller increments of attenuator (1–5 cm acrylic or 2–5 mm Al) while monitoring variation of technique factors and beam filtration as a function of thickness [8]. Attenuator should be added until maximum technique factors are attained.

9.3 Testing Paradigm and Clinical Implementation

9.3.1 Acceptance Testing and Commissioning

After installation, initial calibration and configuration by the equipment manufacturer, fluoroscopy systems should be tested to verify proper performance and installation of all purchased options. The testing should occur prior to clinical use. Acceptance testing should be comprehensive in nature, including all system performance tests described above with measurements made in all applicable dose modes and FOVs. In addition, testing of connectivity to the modality worklist broker, radiology informatics system (RIS), and picture archiving and communication system (PACS) should be conducted at this time [26].

Commissioning of an imaging equipment involves evaluation of the system configuration to ensure it meets the user's clinical requirements. This includes review of the manufacturer's default settings for adjustable parameters such as dose settings, factors affecting technique selection and image processing. If adjustment of defaults settings is needed, collaboration with manufacturer application specialists and service engineers is advisable.

9.3.2 Quality Control

Following acceptance testing, a routine quality control (QC) program that includes a subset of tests and operation modes should be established to verify continued equipment performance. Modes to be tested annually should include the most commonly used settings in clinical use. Test results collected during acceptance testing serve as baselines for routine QC. Control limits on these baseline values should be selected so that equipment changes may be detected prior to producing clinically significant degradation in image quality or an increase in radiation exposure.

9.3.3 Manufacturer QC

Some manufacturers provide integrated quality control testing protocols for regular evaluation of image quality. These tests are generally designed for performance by a technologist on a frequent (weekly or monthly) basis, using manufacturer-provided imaging phantoms and analysis software. A test failure alerts the user that possible system degradation has occurred and that service may be required. For example, manufacturer quality control tests have been designed to search for bad pixels or increased image noise in FPD systems. Medical physicists are advised to repeat these tests during routine annual QC and review site records to ensure the tests are being conducted at the designated frequency.

9.3.4 Purchase Specification

The life cycle of imaging equipment begins with purchase specification, followed by installation, acceptance testing, and commissioning. Successful purchase specification requires identification of the clinical needs and selection of equipment that can best address those needs. Without this step, problems that arise from equipment limitations are likely to occur. A detailed description of the imaging equipment acquisition process has been provided by Strauss [27]. In summary, the medical physicist can assist the facility by identifying the type of patients (pediatric, adult, bariatric, ...) and procedures (limited to one specialty group or shared by multiple groups) to be imaged. Then, reviewing equipment specifications for different vendors and models to determine which will be acceptable. Some features specific to fluoroscopy equipment that should be considered include mobile versus fixed C-arms, image receptor FOV, and addition of cone beam CT functions. Site visits can be helpful. The visit should include physicians and technologists who will be operating the equipment so that they can observe clinical image quality and performance, and assess the operation and user interface. Limited performance tests may also be done during a site visit to provide comparison data for later acceptance testing. Once a model has been selected, a careful review of the quotation is necessary to ensure all necessary options are included and unnecessary items eliminated. It is advisable to include user and manufacturer representatives in this review to confirm clinical needs and explanations of various options and features.

9.3.5 Optimization of Use

For many clinical applications of fluoroscopy, the manufacturer-provided imaging protocols provide sufficient image quality at an appropriate radiation dose level. However, in some instances, modifications to the default protocol parameters such as dose setting, pulse rate or image processing settings may be called for. Situations that require modifications may be initiated by the user, such as introduction of a new clinical procedure, dissatisfaction with default image quality, or the need to match image quality to another imaging system. Alternatively, a medical physicist may initiate protocol modifications if they note that default radiation dose settings or image quality measurements are outside the recommended range of performance.

Modification of imaging protocols usually requires access to the service mode and assistance from a service engineer. Before making parameter changes, consider the specific clinical exam being performed: is the clinical study dynamic in nature, like a cardiac study or swallowing study, or is it more static, like a colon exam? Will the contrast material to be imaged be barium or will it be iodine? Is the body part thickness generally large, such as for abdominal fluoroscopy, or is it generally rather thin, such as for most pediatric subjects? What is the principle clinical deficiency – excessive noise, poor contrast, insufficient sharpness or poor dynamic range? Answers to these questions will help guide selections for improved image quality. Note that adjustments that improve image quality may increase patient dose, so additional dose-saving measures may be needed.

9.3.6 Compliance-Related Matters

Fluoroscopic quality control requirements are generally prescribed by local regulations. In the United States, individual states develop regulatory requirements for medical x-ray equipment utilization. These regulations may include required equipment features (such as a five minute cumulative on-time audible signal), minimum performance specifications (such as limiting spatial resolution values) and minimum QC testing frequencies. Though regulations vary from state to state, health departments frequently follow guidelines developed by the Council of Radiation Control Program Directors (CRCPD) which publishes a set of suggested state regulations [28].

All fluoroscopic systems sold in the United States must comply with Food and Drug Administration (FDA) regulations [10, 20]. The International Electrotechnical Commission (IEC) develops voluntary international standards for equipment [21, 22]. Since most imaging equipment today is manufactured and sold world-wide, models are typically designed to comply with both FDA and IEC standards. As a result, knowledge of both standards will aid in understanding design features and performance specifications.

9.3.7 Training

Fluoroscopy equipment is capable of producing high radiation dose to patients and also high radiation dose to support staff that remain in the room during exposure. Therefore, it is important that fluoroscopy operators and staff receive training in radiation effects and safe radiation use. This training should include didactic instruction in radiation management and hands-on training. As described in NCRP Report 168, didactic training should comprise a full day of instruction, including the following topics:

- physics of x-ray production and interaction;
- technology of fluoroscopy machines, including modes of operation;

- characteristics of image quality and technical factors affecting image quality in fluoroscopy;
- dosimetric quantities and units;
- health effects of radiation;
- principles of radiation protection in fluoroscopy;
- applicable federal, state and local regulations and requirements; and
- techniques for minimizing dose to the patient and staff [7].

Hands-on training is needed for each person that will operate or direct operation of the fluoroscopy equipment. Ideally, this training should occur on the same system used clinically or the same model and include use of all controls, modes of operations, dose reduction features and dose displays. Assisting personnel should also receive training specific to their responsibilities and staff dose reduction.

9.4   Medical Physics 1.5

Though fluoroscopic imaging has a long history and its use is well-established in clinical practice, there continue to be advances in hardware and software that extend fluoroscopy system capabilities and performance. These advances require changes to traditional performance testing methods. The replacement of II-video image receptors with FPDs represents a significant advance in fluoroscopic imaging. FPDs are smaller in size allowing for more flexible movement and less visual obstruction. They have a wider dynamic range (less image saturation) and no geometric distortion for improved image quality. Plus, they have greater stability, requiring less time to calibrate and maintain. As a result, system performance evaluation of FPD fluoroscopy systems must be modified as compared to traditional II-video systems to take into account their unique properties. Specifically, FPD HRC may be useful to measure at acceptance testing and after software revisions, but routine annual measurements are not likely to show image degradation. Artifact evaluation with a flat field image is valuable for FPD evaluation, but imaging of a grid for distortion is not needed. Regular monitoring of EDAK values is also of lesser importance since gradual decreases in image receptor efficiency are unlikely. In addition, several factors have led to an increased emphasis on radiation dose reduction in fluoroscopic procedures. Improved x-ray tube heat loading capabilities and increased generator power allow use of high radiation dose rates and the ability to lengthen procedures without equipment heat overload restrictions. Also, improvements in fluoroscopic image quality and interventional procedure device advancement have resulted in longer, more complex interventional procedures. Finally, increased public attention to radiation exposure levels and dose recording regulations and initiatives have highlighted the need for dose reduction. For the medical physicist, this situation requires that additional emphasis be placed on image quality and dose optimization as well as operator education. Additionally, the increased patient radiation dose and dose awareness has resulted in requests for individual patient dose estimation. This currently is generally a manual process, based on manufacturer-provided summary dose reports (see Figure 9.6) and multiple corrections to determine skin dose [29, 30] Automated dose estimation will be discussed in the following chapter.

In conclusion, medical physicists play an important role in supporting fluoroscopic system use, including purchase specification, equipment selection, performance evaluation, image quality and dose optimization and operator education. To achieve optimal results for clinical imaging, the operation and performance capabilities of a system must be well understood. To help ensure the safety of both patients and staff, both radiation dose and image quality need to be optimized for the particular clinical tasks to be performed.

(a)

Examination report

Patient's name:	Test, Patient
Exam. Date and time:	August 12, 2019 9:25 AM

Examination		
Cumulative fluoroscopy time:	1:15:33	hh:mm:ss
Cum. DAP (fluoroscopy)	1332	mGycm²
Cum. DAP (exposure)	902	mGycm²
Total DAP:	2234	mGycm²
Cumulative Air Kerma:	150.32	mGy
Total number of acquired runs:	6	
Total number of acquired images:	82	
Total number of acquired exposure images:	82	

Run	Procedure	Time	Speed fr/sec	kV	mA mAs	ms	Rot	Ang	SID cm	Images
1	Stomach	13;45	3	70	130				98	9
2	Stomach	13:51	3	72	115				98	8
3	Stomach	14:01	3	85	10	15			100	10
4	Kidney	14:30	8	85	10	20	100	23	121	23
5	Kidney	14:43	8	80	10	20	121	45	121	15
6	Kidney	14:57	8	80	10	20	121	45	91	17

(b)

12	DSA		VARIABLE IVC						7s	2F/s	16-Mar-19 17:45:07		
A	117kV	266mA	199.6ms	****	large	0.0Cu	22cm	370.2µGym²	203mGy	31LAO	4CA	13F
13	DSA		VARIABLE IVC						1s	2F/s	16-Mar-19 18:04:07		
A	102kV	304mA	199.5ms	****	large	0.0Cu	22cm	174.2µGym²	28.2mGy	34LAO	4CA	2F
14	DSA		VARIABLE IVC						8s	2F/s	16-Mar-19 18:14:25		
A	89kV	529mA	125.0ms	****	large	0.0Cu	42cm	908.9µGym²	158mGy	0LAO	1CR	14F
15	DSA		VARIABLE IVC						1s	2F/s	16-Mar-19 18:17:49		
A	88kV	531mA	125.3ms	****	large	0.0Cu	42cm	556.8µGym²	22.5mGy	0LAO	1CR	2F
16	DSA		VARIABLE IVC						1s	2F/s	16-Mar-19 18:18:14		
A	93kV	504mA	125.0ms	****	large	0.0Cu	32cm	279.1µGym²	24.3mGy	0LAO	1CR	2F
17	DSA		VARIABLE IVC						9s	2F/s	16-Mar-19 18:22:22		
A	102kV	305mA	199.6ms	****	large	0.0Cu	32cm	336.9µGym²	194mGy	22LAO	2CR	14F
18	DSA		VARIABLE IVC						7s	2F/s	16-Mar-19 18:33:21		
A	102kV	304mA	199.6ms	****	large	0.0Cu	32cm	419.9µGym²	193mGy	22LAO	2CR	14F
*** Accumulated exposure data ***											16-Mar-19 19:26:50		
Phys:			Exposures:	18	Fluoro: 63.2min			Total:	90737.4µGym²			10042mGy

Figure 9.6 Example manufacturer-provided examination reports.

References

1 Seibert, J.A., Barnes, G.T., and Gould, R. (eds.). (1994). Specification, Acceptance Testing, and Quality Control of Diagnostic X-Ray Imaging Equipment. American Association of Physicists in Medicine Medical Physics Monograph No. 20.Woodbury, NY: American Institute of Physics.

2 Chakraborty, D.P. (1994). Routine fluoroscopy quality control. In: *Specification, Acceptance Testing, and Quality Control of Diagnostic X-Ray Imaging Equipment*, American Association of Physicists in Medicine Medical Physics Monograph No. 20 (eds. J.A. Seibert, G.T. Barnes and R. Gould), 569–595. Woodbury, NY: American Institute of Physics.

3 Cowen, A.R. (1994). The physical evaluation of the imaging performance of television fluoroscopy and digital fluorography systems using the Leeds x-ray test objects: a UK approach to quality assurance in the diagnostic radiology department. In: *American Association of Physicists in Medicine*, Medical Physics Monograph No. 20 (eds. J.A. Seibert, G.T. Barnes and R. Gould), 499–568. Woodbury, NY: American Institute of Physics.

4 High, M. (1994). Digital fluoro acceptance testing: the AAPM approach. In: *Specification, Acceptance Testing, and Quality Control of Diagnostic X-Ray Imaging*, American Association of Physicists in Medicine Medical Physics Monograph No. 20 (eds. J.A. Equipment, G.T.B. Seibert and R. Gould), 709–730. Woodbury, NY: American Institute of Physics.

5 AAPM (2001). American Association of Physicists in Medicine Report No. 70. Cardiac Catheterization Equipment Performance. Madison, WI: Medical Physics Publishing, February 2001.

6 IPEM (2005). Institute of Physics and Engineering in Medicine Report 91. Recommended Standard for the Routine Performance Testing of Diagnostic X-ray Imaging Systems. York, United Kingdom: IPEM.

7 NCRP (2010). National Council on Radiation Protection and Measurements. Report No. 168. Radiation Dose Management for Fluoroscopically Guided Interventional Medical Procedures. Bethesda, MD: NCRP.

8 AAPM (2012). American Association of Physicists in Medicine Report No. 125. Functionality and Operation of Fluoroscopic Automatic Brightness Control/Automatic Dose Rate Control Logic in Modern Cardiovascular and Interventional Angiography Systems, AAPM, College Park, Maryland.

9 EC (2012). European Commission Radiation Protection No. 162 Criteria for Acceptability of Medical Radiological Equipment used in Diagnostic Radiology, Nuclear Medicine and Radiotherapy. Luxembourg, Publications Office of the European Union. https://ec.europa.eu/energy/sites/ener/files/documents/162.pdf.

10 FDA (2010a). U.S. Food and Drug Administration. Center for Devices and Radiological Health. Code of Federal Regulation, Title 21 Part 1020, Section 1020.30 "Performance standards for ionizing radiation emitting products: Diagnostic x-ray systems and their major components." http://www.accessdata.fda.gov/scripts/cdrh/cfdocs/cfcfr/CFRSearch.cfm.

11 AAPM (2005). American Association of Physicists in Medicine On-line Report No. 3. Assessment of Display Performance for Medical Imaging Systems, AAPM, College Park, Maryland.

12 Nickoloff, E.L. (2011). AAPM/RSNA physics tutorial for residents: physics of flat-panel fluoroscopy systems: survey of modern fluoroscopy imaging: flat-panel detectors versus image intensifiers and more. *Radiographics* 31: 591–602.

13 Wagner, A.J., Barnes, G.T., and Xizeng, W. (1991). Assessing fluoroscopic contrast resolution: a practical and quantitative test tool. *Med. Phys.* 18 (5): 894–899.

14 Wilson, C.R., Dixon, R.L., and Schueler, B.A. (2001). American College of Radiology Radiography Fluoroscopic Phantom. In: RL Dixon, P Butler, WT Sobol. Accreditation Programs and the Medical Physicist. Proceedings of the AAPM 2001 Summer School. AAPM Monograph No. 27 Madison, WI: Medical Physics Publishing; p. 183–189.

15 Balter, S., Heupler, F.A., Lin, P.P., and Wondrow, M.H. (2001). A new tool for benchmarking cardiovascular fluoroscopes. *Catheter. Cardiovasc. Interv.* 52: 69.

16 Suleiman, O.H., Conway, B.J., Quinn, P. et al. (1997). National survey of fluoroscopy: radiation dose and image quality. *Radiology* 203: 471–476.

17 Wang, J. and Blackburn, T.J. (2000). The AAPM/RSNA physics tutorial for residents: X-ray image intensifiers for fluoroscopy. *Radiographics* 20: 1471–1477.

18 Anderson, J.A., Wang, J., and Clarke, G.D. (2000). Choice of phantom material and test protocols to determine radiation exposure rates for fluoroscopy. *Radiographics* 20: 1033–1042.

19 Strauss, K.J. (2006). Pediatric interventional radiography equipment: safety considerations. *Pediatr. Radiol.* 36 (Suppl 2): 126–135.

20 FDA (2010b). U.S. Food and Drug Administration. Center for Devices and Radiological Health. Code of Federal Regulation, Title 21 Part 1020, Section 1020.32 "Performance standards for ionizing radiation emitting products: Fluoroscopic equipment, http://www.accessdata.fda.gov/scripts/cdrh/cfdocs/cfcfr/CFRSearch.cfm.

21 IEC (2000). International Electrotechnical Commission. Medical Electrical Equipment – Part 2-43: Particular Requirements for the Safety of X-Ray Equipment for Interventional Procedures, IEC 60601-2-43. Geneva, Switzerland: IEC, 2000.

22 IEC (2010). International Electrotechnical Commission. Medical Electrical Equipment – Part 2-43: Particular Requirements for the Basic Safety and Essential Performance of X-Ray Equipment for Interventional Procedures, IEC 60601-2-43, 2nd ed. (International Electrotechnical Commission, Geneva).

23 AAPM Report 190 (2015). American Association of Physicists in Medicine Report No. 190. Accuracy and Calibration of Integrated Radiation Output Indicators in Diagnostic Radiology, AAPM, College Park, Maryland.

24 ICRU (2005). International Commission on Radiation Units and Measurements. Report 74. Patient dosimetry for x-rays used in medical imaging. J. ICRU 5:65-66.

25 Laskey, W.K., Wondrow, M., and Holmes, D.R. (2006). Variability in fluoroscopic x-ray exposure in contemporary cardiac catheterization laboratories. *J. Am. Coll. Cardiol.* 48: 1361–1364.

26 Kinzel, S., Langer, S.G., Stekel, S., and Walz-Flannigan, A. (2012). Operational issues. In: *Informatics in Medical Imaging* (eds. G.C. Kagadis and S.G. Langer), 275–288. Boca Raton, Florida: CRC Press.

27 Strauss, K.J. (2006). Interventional suite and equipment management: cradle to grave. *Pediatr. Radiol.* 36 (Suppl 2): 221–236.

28 CRCPD (2014). Conference of Radiation Control Program Directors, Inc. Suggested State Regulations for the Control of Radiation, Part F, Frankfort, KY. https://www.crcpd.org/.

29 Jones, A.K. and Pasciak, A.S. (2011). Calculating the peak skin dose resulting from fluoroscopically guided interventions. Part I: methods. *J. Appl. Clin. Med. Phys.* 12: 231–244.

30 Jones, A.K. and Pasciak, A.S. (2012). Calculating the peak skin dose resulting from fluoroscopically guided interventions. Part II: case studies. *J. Appl. Clin. Med. Phys.* 13: 174–187.

10

Clinical Fluoroscopy Physics: Emerging Practice

Keith J. Strauss[1] and Beth A. Schueler[2]

[1] Department of Radiology and Medical Imaging, Children's Hospital Medical Center, Cincinnati, OH, USA
[2] Department of Radiology, Mayo Clinic Rochester, Rochester, MN, USA

10.1 Philosophy and Significance

Quantification of system performance of fluoroscopes by the medical physicist at an elevated level is necessary to provide useful, clinically relevant information to the fluoroscopist. Regardless of the type of examination performed and the unique size of the patient, the fluoroscopist needs assurance that good diagnostic image quality will be provided at a well-managed patient dose rate. First, the lowest air KERMA rate at the skin surface of the patient (ESAK) that delivers the necessary air KERMA rate at the surface of the detector (EDAK) to provide good quality diagnostic images should be used. Second, the image quality must be adequate for the fluoroscopist to effectively and efficiently complete the examination. Providing better image quality than necessary for a given examination and patient size should be avoided to ensure that the patient's radiation dose is not higher than necessary.

Performance testing of fluoroscopic/angiographic imaging equipment needs to follow the newer quantitatively based model of other areas of medicine. Medical physicists need to focus on tasks that have a direct impact on patient care. Design improvements of state-of-the-art units have essentially eliminated the types of issues identified in Figure 10.1, typically found more than 15 years ago during thorough acceptance testing [1]. Exhaustive acceptance testing used previously is no longer good stewardship that provides value-based medicine. Streamlined performance checks should allow the medical physicist to focus more on the clinical needs of the patient, which are driven by the type of study performed and the physical size of the patient.

The dramatic improvement in capabilities and performance of state-of-the-art fluoroscopic/angiographic imaging devices, Figure 10.2(a)–(i), has created four new paradigms for the medical physicist. First, the more accurate control of the multitude of acquisition parameters has dramatically improved the consistency and reliability of the fluoroscope's performance, Figure 10.1(c). This should allow the medical physicist to spot check the accuracy of acquisition parameters, e.g. high-voltage, tube current, pulse widths, pulse rates, etc. as opposed to testing this performance over the entire operational range of the unit. At the same time, better methods are needed to test the performance of the digital detector, i.e. analysis of "for processing images."

Second, the variety and complexity of the operational acquisition modes of the fluoroscope have exploded in recent years. Careful operational testing of the different configurations of the multiple

Clinical Imaging Physics: Current and Emerging Practice, First Edition. Edited by Ehsan Samei and Douglas E. Pfeiffer.
© 2020 John Wiley & Sons, Inc. Published 2020 by John Wiley & Sons, Inc.

(a)

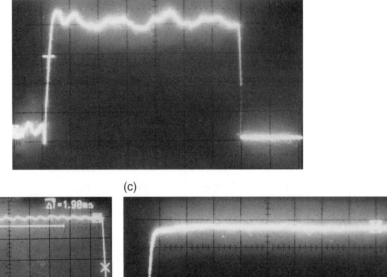

(b)   (c)

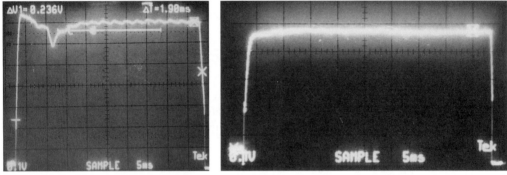

Figure 10.1 Photographs of three high voltage waveforms. Voltage and exposure time is on the vertical and horizontal axes, respectively. (a) 80 kVp waveform of a 12 pulse three-phase generator of a major imaging equipment vendor manufactured in the late 1970s measured with an invasive high voltage divider. Major ripple indicates that the high voltage during the exposure was not well controlled. (b) Similar measurement as in first image except 140 kVp waveform and generator manufactured in 1996. The irregular voltage drop probably would not have been identified without an oscilloscope connected to the invasive high voltage divider. The repair required the replacement of the entire high voltage tank of the generator; a high voltage tank that should have been identified as faulty and discarded prior to leaving the factory. (c) 80 kV waveform of mid frequency three-phase generator manufactured after 2009. Minimum ripple results in a constant potential high voltage during the exposure, greatly improving the consistent production of x-rays.

parameters of the Automatic Exposure Rate Control (AERC) and Dose Management System is necessary to verify the leveraging of these parameters to the type of examination and the size of the patient. The medical physicist must develop an understanding of the design strengths and weaknesses of the fluoroscope in consultation with the manufacturer. This allows them to help develop configurations that enhance the unique clinical work of their department. The best methods to improve the efficiency of the image acquisition process at a reduced dose rate to the image receptor cannot be identified by the manufacturer without the help of clinical staff.

Third, the large variety of images created today by fluoroscopes must be monitored for appropriate quality. These types of images include fluoroscopic, angiographic (typically cardiac), digital subtraction angiographic, rotational angiographic, cone beam CT, 3D reconstructions, registration with other modalities, etc. Additional testing tools that are sorely needed to address image quality and patient dose will be discussed.

Finally, the high degree of image processing available today allows state-of-the-art fluoroscopy units to create better image quality than is clinically required in significant portions of numerous

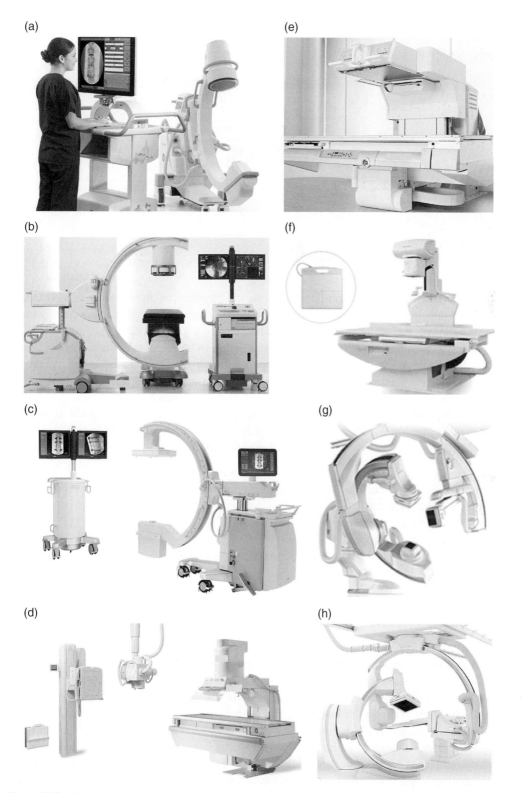

Figure 10.2 Examples of state-of-the-art-fluoroscopes: (a) Base mobile c-arm fluoroscope with image intensifier; (b) Mobile c-arm fluoroscope with image intensifier designed with cone beam capability; (c) Mobile c-arm fluoroscope with flat panel detector with cone beam capability; (d) Traditional configuration of tilt table general fluoroscope with over table image intensifier and ceiling suspended x-ray tube for imaging at the table or vertical wall stand; (e) Tilt table general fluoroscope with over table flat panel detector; (f) Remote tilt table general fluoroscope with over table x-ray tube and flat panel digital detector; (g) Biplane interventional cardiac fluoroscope with smaller flat panel detectors for imaging the heart; (h) and (i) Biplane interventional radiology angiographic fluoroscopes with larger flat panel detectors;

(i)

Figure 10.2 (Continued)

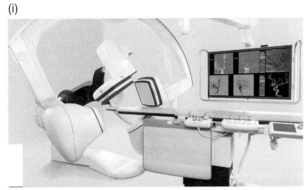

procedures. This provides opportunities for the medical physicist and fluoroscopist to work closely with their equipment manufacturer to alter the acquisition process to reduce image quality to the necessary clinical level while reducing the radiation dose to the patient [2].

What are the ramifications of these four paradigm shifts on the technical management of fluoroscopes? First, acceptance testing is just as important as in the past, but for different reasons. Formerly, acceptance testing primarily identified calibration or installation errors and substandard components requiring replacement. These types of failures are much less likely today. However, more limited performance testing of the fluoroscope prior to first clinical use provides opportunities to identify rare installation or calibration errors. Part of the saved testing time can be used to adequately investigate newer capabilities of state-of-the-art fluoroscopes such as:

a) baseline radiation output measurements for each added filter thickness
b) internal dose display accuracies: interventional reference point (IRP)
    i) air KERMA rate at IRP ($K_{a,r}$)
    ii) KERMA-Area-Product rate at IRP (KAP)
    iii) displays of real time peak skin dose at IRP (PSD)
c) image quality of flat panel detectors prior to image processing
d) cone beam CT and/or 3-D imaging
    i) image quality
    ii) patient dose
e) measurements of EDAK.

The baseline performance data measured when the unit is new is also needed to support an ongoing quality control program during the lifetime of the unit [3].

While the equipment spot performance testing described above is important, functional testing of the fluoroscope's ability to meet the clinical needs of the patient and fluoroscopist, during both acceptance testing and periodic checks, is equally important. Is the fluoroscope adapted to the clinical needs of the patient? First, medical physicists must serve as interpreters between the fluoroscopists and the equipment manufacturer. This dialog helps to ensure that the fluoroscope is properly configured for the department's unique clinical practice prior to first clinical use. This means that acquisition parameters and programmed image processing should be appropriate and unique for the type of clinical examination performed and the actual size or thickness of the body part examined. The manufacturer must understand the unique clinical objectives of each site to offer methods to leverage the strengths and minimize the weaknesses of their product's design. The operator needs a fundamental understanding of the design capabilities of the fluoroscope to make appropriate operational choices during an examination. A customized configuration of the fluoroscope is necessary to provide good diagnostic image quality at a well-managed patient dose – a fundamental aspect of good patient care.

Establishing a validated customized configuration can be very time-consuming depending on the uniqueness of the clinical practice. Yet, it can dramatically affect patient care. Typically, the "out-of-the-box" fluoroscope is reasonably configured for patients that range in size from small to large adults. These recommended configurations, however, most likely will not achieve both good diagnostic image quality at well managed patient doses when the patient is less than 30 kg or larger than 100 kg. A fluoroscope properly configured for a unique practice orchestrated by radiologists, manufacturer, and medical physicist working as a team will probably impact patient care today more than elimination of the rare equipment performance issues identified by traditional compliance testing methods.

10.2 Metrics and Analytics

10.2.1 Intrinsic Performance

The intrinsic capabilities of fluoroscopy have dramatically changed over the past 35 years and created the four new paradigms previously mentioned. In 1980, only a two-dimensional image could be acquired either in the fluoroscopic or angiographic mode. The fluoroscopic images could be reviewed only during live fluoroscopy during exposure of the patient to radiation. Angiographic images, stored on photographic film, were typically acquired at a dose/image approximately 10 times that of fluoroscopy. Since all images were in analog format, image processing to improve image quality was non-existent. The limited image quality limited the scope of angiographic procedures to only diagnostic studies, as opposed to complex interventional procedures. Despite this dramatic evolution of fluoroscopy over the past 35 years, many of the performance tests completed today by medical physicists were developed in the era of analog fluoroscopy [4–6]. Continued use of these outdated tests is not good stewardship and does not provide value-based medicine.

The AERC of analog continuous fluoroscopy changed the EDAK produced by the fluoroscope in response to changes in brightness of the TV monitor as a result of changes in thickness or density of patient anatomy. The generator either increased or decreased the high voltage and tube current in parallel. The minimum tube current was used with the minimum high voltage for a neonate or distal appendage of an adult and both acquisition parameters, the only two available, increased linearly as patient thickness increased. The maximum high voltage and tube current combination was chosen not to exceed either 88 or $176 \, \text{mGy/min}^{E-1}$, the maximum allowed fluoroscopy dose rate in the normal or high dose rate mode, respectively [7].

Coupled with AERC is Automatic Brightness Control (ABC), in which adjustment of the brightness gain is applied to the image from the detector prior to display on the monitor. This is performed independently of the AERC function and helps to eliminate saturation veiling glare or images that are too dark on the display. This function can be observed by slowly moving a highly attenuating object into the field. It will be observed, if the ABC is engaged, modification of the visual presentation while the technical factors remain constant. Only when the object reaches the region of the image used by the AERC system will the technical factors change.

State-of-the-art AERC systems have become more complex Automatic Brightness Control/Dose Management Systems (ABCDMS) with a twofold goal. The acquisition parameters are modulated in response to patient size to maintain a prescribed EDAK to manage the desired quantum mottle in the image. The variable x-ray beam filter thickness and pulse width join the high voltage and tube current as acquisition parameters that must be managed by the ABCDMS in response to changes in patient thickness. The ABC is applied to the image from the detector prior to display to provide the correct brightness on the operator's monitor. The scheme used by one manufacturer to manage these parameters is illustrated in Figure 10.3. ([8]). Clearly, the modulation of the high-voltage, filter thickness, pulse width, and tube current are not modulated in a linear fashion in the same direction. More information concerning the design and performance of the ABCDMS can be found for adult sized patients [8] and small pediatric patients [9] elsewhere.

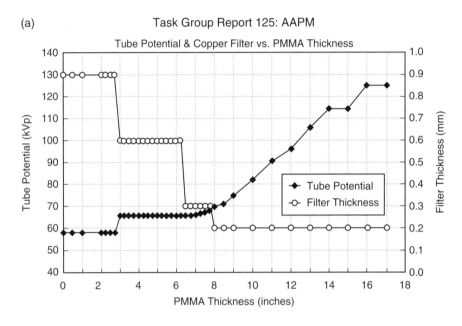

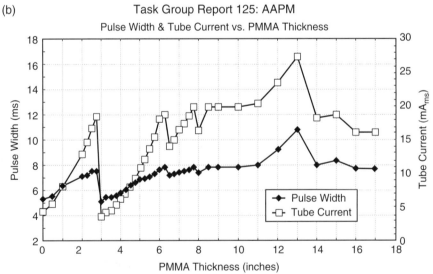

Figure 10.3 Modulation of high voltage, filter thickness (a), tube current, and pulse width (b) of a state-of-the-art ABCDMS of a pulsed fluoroscope in response to a change in patient thickness. Appropriate changes for these four parameters are more complex than the simple two factor AERC systems on continuous fluoroscopes. *Source:* Reprinted with permission [8].

Today, fluoroscopic and angiographic images are digitized from initial production of the unprocessed image by the detector to storage of the highly processed "for presentation" images. Extensive image processing, both real-time during acquisition and after the acquisition sequence for more complex processes, has dramatically improved image quality and its presentation, e.g. 2-, 3-, and 4-dimensional presentations. Improvements in the hardware of the x-ray generator, the gantry, x-ray tube, and image receptor were required to support these advancements.

The recent dramatic improvement in image quality has created a new challenge for the medical physicist, fluoroscopist, and manufacturer. Previously, the best image quality the fluoroscope could produce at a reasonable dose to the patient limited the complexity of performed procedures. Today, advanced image processing may result in better image quality than clinically necessary in portions of procedures. Clearly, the fluoroscopist should have simple, straightforward controls with which the image quality and patient dose can be decreased for less difficult portions of the examination. These controls should be developed by alterations to the configuration of the fluoroscope after consultation between the fluoroscopist, medical physicist, and manufacturer. After procedures, the fluoroscopist should be given feedback by the medical physicist on the degree of dose reduction achieved by the use of alternate configurations. This provides incentive for the fluoroscopist to identify portions of their procedures where dose reduction is possible. The medical physicist should test any configuration changes to the fluoroscope with appropriate phantoms prior to first clinical use.

10.2.2   Qualimetry

Limited measurements of the accuracy of acquisition parameters, high-voltage, tube current, pulse width, frame rate, beam quality, rates of x-ray production, and accuracy of collimation should be performed at acceptance testing and periodic performance testing with physics 1.0 test protocols. The performance data at acceptance testing provides a baseline of equipment performance when new. Repeated spot checks of these accuracies during the lifetime of the unit should be compared to baseline data.

As detailed in Chapter 9, high contrast resolution (HCR), low contrast resolution (LCR), and temporal resolving capability (TRC) of the fluoroscope's images, have typically been checked qualitatively using the phantoms described there. This presents several difficulties. First, qualitative evaluation of image quality by observing images created with relatively complex and expensive phantoms, Figure 10.4, is too subjective. Second, the only available images for testing are highly processed images. This evaluation provides little information about performance of the flat-panel image receptor because the "for processing" image produced by the image detector is not available.

It is highly desirable and expected that qualitative image quality assessment will be extended to a quantitative paradigm. Measurement of an impulse function in images prior to image processing is followed by calculating the Fourier Transform of the impulse function to create the Modulation Transfer Function (MTF) of the image receptor, Figure 10.5(b), ([10]) a quantitative evaluation of HCR. Small degradations in the performance of the image receptor can be tracked over time by periodically repeating the measurement with the exact same protocol. Likewise, by separating the noise power content of the image as a function of spatial frequency and plotting the results creates the Noise Power Spectrum (NPS) Figure 10.6, ([10]) which quantifies LCR of the image receptor when "for processing" images are analyzed. Again, repeating the measurement over time would allow tracking of any deterioration of performance. The Detector Quantum Efficiency (DQE), Figure 10.7, which is a measure of the detector's ability to preserve information in the image relative to the incident x-ray information presented at the image receptor [11] can also be calculated.

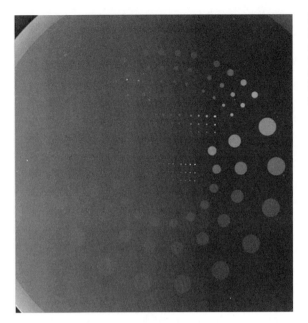

Figure 10.4 Image of popular qualitative LCR phantom developed in the 1990s. The required intricate detail of construction results in high purchase prices. Qualitative results are very dependent on the observer's interpretation of the image resulting in a distribution of results.

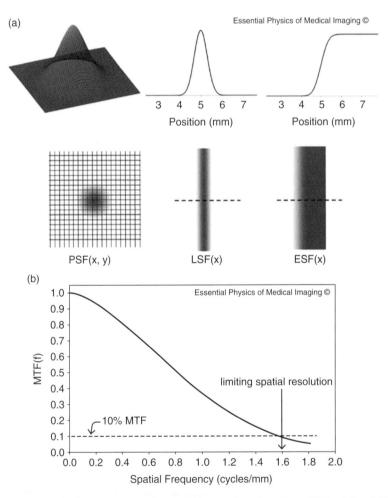

Figure 10.5 Measuring the image processor's response to an impulse object, PSF(x, y), line, LSF(x), or an edge, ESF(x) (a) allows one to quantitate the HCR by calculating the MTF(f) (b). *Source:* Reprinted with permission [10].

Figure 10.6 The NPS(f) analyzes the noise content, vertical axis, within an image based on individual spatial frequency components of the noise, horizontal axis. This allows quantification of LCR. *Source:* Reprinted with permission [10].

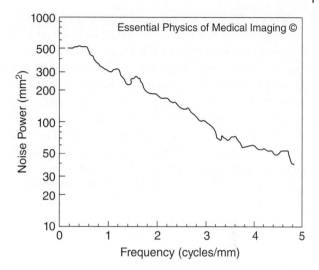

Figure 10.7 The DQE(f) analyzes the detector's ability to accurately record information (output) in the image relative to the input. *Source:* Reprinted with permission [10].

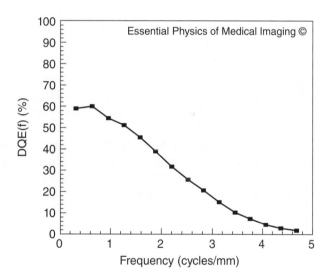

DQE, conceptually, is the square of the ratio of output performance of the detector to signal input (x-ray pattern in space):

$$DQE = \left[SNR_{out} / SNR_{in} \right]^2 \tag{10.1}$$

Since the performance of the detector is dependent on its MTF(f) and NPS(f), it is easy to show that: [12]

$$DQE = k \left[MTF(f) \right]^2 / N\,NPS(f) \tag{10.2}$$

Where k = a constant
N = mean photon fluence (photons mm^{-2})

Quantitative measurements of HCR and LCR of the image receptor can be achieved with a relatively inexpensive phantom. Multiple Plexiglas slabs (approximately 5 cm thick) create the necessary uniform attenuation phantom for measuring the NPS. If one adds a thin sheet of Plexiglas containing a high contrast impulse object, one can measure the point-spread function of images from the image receptor. This phantom construction allows positioning of the impulse object at different levels between the uniform slabs. This allows calculation of the MTF of the image receptor (impulse adjacent to image receptor) or of the "system" MTF (impulse object at center of phantom depth), the composite MTF of the image receptor and focal spot.

With this relatively inexpensive phantom and appropriate computer code, a medical physicist could calculate a quantitative LCR and HCR of the image receptor by calculating NPS and MTF of unprocessed images. A standard should be developed containing specific construction details of the phantom and computer algorithm for data analysis to minimize the variation in calculated values of HCR and LCR by different medical physicists. A requirement for such measurements, National Electrical Manufacturers Association (NEMA) publication XR-27, [13] discussed later in this chapter, should make "for processing" images available on interventional fluoroscopes by all manufacturers.

The quantitative metrics described above can then be used to determine the detectability index (d') for a particular diagnostic task. Other chapters provide more detail regarding the detectability index, so it will not be described here further. The important point is that the detectability index relates directly to physician performance. This means that use of d' can help to quantitatively adjust the equipment to optimize dose versus clinical performance.

TRC is the ability of the imaging system to sharply image edges and structures within moving objects in the image. This is an important consideration in pediatric fluoroscopy with involuntary patient motion or cardiac fluoroscopy with the rapid motion of the heart wall. Relatively short pulse widths (<3–4 msec) during either fluoroscopy or the acquisition of recorded images improves TRC. However, this is not possible during imaging of thicker body parts, which require higher ESAK to deliver a sufficient EDAK at the image receptor.

A multiplicity of temporal filtering techniques (most commonly, frame averaging) is available on most interventional fluoroscopes in the field today. Frame averaging, which reduces the perceived quantum mottle in the clinical image, degrades TRC. Manufacturers tend to overuse this feature ("out-of-the-box" configurations) because it reduces the perceived noise in the image and improves images created with motionless phantoms. Degradation of image sharpness due to motion of the patient's anatomy and over-used frame averaging is not detected with a motionless phantom.

Robert Moore understood the need to evaluate the degradation of image quality due to motion in the 1980s and developed a simple test tool, Figure 10.8(a), [14] to allow qualitative evaluation of TRC. The device is placed on 15–25 cm of Plexiglas to simulate the clinical scatter present in the image and to drive the ABCDMS controlled acquisition parameters to typical clinical values. The wires are moving at 200 mm s^{-2}, approximate speed of the heart wall, at the full disk diameter [14]. If one doubles the diameter of the disc and halves the rotational speed, the maximum motion is unchanged. However, the motion of each wire is less rotational which is a better model of the clinical motion of a guide wire within the patient Figure 10.8b. Ideally, the rotational speed of the phantom should be adjustable to allow the simulation of clinical motions of different regions of the body. TRC is improved when the diameter of the wire that can be identified during motion is not more than one step larger than the diameter of the identified stationary wire. When frame averaging of the fluoroscope is minimized or turned off to improve TRC, the perceived quantum mottle increases. This may require an increase in the EDAK to satisfy the clinical needs of the

(a)

(b)

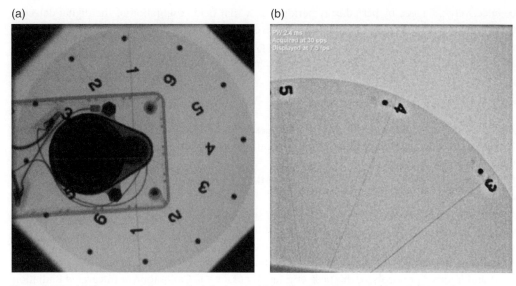

Figure 10.8 (a) Fluoroscopic image of original rotatable spoke test pattern phantom. A 13 cm diameter plexiglas disk that rotates at 30 rpm holds six 25 cm long piano wires of different diameters from 0.127– 0.559 mm. The phantom simulates different diameter guide wires and allows qualitative analysis of TRC [14]. (b) Fluoroscopic image of modified Moore TRC phantom in Figure 10.8(a). The modifications result in a more translational motion of the simulated guide wires.

operator. This is just one example of the need to balance both clinical image quality and patient radiation dose.

For a fuller characterization of the fluoroscopic system performance in the presence of motion, the static performance of the system in terms of the MTF, the NPS, and the DQE, can be extended into the temporal domain. A moving test object (wire or edge), depending on the speed of the motion, would not be as precisely depicted within the time dimension across an ensemble sequence of fluoroscopic images. The "blur" along that dimension can be characterized as a temporal MTF. Similarly, correlation of noise across an ensemble of otherwise uniform fluoroscopic images (at a specific targeted dose rate level) can be characterized in terms of the temporal NPS. Temporal filtering (e.g. frame averaging) influences both the temporal MTF and the temporal NPS. As such, they can be used to compare different filtering techniques. It is also possible to combine the complete MTF and NPS (spatial and temporal) with a definition of a spatio-temporal task (a moving object of certain morphology, contrast, and speed), and spatio-temporal attributes of the human visual system via an observer model to derive a d' specific to the targeted task. The d' can be used as a comprehensive surrogate of imaging performance for characterization, comparison, and optimization purposes of different fluoroscopic systems and techniques.

The extension of the metrology to a third dimension can also be applied to 3D imaging, and possibly even to 4D. Options are available for some fluoroscopes with a true isocenter between the focal spot and image receptor to provide cone beam CT acquisitions. These volumetric CT images require assessment. While the test methods described in Chapter 13 may be useful for some tests, the characteristics of cone beam volumetric CT images are not identical to images created by CT techniques [15]. The geometry of the detectors and the reconstruction algorithms of the two methods are significantly different, [16, 17] necessitating adjustments to the test methods [18]. Image uniformity may be more problematic during cone beam acquisitions. Managing image artifacts from cone beam acquisitions are also unique [19]. Many artifacts in 2D conventional images can be effectively managed by periodically performing a "flat field" calibration of the digital detector. Cone beam acquisitions contain additional sources of artifacts, e.g. additional patient motion, limited rotation of the c-arm gantry, cone beam geometry, x-ray scatter, beam hardening, partial volume effects, etc. making the management of these image artifacts more difficult.

10.2.3 Radiometry

At a minimum, compliance testing of fluoroscopes, Medical Physics 1.0, involves measurement of the ESAK at the maximum output limit of the unit. This only provides clinical information about the ESAK for the largest patients. It provides no information about the appropriateness of the configuration of the ABCDMS of the fluoroscope for the types of examinations and size of the patients examined in the department.

Fluoroscopes manufactured since 2006 display the rate of ESAK or KAP during live fluoroscopy and acquisition [20]. The medical physicist should make radiation output measurements that allow calculation of the correction factor used to convert the displayed dose indices to calibrated values. Task group 190 of the American Association of Physicists in Medicine (AAPM) has developed standardized protocols for this task, entitled Accuracy and Calibration of Integrated Radiation Output Indicators in Diagnostic Radiology [21]. Application of calibration factors to subsequently displayed dose indices allow simple determination of ESAK or KAP rates during subsequent testing.

An effective and efficient way to spot check the configuration of the ABCDMS is the measurement of the EDAK. This measured parameter should fall within a limited range to provide good diagnostic image quality at a well-managed patient dose based on the type of examination and the thickness of the body part that is examined.

The Fluoroscopy 1.0 discussion includes methods to make this measurement. Grid removal eliminates its Bucky factor. A non-attenuating dosimeter covering the sensing area of the ABCDMS avoids alteration of the performance of the ABCDMS. Alternatively, attenuating dosimeters must be placed outside of the sensing area. Positioning dosimeter probes sensitive to backscatter radiation 10–15 cm in front of the image receptor minimizes recording of backscatter radiation. 1 mm thick copper sheets with a cross-sectional area sufficient to cover the area of the x-ray beam are placed on collimator face to activate the ABCDMS and provide an x-ray beam of approximately 70–80 kV. The location of the copper sheets as opposed to a thicker plastic phantom resting on the patient table reduces the amount of scatter radiation in the beam where the air KERMA rate is measured.

If the manufacturer's "out-of-the-box" acquisition algorithms of the ABCDMS are inappropriate for a specific patient population or type of examination, changes to the configuration should be made and tested over the range of exam types and patient sizes performed in the department to confirm appropriate performance prior to first clinical use. Specifically, how does the EDAK change:

1) With the selection of each different Field of View (FoV) of the image receptor? [22]
2) With the selection of each different available pulse rate? [23]

Using different thicknesses of copper to model the clinical range of patient sizes and a dosimeter to measure the EDAK, the medical physicist should monitor and record the nominal acquisition parameters used by the fluoroscope, e.g. high-voltage, tube current, pulse width, pulse rate, and added filter thickness. In addition, the $K_{a,r}$ and KAP displayed by the fluoroscope should be corrected to calibrated values at the entrance plane of the patient.

Do the acquisition parameters automatically selected by the fluoroscope result in a reasonable EDAK and ESAK (diagnostic image quality at well managed patient dose rates)? While the reduction of the ratio of ESAK:EDAK is desired, choices that minimize this ratio may not result in acceptable image quality. For example, an increase in high voltage or added filter thickness reduces the ratio, but the loss of contrast in the image may be unacceptable. The appropriate value of this ratio depends on the type of examination and the actual thickness of the body part. The fourth paradigm, possible image quality that exceeds clinical requirements, may allow reduction of the ESAK by reducing the EDAK.

This type of functional testing of the ABCDMS is time consuming, but necessary to confirm quality imaging at well managed patient doses. Its importance grows when a department performs a large variety of both examinations and patient sizes. Spot checks during periodic testing of the functional testing completed at acceptance testing are necessary if modifications to the manufacturer's "out-of-the-box" configurations were made. Subsequent routine software upgrades by the manufacturer may revert a site's selected modified configuration to default values. A few spot checks during periodic performance testing should be sufficient to verify the presence of unauthorized configuration changes.

If the above described functional testing of both EDAK and ESAK is not performed, the medical physicist should measure the ESAK for both the fluoroscopy and angiographic modes of operation of the fluoroscope. This should be accomplished at the most frequently clinically used range of frame rates and FoVs. Measurements with a varying number (4–6) of Plexiglas plastic slabs each 5 cm thick should model the range of sizes of patients seen in most departments.

At a minimum, the medical physicist should measure and monitor the radiation production of a fluoroscope in cone beam mode over time [24]. One could scan a standard phantom located at isocenter with various combinations of acquisition parameters while noting the machine's displayed $K_{a,r}$ or KAP. While this method allows verification of consistency of the machine's radiation at specified intervals, it does not measure the radiation production of the machine. A more complete approach might involve measuring the radiation dose free-in-air with a radiation detector with no angular dependence [25, 26]. It is hoped that AAPM Task Group 238 are developing more rigorous standards of dose measurement within or without phantoms that follow the conventions of standard CT dosimetry for the future introduced by AAPM TG 111 [27].

It is anticipated future interventional fluoroscopes will have real-time indicators of PSD on the skin of the patient as illustrated by a current prototype unit in Figure 10.9. ([28]). The level of dose to the skin in each area of the patient is illustrated by different shades of gray. The patch of skin receiving the highest summed dose during the case is the location that received the PSD. The skin dose to any single patch of skin is a function of the summation of each exposure rate of the x-ray beam and the duration that it is applied during the procedure. Late in the case (part (a)) the region of skin within the white square (x-ray beam originating from lower right) has received the PSD to that point in the case since the "FoV PSD" (skin dose of current x-ray beam projection = PSD). Part (b) of the figure occurs later in the case since the PSD is approximately 6% greater than in part (a). Part (b) represents a time when the x-ray beam is originating from the lower left of the patient, a little used projection since the FoV PSD is 10% of the cumulative PSD of the case. Once this type of indication is provided on a fluoroscope, the medical physicist should test this feature with phantoms and dosimeter to determine any calibration factors that need to be applied to the displayed values to more accurately reflect the PSD at the entrance plane of the patient's skin.

(a)   (b)

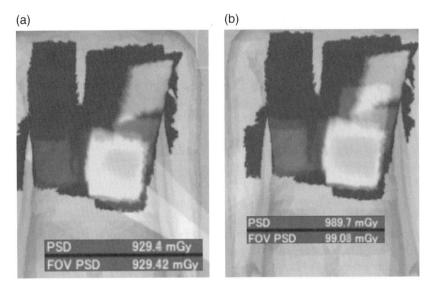

Figure 10.9 PSD Real Time Display: Image of patient's back used to illustrate real time build-up of peak skin dose (PSD) from radioscopy and radiography. Different shades of gray display the level of PSD from 0–200 mGy, to 450–550 mGy in white, to 800 mGy, and up to ~2000 mGy. Shaded white indicates the direction of the x-ray beam. PSD is the maximum level of skin dose any patch of skin has received during the case. FoV PSD is the PSD of the skin irradiated by the current indicated projection of the x-ray beam. (a) Late in case, x-ray beam originating from lower right is irradiating patch of skin that has received the highest level of PSD (FoV PSD = PSD). (b) Later in case since PSD has increased ~6%. FoV PSD is significantly less than PSD since beam originating from lower left relative to patient [28].

10.3 Testing Implication of New Technologies

Improvements in technology of more recent capabilities the fluoroscope result in a number of implications with respect to properly testing state-of-the-art equipment. Some of these implications are described below.

10.3.1 Hardware

In the last 20 years, closed loop control of the high-voltage and tube current by the x-ray generator have significantly improved the accuracy, consistency, and reliability of these two acquisition parameters. Figure 10.10 illustrates this effect on the tube current of an early vintage closed loop generator. The accuracy of the tube current during the first 15 msec of the exposure, left of the vertical arrows, was dependent upon the calibration of the filament current of the x-ray tube. After the first 15 msec of the exposure, the feedback mechanism activated and adjusted the filament current to provide the calibrated tube current. Closed loop generators today apply the correction much earlier in the exposure. This feature of the generator eliminates most calibration errors commonly found during acceptance testing of fluoroscopes without closed loop control.

Many C-arm gantries today have a true isocenter about which the x-ray tube and image receptor rotate. This is mandatory for cone beam CT. This volumetric computed tomography capability is an important addition to simple projection fluoroscopy in the interventional procedure room. Cone beam CT capabilities of the c-arm provide rapid production of 3D imaging with higher spatial resolution and lower dose than conventional CT exams with multi detector technology.

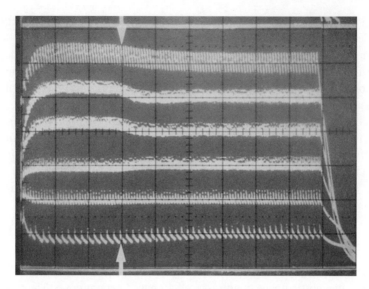

Figure 10.10 Six different tube current waveforms of a closed loop generator illustrate the improvement in the accuracy of the tube current when the closed loop feedback is applied (location of vertical arrows). Prior to the feedback, calibration of tube current is limited to the calibration of the initial filament current of the x-ray tube. The horizontal axis is exposure duration in units of 5 msec per division on the oscilloscope trace. The vertical axis is tube current in units of 100 mA per division.

Flat-panel digital detectors have replaced analog image intensifiers and TV cameras on most interventional fluoroscopes. The analog image receptor was bulky in size, provided a round rather than a rectangular image, saturated over a limited dynamic range, had pincushion distortion, had S distortion (problematic for cone beam applications), had vignetting (less light intensity at the image's periphery), demonstrated veiling glare (due to light scatter), and had a nonlinear TV camera. [11] Testing in the field to quantify these deficiencies was difficult. Fortunately, this type of performance testing is no longer necessary. In its place, the medical physicist can focus on identifying and eliminating artifacts in digital images before they affect the clinical interpretation of the images.

In addition to the advantages above over the analog image receptor and camera, the flat-panel digital detector also has a higher DQE at EDAKs during the creation of angiographic images. However, the digital detector's DQE at low EDAKs associated with continuous fluoroscopy is inferior to that of the image intensifier. The significant amplification gain required by the signal from the flat-panel detector prior to digitization amplifies the electronic and other noise sources, resulting in images with a relatively low signal-to-noise ratio (SNR) [11]. The medical physicist should be determining the DQE of the flat-panel detector. Fortunately, this problem is partially mitigated by the replacement of continuous fluoroscopy with a pulsed x-ray beam with higher intensity within each pulse.

10.3.2 Acquisition Methods

Section 10.2.3, discussed the need for functional testing of ABCDMS, due to the wide variety of acquisition techniques that are available. The limited availability of the clinical fluoroscope makes it impossible to check the response of the ABCDMS to all combinations of clinical examinations and thicknesses of patient. The medical physicist needs information from the manufacturer on expected EDAKs for different types of examinations for average sized adult patients. The manufacturer also needs to provide information on how these rates change, if at all, as a function of patient size.

The medical physicist should also determine the ratio ESAK:EDAK as a function of patient thickness, which is affected by the high-voltage/added filtration selected by the ABCDMS. While the ESAK to an average size adult abdomen is generally known for a given fluoroscope model, the appropriate rate for newborn, one-year-old, five-year-old, etc. abdomens of children most likely is not as well known. AAPM Task Group 251, is currently collecting data on typical fluoroscopes to provide this type of information in the near future.

Spot checks of the EDAK should be repeated at least annually and if the configuration of the fluoroscope has been altered to address the unique clinical needs of a specific department. Mandatory software upgrades installed by the manufacturer periodically to correct identified problems may reset the configuration of the fluoroscope back to its default settings. The medical physicist should not assume the manufacturer will always inform them of a software upgrade that may produce this undesired effect.

10.3.3 Image Processing and Analysis

Image processing should be selected based on examination type and thickness of the body part imaged to ensure diagnostic image quality at well-managed patient doses. The medical physicist has not been able to effectively influence image processing for either a given type of examination or thickness of body part. This has occurred for two reasons. First, the manufacturer has provided few technical details about their image processing routines. Second, only extensively processed images interpreted by the radiologist have been available.

This makes the analysis of the performance of the image receptor impossible. Is a substandard image on the operator's monitor in the procedure room due to problems with the image receptor or due to inappropriate image processing applied to detector's images? Better education of medical physicists about fundamental image processing routines should allow them to ask more focused questions of the manufacturer resulting in a better understanding. Lack of non-processed images from the image receptor should soon be addressed by the implementation of a new standard, NEMA XR 27, described in the following section.

10.3.4 New System-Wide Technologies

The evolution of the fluoroscope in the last 30 years has greatly

1) improved the accuracy in control of acquisition parameters,
2) increased the complexity of the ABCDMS,
3) increased the variety of types of images produced, and
4) increased image quality to levels that exceed clinical needs for some portions of most examinations.

Due to these changes, acquisition parameters need adjustment within the ABCDMS to provide better manage image quality and patient dose.

In some instances, excellent image quality can be degraded to acceptable diagnostic quality by reducing the EDAK. The increased quantum mottle of images may be acceptable if initial image quality exceeded clinical needs. This change reduces patient dose per image and creates opportunities to improve image quality by adjusting acquisition parameters, especially for smaller body parts. For example, if the pulse width is reduced due to a reduced exposure rate, blurring in the image due to patient motion may be reduced.

An increase in the high-voltage may provide adequate image quality despite some loss of subject contrast. This change reduces both patient dose and required exposure rates; this may allow additional copper filtration in the x-ray beam to further reduce the ESAK:EDAK. However, only small increases in additional beam filtration (~0.1 mm copper) can be made without requiring excessive pulse widths.

Reducing the frame rate reduces ESAK without increasing the absolute quantum mottle in the image. However, this degrades TRC of the images. Acceptable reduction of the frame rate depends on speed of moving objects in the images. Most fluoroscopists can perform a portion of their fluoroscopic studies at frame rates lower than the default frame rates. However, this is a skill that most fluoroscopists develop with practice as they learn to adapt to the lag in the image and its effect on the devices they manipulate.

The previous three paragraphs describe more clinical presence and impact for the medical physicist than in the past. The medical physicist needs additional tools to allow testing of the functionality of the fluoroscope to help develop better configurations. NEMA XR 27 published in 2012 [13] defines one such tool. This standard will establish the following access and controls on interventional fluoroscopes:

1) user quality control mode
2) manual control of high voltage, tube current, pulse width, added beam filtration, and focal spot size for single shot exposures
3) direct access to "For Processing Images," Figure 10.11(a), ([10]) with control of high voltage, spectral filtration, and EDAK during:
   a) radioscopy
   b) radiography

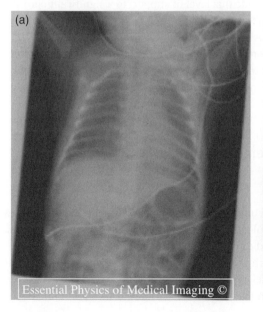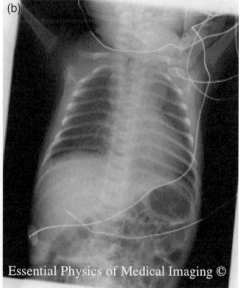

Figure 10.11 (a) For Processing Image of a small child which represents the image quality produced by the flat panel detector without image processing. (b) For Presentation Image of the same child after the application of image processing prior to interpretation of the image. *Source:* Reprinted with permission [10].

4) direct access to "For Presentation Images," Figure 10.11b, ([10]) with control of high voltage, spectral filtration, EDAK during:
   a) radioscopy
   b) radiography
5) electronic documentation of system configuration
6) access to Radiation Dose Structured Reports (RDSR).

This tool allows trial and error testing that helps identify improved configurations for a given fluoroscope, allows access patient dose information, allows accurate documentation of configuration changes, and provides access to non-processed images from the image receptor and to images that will be interpreted.

A number of task groups are working within the AAPM to establish additional information needed to support fluoroscopic units. TG 190 standardizes protocols to determine calibration factors for $K_{a,r}$ and KAP [21]. TG 251 is currently collecting data to establish Diagnostic Reference Levels (DRL) for ESAK of fluoroscopes during radioscopy and radiography as a function of patient thickness. TG 238 is currently developing standardized testing for both image quality assessment and patient dose determination associated with cone beam CT functionality.

Few of the changes described in this section will happen without leadership and support of the medical physicist in the clinic. Few fluoroscopists will experiment on their own to implement the changes described above since some loss of image quality will likely occur. The medical physicist can help fluoroscopists understand which changes reduce patient dose rates the most with the smallest impact on image quality. The fluoroscopist needs assurance from the medical physicist that the planned changes will provide good clinical image quality at reduced doses to the patients.

Some departments still believe that the leadership described above typically comes from the manufacturer of their fluoroscopes. This is not likely. First, the manufacturers are not staffed with an adequate number of medical physicists to provide this level of support to a significant percentage of their customers. Second, a configured state-of-the-art fluoroscope that provides good, diagnostic image quality at well-managed patient doses probably produces less attractive images than the manufacturer's "out-of-the-box" configuration. While the primary goal of the operator and the medical physicist should be improved patient care, this may be at odds with the manufacturer's primary goal of selling more equipment. The manufacturer has no incentive to reduce image quality on an installed unit unless specifically requested by the customer.

10.4 Clinical Integration and Implementation

10.4.1 Training and Communication

The medical physicist should build their clinical understanding of typically performed procedures closer to the level of their understanding of radiologic physics of imaging. Clinical cases should be observed; subtle findings that must be identified during the interpretation of the images to accurately manage the case should be discussed with the fluoroscopists. The medical physicist must understand the design strengths and weaknesses of the individual fluoroscopes available in the department based on information from the manufacturer and experience from performance testing the imagers.

Three areas of knowledge – clinical requirements of procedures, strengths and weaknesses of available fluoroscopes, and knowledge of radiological imaging physics – allow the development of a plan and strategy to properly manage image quality and radiation dose. This may involve changes in the configuration of acquisition parameters, changes in applied image processing, and recommendations for the fluoroscopist to follow when manipulating the controls of the fluoroscope.

The following is a brief description of a training intervention to improve image quality and reduce patient dose for common pediatric fluoroscopic procedures. All fluoroscopists and technologists were asked to complete three web modules [29] that discussed the basic goals of pediatric fluoroscopy:

1) enhancing radiation protection during pediatric fluoroscopy
2) steps to manage radiation dose during the examination
3) steps to manage radiation dose and possible tissue effects after a fluoroscopic procedure.

The above modules explain the basic "what" of pediatric fluoroscopy. The medical physicist developed a one-hour presentation on the details of the controls of the models of fluoroscopes within the department: the "how" of pediatric fluoroscopy with a specific fluoroscope. All fluoroscopic staff members were required to attend this lecture. The medical physicist followed up the intervention by working individually with staff members who had additional questions. As a quantitative evaluation of the effectiveness of the educational intervention, the medical physicist analyzed the clinical patient doses for four months prior to and after the intervention.

10.4.2 Optimization

Complete imaging protocols for all clinical examinations help manage radiation dose and image quality. While developing techniques to manage patient dose is important, additional steps are necessary to ensure that the desired dose rates are consistently delivered to all patients of a given size for a given type of fluoroscopic examination regardless of the operator or the unit on which the procedure was performed [30]. This requires a protocol that details:

1) configuration of the acquisition parameters of the fluoroscope
2) applied image processing
3) guidance for the fluoroscopist with respect to operation of the manual controls during the procedure.

The medical physicist should study the "out-of-the-box" protocols recommended by the fluoroscope's manufacturer to gain insights into the strengths and weaknesses of the fluoroscope's design. Aspects of the fluoroscope's design that need clarification should be discussed with the manufacturer. Reading the literature and testing the performance of available fluoroscopes with phantoms or possibly animals that model the thickness of average sized patients may be helpful. Well-designed protocols for the unique types of exams and patients within the department require an understanding of the design of the available fluoroscopes.

Once the protocol is developed, the medical physicist should test it and monitor the values of the acquisition parameters as the range of patient sizes is modeled with phantoms. The ESAK and EDAK are good metrics for monitoring the appropriateness of the acquisition parameters.

After the protocol is properly tested and implemented, the imaging process and workflow of future studies should not be overlooked. Continued dialog with the fluoroscopists allows identification of protocol weaknesses that need improvement. The two most promising image processing algorithms might be trialed on a handful of patients before selecting the final image-processing algorithm. Best patient care is achieved when the radiologists, technologists, and the medical physicist work together as a team to improve the performance of the fluoroscope and each team member. The following are some examples on the possible management of EDAK.

The fluoroscope should be configured to manage EDAK for the range of patient sizes for each type of study performed in the department. The operator typically selects an anatomical program setting that matches the type of study and patient size. A minimum of two levels of ESAK should be available to the operator to adjust the level of quantum mottle in the images depending on the complexity of each phase of the fluoroscopic exam. Typically, the low dose setting $= 0.5 \times$ medium dose setting $= 0.25 \times$ high dose setting. Establishing the EDAK of a flat panel detector is an example of clinical integration and implementation optimization. Good image quality is achieved by maintaining an appropriate EDAK for each created image during a variety of operational modes during either radioscopy or radiography.

In addition to these operator controls of ESAK, the fluoroscope should automatically adjust the EDAK when the operator changes other acquisition parameters. These include the FoV of the image receptor, the pulse rate during fluoroscopy, the added filter thickness in the x-ray beam, the operational mode, e.g. fluoroscopy, digital angiography, digital subtraction angiography, and cardiac angiography. Patient care, in some situations, may be improved by the following configuration changes when originally configuring the unit. These three changes illustrate that properly managing (lowering overall) patient dose may be counterintuitive since all three examples increase the EDAK at the image receptor to maintain image quality.

10.4.2.1 FoV

The EDAK should change when the operator selects a different FoV of the image receptor. The EDAK was historically proportional to $1/\mathrm{FoV}^2$ or $1/\mathrm{FoV}$ depending on equipment design [22]. These designs respectively increase the EDAK per image fourfold or twofold as the FoV dimension is cut in half. The total noise in the image is relatively unchanged as a function of FoV if the EDAK is constant. However, since the image becomes sharper as the FoV decreases (image intensifier, flat panel receptor when pixel size decreases), perceived noise increases despite constant total noise. Therefore, EDAK $\propto 1/\mathrm{FoV}$ is a good choice for image intensifiers. EDAK remaining constant [22] or $\propto 1/\mathrm{FoV}^{0.5}$ may be a reasonable choice for imaging with flat panel detectors when the FoV decreases without a change in binning of the flat panel's detector elements. At the point of a large FoV flat panel detector where a reduction of the FoV eliminates binning of the individual detectors, EDAK $\propto 1/\mathrm{FoV}$ may not be a large enough change [9].

10.4.2.2 Pulse Rate

The EDAK per image should automatically increase relative to EDAK at 30 pulses/second, according to Eq. (10.3), when the operator reduces the pulse rate during pulsed fluoroscopy from 30 to 7.5 pulses/second. This change in dose per image is required to maintain a constant perceived noise level in the image [23].

$$\text{Increase in EDAK / pulse} = \left(30 / \text{pulse rate}\right)^{0.5} \tag{10.3}$$

Perceived noise in the image is a function of the number of images averaged together by the operator's brain for 0.2 seconds. At 30 pulses/second the human eye integrates six fluoroscopic images which reduces the perceived noise; dose per pulse should increase for slower pulse rates to compensate for the loss of physiological integration of the images. Equation (10.3) applies only to pulse rates >7 pulses/second. For pulse rates at or less than 7 pulses/second, the dose per pulse should be unchanged since regardless of the pulse rate (0.5–5 pulses/second) physiological integration of images is not possible.

$$\text{EDAK / pulse} = \text{constant} \tag{10.4}$$

10.4.2.3 Spectral Filter Thickness

When spectral filters (materials with $z > 13$) are added to the x-ray beam, the effective energy of the beam increases. This delivers the prescribed energy to the image receptor with fewer photons since each photon is carrying more energy. Therefore, the quantum mottle in the image increases unless an increase in EDAK restores the number of photons to their original level. When copper filters with thicknesses of 0.1 or 0.2–0.9 mm are used, increasing the EDAK by a factor of 1.4 and 2 [31] respectively, mitigates the loss of image quality due to increased quantum mottle.

10.4.3 Automated Analysis and Data Management

Few, if any, automated quality control methods are provided by the fluoroscope system manufacturers. Third-party test tools are available, some with software included to analyze collected data, but these tools typically are not automated. Third-party radiation dose databases are available that can be interfaced to fluoroscopes with RDSR capability; once the procedure is complete the RDSR data is automatically transmitted to the central database. This data is then available for quality control analysis, but little of this analysis is currently automated. While the capabilities added to interventional fluoroscopes in the near future by the NEMA XR 27 standard are a huge advancement, this standard does not develop automated analysis.

Many of the metrics previously discussed in this chapter are appropriate for automated collection and analysis of performance data. Section 10.2.2. of this chapter suggested standardized phantoms and software analysis tools that allow quantitative analysis of both HCR (MTF) and LCR (NPS). With the capabilities created by the NEMA XR 27 standard, these analyses can be performed on "For Processing" images to test the performance of the image receptor. Additional analyses of "For Presentation" images would allow analysis of the effectiveness of available image processing algorithms. This type of analysis should also be applied to TRC of different configurations provided a more robust phantom with moving objects is developed.

QC data from all fluoroscopes in the department should be automatically transferred and stored in a central database; it could be the same database used to store the $K_{a,r}$ and KAP. Protocols should be set up so that the technologist positions the appropriate phantom and collects data either at the end or beginning of the clinical day. Since the thickness of the phantom suggested in this chapter is variable, a schedule could be created for the technologist to follow so that periodically the HCR and LCR would be tested for the entire range of sizes of patients imaged. Transmitted data should be plotted to identify trends in equipment performance. Access to the results in the central database should be web-based to allow any authorized individual easy access. Since this proposal would monitor ongoing performance of the fluoroscope, the medical physicist should require less testing time within each procedure room. This would provide more time for the medical physicist to review trends and help identify solutions to discovered problems.

10.4.4 Meaningful QC

The principle of stewardship dictates that if a QC procedure does not directly maintain or improve patient care, it should be abandoned. While everyone agrees that attempting to reduce patient dose while maintaining image quality is important, too often little effort is expended to ensure that this is consistently achieved for all exams on all fluoroscopes within the department. Collection of quantitative QC data by technologists with an extensive assistance of computational routines built into each fluoroscope by the manufacturer, coupled with computational analysis and plotting of performance trends within a central database is a key first step. This should dramatically reduce equipment performance testing time of the medical physicist and allow them to focus on solving identified problems. This also allows the medical physicist to focus on clinical operational issues. Is the patient dose, detector dose, and image quality appropriate for each exam regardless of the type of exam, size of the body part imaged, the actual fluoroscope used, or the individual fluoroscopist? The medical physicist must be given adequate time to interpret and respond to equipment configuration issues and/or misunderstanding of operators to improve patient care by properly managing patient radiation doses and the quality of the images produced.

References

1 Strauss, K.J. (2002). Interventional equipment acquisition process: cradle to grave. In: *Intravascular Brachytherapry Fluoroscopically Guided Interventions* (eds. S. Balter, R.C. Chan and T.B. Shope), 797–848. Madison, WI: Medical Physics Publishing.

2 Strauss, K.J., Nachabe, R.J., and Racacio, J.M. (2015). Estimates of diagnostic reference levels for pediatric peripheral and abdominal fluoroscopically-guided procedures. *American Journal of Roentgenology* 204 (6): W713–W719.

3 Strauss, K.J. (2006). Interventional suite and equipment management: cradle to grave. *Pediatric Radiology* 36 (Suppl 2): 2221–2236.

4 Rossi, R.P. (1982). Acceptance testing of radiographic x- ray generators. In: *Acceptance Testing of Radiological Imaging Equipment*, AAPM Symposium Proceedings, No 1 (eds. P.J.P. Lin, R.J. Kriz, P.L. Rauch, et al.), 110–125. New York, NY: American Institute of Physics.

5 Rauch, P.L. (1982). Performance characteristics of diagnostic x-ray generators. In: *Acceptance Testing of Radiological Imaging Equipment*, AAPM Symposium Proceedings No 1 (eds. L. PJP, R.J. Kriz, P.L. Rauch, et al.), 126–156. New York, NY: American Association of Physicists in Medicine.

6 Rauch, P.L. and Strauss, K.J. (1998). X-ray generator, tube, collimator, positioner, and table. In: *Syllabus: Categorical Course in Diagnostic Radiology Physics: Cardiac Catheterization Imaging* (eds. E.L. Nickoloff and K.J. Strauss), 61–82. Oak Brook, IL: RSNA Publications.

7 FDA (2010). US Food and Drug Administration, Center for Devices and Radiological Health. Code of Federal Regulation, Title 21 Part 1020, Section 10230.32. Performance standards for ionizing radiation emitting products: Fluoroscopic equipment. http://www.accessdata.fda.gov/scripts/cdrh/cfdocs/cfcfr/CFRSearch.cfm.

8 Rauch, P., Lin, P.J., Balter, S. et al. (2012). Functionality and operation of fluoroscopic automatic brightness control/automatic dose rate control logic in modern cardiovascular and interventional angiography systems: a report of Task Group 125 Radiography/Fluoroscopy Subcommittee, Imaging Physics Committee, Science Council. *Medical Physics* 39: 2826–2828.

9 IAEA (2013). *Dosimetry in Diagnostic Radiology for Paediatric Patients*, IAEA Human Health Series No 24 (ed. IAEA). Vienna, Austria: IAEA.

10 Bushberg, J.T., Seibert, J.A., Leidholt, E.M. Jr., and Boone, J.M. (2002). *The Essential Physics of Medical Imaging*, 2nd edition. Philadelphia: Lippincott Williams & Wilkins.

11 Seibert, J.A. (2006). Flat-panel detectors: how much better are they? *Pediatric Radiology* 36 (Suppl 2): 173–181.

12 IEC (2003). Characteristics of digital x-ray imaging devices, Part 1: Determination of the detector quantum efficiency. In: IEC (ed) 62220-1, Switzerland.

13 NEMA (2013). NEMA XR 27: Xray equipment for interventional procedures: User Quality Control Mode. In: NEMA (ed). National Electrical Manufacturers Association XR 27.

14 Moore, R.J. (1990). *Imaging Principles of Cardiac Angiography*. Rockville, Md: Aspen Publishers.

15 Siewerdsen, J.H. (2011). Cone-beam CT with a flat-panel detector: from image science to image-guided surgery. *Nuclear Instruments & Methods in Physics Research Section A, Accelerators, Spectrometers, Detectors and Associated Equipment* 648: S241–S250.

16 Sisniega, A., Zbijewski, W., Badal, A. et al. (2013). Monte Carlo study of the effects of system geometry and antiscatter grids on cone-beam CT scatter distributions. *Medical Physics* 40: 051915.

17 Daly, M.J., Siewerdsen, J.H., Cho, Y.B. et al. (2008). Geometric calibration of a mobile C-arm for intraoperative cone-beam CT. *Medical Physics* 35: 2124–2136.

18 Friedman, S.N., Fung, G.S., Siewerdsen, J.H. et al. (2013). A simple approach to measure computed tomography (CT) modulation transfer function (MTF) and noise-power spectrum (NPS) using the American College of Radiology (ACR) accreditation phantom. *Medical Physics* 40: 051907.

19 Chan, Y., Siewerdsen, J.H., Rafferty, M.A. et al. (2008). Cone-beam computed tomography on a mobile C-arm: novel intraoperative imaging technology for guidance of head and neck surgery. *Journal of Otolaryngology – Head & Neck Surgery = Le Journal d'oto-rhino-laryngologie et de chirurgie cervico-faciale* 37: 81–90.

20 FDA (2005). US Food and Drug Administration, Center for Devices and Radiological Health. Code of Federal Regulation, Title 21 Part 1020, Section 10230; Electronic Products; Performance standards for diagnostic x-ray systems and their major components; final rule. In: Health CfDaR (ed). FDA.

21 AAPM (2015). Accuracy and Calibration of Integrated Radiation Output Indicators in Diagnostic Radiology. In: AAPM (ed) AAPM report no 190. AAPM.

22 Strauss, K.J. (2006). Pediatric interventional radiography equipment: safety considerations. *Pediatric Radiology* 36 (Suppl 2): 126–135.

23 Aufrichtig, R., Xue, P., Thomas, C.W. et al. (1994). Perceptual comparison of pulsed and continuous fluoroscopy. *Medical Physics* 21: 245–256.

24 Kyriakou, Y., Deak, P., Langner, O. et al. (2008). Concepts for dose determination in flat-detector CT. *Physics in Medicine and Biology* 53: 3551–3566.

25 Daly, M.J., Siewerdsen, J.H., Moseley, D.J. et al. (2006). Intraoperative cone-beam CT for guidance of head and neck surgery: assessment of dose and image quality using a C-arm prototype. *Medical Physics* 33: 3767–3780.

26 Fahrig, R., Dixon, R., Payne, T. et al. (2006). Dose and image quality for a cone-beam C-arm CT system. *Medical Physics* 33: 4541–4550.

27 AAPM (2010). Comprehensive methodology for the evaluation of radiation dose in x-ray computed tomography. In: AAPM (ed). AAPM Report No 111. AAPM.

28 Bednarek, D.R., Barbarits, J., Rana, V.K. et al. (2011). Verification of the Performance Accuracy of a Real-Time Skin-Dose Tracking System for Interventional Fluoroscopic Procedures. SPIE vol. 7961-78. In: Proceedings from Medical Imaging 2011: Physics of Medical Imaging, Orlando, FL, paper 796127:1-8. NIHMSID 303276. https://www.ncbi.nlm.nih.gov/pcm/articles/PMC3127243/.

29 Image Gently Educational Modules Section I: An introduction to image gently: enhancing radiation protection in pediatric fluoroscopy: Section II: Steps to manage radiation dose during the examination; Section III: Steps to manage radiation dose and possible tissue effects after a fluoroscopic procedure. In: Image Gently I (ed) Image Gently Training Modules. www.imagegently.org.

30 Larson, D.B., Strauss, K.J., and Podberesky, D.J. (2015). Toward large-scale process control to enable consistent CT radiation dose optimization. *AJR American Journal of Roentgenology*: May: 959–966. PMID: 25730157.

31 Rauch, P. (2010). The "30-30-30 rule", a practical guide to setting the detector input exposure rate for a fluoroscopic imager. *Medical Physics* 37: 3123.

Part IV

Computed Tomography

11

Clinical CT Physics: Perspective

Douglas E. Pfeiffer[1] and Mahadevappa Mahesh[2]

[1] Boulder Community Health, Boulder, CO, USA
[2] The Russell H. Morgan Department of Radiology and Radiological Science, Johns Hopkins University, Baltimore, MD, USA

As with other modalities, computed tomography (CT) has evolved significantly since its invention in the 1970s. CT is unique among the x-ray modalities in that it has always been digital. From the first EMI head scanner, technological advances in other areas allowed CT scanner technology to advance as well. Computer power and speed increased significantly, allowing for the processing of greater amounts of data. Slip ring technology allowed for the development of helical scanning. X-ray tubes advanced, becoming much larger and more robust, high power tubes permitting longer scans at higher mA settings. Multiple row detectors allowed for acquisition of multiple slices in one rotation in axial mode, or greater volumes of data in helical mode.

11.1 Changing Technologies

Much of the advancement in recent years has been in improved detectors to be more efficient, smaller, and faster. Rotation times have been reduced to as low as 0.3 s. But perhaps most importantly, the number of detector rows has grown significantly, with arrays now wide enough to image the entire heart in just one rotation. All modern scanners have automatic mA control, changing the mA per rotation based on the attenuation properties of the tissue being imaged. Many are automatically selecting a kV setting appropriate for the body habitus and purpose of the scan. Dual energy is becoming more common, allowing for many advanced functions including selection of soft tissue or dense material contrast, virtual non-contrast, renal stone evaluation, and gout differentiation. With such powerful technology, the clinical physicist is in a position to provide important guidance for building protocols that use the features of the scanner at doses as low as diagnostically appropriate.

11.2 Quantitative Metrics

CT scanners offer the physicist a unique opportunity for quantification that is just now being realized in other modalities. Being inherently digital, the modulation transfer function (MTF), the noise power spectrum (NPS) and detectability indices are readily measurable with a relatively simple phantom. These metrics would assist in the design and optimization of protocols, providing task-based information. They would be valuable as the scanners become used more for 3D and even 4D imaging (e.g. perfusion imaging). Such metrics can be easily tracked over time for more sensitive management of image quality. Comparison between scanners is simplified. Subjective analysis of traditional image quality phantoms cannot provide quantitative management.

Quantitative metrics would be of great assistance in the establishment of automatic kV and mA response curves, specific to the diagnostic task. At this time, selection of these parameters is based on basic metrics such as noise. However, the reconstruction kernel selected has a great impact on the noise in the images, independent of dose. The clinical physicist, with robust metrics at hand, can offer invaluable advice balancing all of these factors impacting the final image. Current phantoms allow for ensuring consistent performance of the scanner, but their properties limit their application to protocol optimization as there is no direct tie between the measured values and clinical demands.

Dosimetry of CT scanners is evolving in theory [1], but clinical measurement of dose or dose indexes has not changed, as it is not clear how to implement the new theoretical descriptions of CT dosimetry. Given that the science has demonstrated that the current computed tomography dose index (CTDI) methodology does not properly reflect CT dose [2, 3], a new clinical methodology must be advanced. Clinical physicists must understand the new theories and work to have an appropriate implementation for the clinic.

11.3 Emerging Applications

There are a host of new and advanced CT technologies coming to practice. Perfusion imaging is an area that needs better optimization of image data while lowering dose, which tends to be high. Likewise, spectral imaging through dual energy or photon-counting presents a significant challenge in a clinic in terms of optimization of implementation and relevance of the data, a challenge that can be tackled by the physicist. As more spectral applications become mainstream, the physicist will be required to learn how a specific spectral system works and develop image quality and dosimetry methods. This situation is very similar to the early days of CT scanning when there were no phantoms or dosimetry methods.

11.4 Performance Monitoring

Frequent quality control scanning is common in CT. Daily measurement of water CT number and noise is required by accrediting bodies. The images are viewed to look for artifacts. Measurement of CT number and noise is easily performed by automated systems. Computer algorithms exist to analyze the texture of the image and can be more sensitive to subtle artifacts than a quick perusal by a busy technologist with patients waiting. Clinical physics should have systems to perform the analysis, keep the database, and alert when action limits are passed. At this time, such systems are found mainly only at certain academic institutions. The MP 3.0 approach can become a reality when the systems are available for all clinical physicists to adopt and implement in their own departments or for small, single scanner practices. With an appropriate phantom, such automated analysis could include image quality metrics such as detectability for quality control of system performance.

Chapters 12 and 13 describe both the current practice as well as the emerging development for clinical CT physics. The transition from the 1.0 practice of CT to 3.0 can be summarized in Table 11.1, some details of which are highlighted in the following chapters.

Table 11.1 Comparison of Medical Physics 1.0 and emerging 3.0 paradigms in CT physics.

Computed Tomography	1.0	3.0
Focus of medical physicist's (MP) attention	Equipment, focused on individual systems and isolated performance	Patient, focused on consistency of care across practice
Image quality evaluation	Specification verification focused, in and through phantoms	Clinical performance-focused, in and through phantoms and patient cases
Evaluation condition	Standardized protocols	Standardized protocols and representative protocols closely reflecting clinical use
MP "tools of the trade" for image quality evaluation	Visibility of line pairs, manual region-of-interest (ROI)-based measurements	MTF, NPS, detective quantum efficiency (DQE), task-based detectability and estimability, radiomics quantification
Routine QC	Task-generic, HU accuracy focused	Task-specific, performance-focused
Patient dosimetry	CTDI, size-specific dose estimate (SSDE), dose length product (DLP) Hounsfield unit (HU)	Patient-focused, organ dose, risk index
CT applications	Focused on few "easy to test" applications	Include advanced applications including perfusion, spectral, and cardiac applications
Protocols	Focused on few protocols devised based or peer benchmarking	Incorporating all protocols optimized based on expected image quality, dose, and consistency across patients and systems

While a 3.0 paradigm is fairly easily to envision, the transition from 1.0 methodology to this new paradigm is non-trivial. In many ways it harkens back to the early days of CT. Research-oriented physicists worked to develop meaningful ways of testing scanner capabilities and dose indexes. These methods were adopted by clinical physicists and regulatory bodies as they became available. With the move of the clinical physicist from the low-yield 1.0 testing to the patient-centered 3.0 approach, we would be able to realize the benefits in the improved care of the patients.

References

1 American Association of Physicists in Medicine (2010). Comprehensive methodology for the evaluation of radiation dose in x-ray computed tomography, *Report of AAPM Task Group 111: The Future of CT Dosimetry* (American Association of Physicists in Medicine, College Park, MD).
2 Boone, J.M. (2007). The trouble with CTDI100. *Med. Phys.* 34 (4): 1364–1371.
3 Dixon, R.L. (2003). A new look at CT dose measurement: beyond CTDI. *Med. Phys.* 30 (6): 1272–1280.

12

Clinical CT Physics: State of Practice

Douglas E. Pfeiffer

Boulder Community Health, Boulder, CO, USA

12.1   Introduction

Computed tomography systems have seen dramatic evolution since their inception in 1972 by EMI. As described in Chapter 11, scanners have developed from very slow translate-rotate technology with simple back-projection reconstruction to 120 detector row arrays with 0.3 second rotation times and computationally-intensive iterative and model-based reconstruction.

The simple translate-rotate generation was replaced with the much faster rotate-rotate geometry, which allowed for helical scanning. While the first EMI scanner was indeed a dual slice unit, the rapid implementation of multiple detector rows took place after the introduction of slip-ring technology in 1989. Dual source scanners were introduced in 2005.

In the early days of computed tomography, it was not clear what the typical failure modes were going to be. Geometric, mechanical, and reconstruction factors led physicists to focus attention on computed tomography (CT) number accuracy, CT number uniformity, slice thickness, spatial resolution, low contrast performance, and dose.

The unique geometry of CT scanners makes regular measurement of kV accuracy and half-value layer problematic. Therefore, generator performance was typically limited to output measurements.

While scanners developed very rapidly, the development of how we test these systems has been less remarkable. Most of the testing performed on early scanners is still the basis of testing modern scanners, with few modifications.

Unlike most x-ray systems, the regulatory environment has not driven the medical physics testing. With few exceptions, federal and state regulations have called for not much more than documentation to be provided to the end user. Some states have mandated technologist and medical physicist testing, but these are in the minority.

Lacking regulatory mandate, physicists have relied upon recommendations by professional organizations, particularly the American Association of Physicists in Medicine and its Report 39 [1] and 1995 Summer School [2]. International organizations also established quality control (QC) programs for their member organizations. In 2002 the American College of Radiology (ACR) established its CT Accreditation Program (CTAP). The CTAP suggested that each accredited facility

Clinical Imaging Physics: Current and Emerging Practice, First Edition. Edited by Ehsan Samei and Douglas E. Pfeiffer.
© 2020 John Wiley & Sons, Inc. Published 2020 by John Wiley & Sons, Inc.

should have a QC program in place [3], but the exact components of that program were not mandated until the ACR CT Quality Control Manual was published in December 2012 [4, 5].

In 2008, the United States passed the Medicare Improvements for Patients and Providers Act of 2008 (MIPPA), which mandated that outpatient providers of advanced imaging modalities (CT, magnetic resonance imaging (MRI), positron emission tomography (PET), and nuclear medicine) that bill under part B of the Medicare Physician Fee Schedule must be accredited by an authorized agency in order to receive technical component reimbursement from Medicare. Four according bodies are currently approved under MIPPA: The ACR, The Joint Commission (TJC), RadSite, and the Intersocietal Accreditation Commission (IAC) [6].

As of July 1, 2015, each of these bodies explicitly requires annual testing and specifies the tests to be performed. All four base their requirements on the aforementioned documents.

Therefore, while the complexity and capabilities of CT scanners has increased dramatically over the last two decades, the typical testing has remained essentially unchanged.

12.2   System Performance

12.2.1   Intrinsic Performance

As alluded to earlier, the rotational geometry of CT systems limits the degree to which the intrinsic performance can be evaluated. Images are only accessible as reconstructions; evaluation of the underlying raw data in the sinogram is of little use from a quality control standpoint. Therefore, intrinsic performance measurements are mostly limited to aspects of generator performance.

12.2.1.1   kV Measurement

Tube potential accuracy poses particular problems. Typical non-invasive kVp measurement devices depend on varying filtration to infer the kVp of the incident beam. A rotating beam will yield varying beam intensity and varying apparent filtration due to trigonometric effects. Both of these nullify the underlying assumptions required to determine kVp non-invasively.

All CT scanners provide a mode in which the tube is fixed while the table translates through the beam, known variously as a scout, scanogram, or other moniker. In this mode, the fixed tube position does allow for most non-invasive meters to function properly, though it might be necessary to fix the kV detector in place relative to the CT gantry, depending upon the specific performance specifications of the kVp measurement device.

Given the stability of modern CT scanner generators, it is extremely rare to detect any kV calibration issues, so this measurement is rarely made in clinical situations. None of the accreditation programs mandates performance of this test.

12.2.1.2   Tube Output

Measurement of dose and indexes of dose in CT has been the topic of much discussion and debate since the inception of the modality [7–11]. A full discussion of the topic can be found in the cited references and others. Suffice it to say here that none of the typically reported quantities reflects patient dose. The most commonly used is the Computed Tomography Dose Index (CTDI), which represents the average dose along the z direction at a given point in the x, y scan plane over the central scan of a series of scans, when the series consists of a large number of scans separated by the nominal beam width. Typically, a derivative known as $CTDI_{vol}$ is used. This value is determined from measurements made in phantom at the central axis and at least one peripheral location (typically 12:00), and accounts for the finite length of the pencil chamber and the pitch of the scan protocol. All CTDI measurements are made in axial mode.

Note that, since most measurements are made in phantom, they are not even strictly tube output by the typical definition. Air kerma can be measured, but care must be taken to understand exactly how the ionization chamber used is calibrated, for the displayed result might include a length dimension due to the pencil chamber geometry.

Typical indicators of tube output performance, mA linearity and timer accuracy, can be inferred from CTDI measurements. Readings must be taken at varying mA and time settings. The resultant CTDI should vary linearly with both mA and time. While most regulations specify performance standards for these metrics for radiographic units, they are not typically applied to CT scanners, though one would expect similar performance. As with kV accuracy, it is very rare that a performance issue will be detected in these metrics.

Of increasing importance is the accuracy of the displayed $CTDI_{vol}$ value for the selected protocol. The ACR CT QC Manual requires this to be accurate to within 30%, while TJC requires it to be accurate to within 20% [12]. On most scanners with original equipment manufacturer (OEM) x-ray tubes, these requirements are not a problem. However, some third-party tubes do not meet OEM standards and may lead to discrepancies between the measured and reported values in excess of these standards. In most cases, this can only be rectified by replacing the x-ray tube.

12.2.1.3 Collimation

Proper collimation of the fan beam is of great importance in CT, due both to the relatively high exposures used and the impact that the additional scatter radiation can have on image quality. Historically, measurements have highlighted slice thickness, a reconstructed quantity, rather than on the radiation beam width. AAPM Report 39 does include measurement of the radiation beam width.

The measurement is not trivial to make. When film processors were more readily available, measurement could be made by placing Ready-Pack (Kodak trademark) film at isocenter. The beam width is the full width at half-maximum of the center of the darkened band (Figure 12.1). This technique can be replicated using radiochromic film that darkens upon exposure. Electronic methods are also available from several manufacturers (Figure 12.2).

12.2.2 Qualimetry

Image quality metrics are central to the evaluation of CT scanner performance. Specialized phantoms designed specifically for CT facilitate these measurements. At the heart of all phantoms are tools for the following metrics: CT number accuracy and uniformity, image thickness, spatial resolution, low contrast performance, and artifact analysis.

12.2.2.1 CT Number Accuracy and Uniformity

CT numbers are reported using the Hounsfield Unit scale,

$$HU\left(CT\,\#\right) = CF \times \frac{\mu - \mu_{water}}{\mu_{water} - \mu_{air}}$$

where

CF = calibration factor
μ_x = the linear attenuation coefficient of the material in the voxel

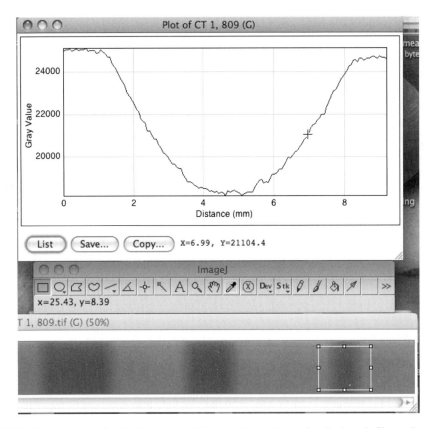

Figure 12.1 Measurement of radiation beam width using the method of radiochromic film and measuring full width half max of the resultant image.

μ_{water} = the linear attenuation coefficient of water
μ_{air} = the linear attenuation coefficient of air

By definition, the CT number of water is zero. Air is typically a calibration point with CT # = −1000, as the CF is typically defined to be 1000. Some scanners may use a calibration factor different from 1000. While this is technically permissible, it can lead to confusion when quantitative information is used for diagnosis and comparison, and may make compliance with testing protocols problematic.

Most CT phantoms provide several different materials for CT number verification. Regions of interest (ROIs) are placed on the image over the area to be measured. The manufacturer of the phantom, or another agency, must provide evaluation criteria for the specific phantom. It is important to note that CT number accuracy is highly dependent upon beam energy. Most limits assume that the scan was performed at 120 kV. While it is important to measure to assess and report to the facility the performance at other beam energies, the pass/fail decisions are typically made only at 120 kV.

CT number uniformity must be measured in a homogeneous image. To avoid beam hardening effects, the uniformity image material is typically water, water equivalent, or soft tissue equivalent. ROIs are placed at the center of the field and at four points around the periphery of the phantom. Comparison is made between the peripheral values and the center, with typical quality control limits of approximately ±5 IIU.

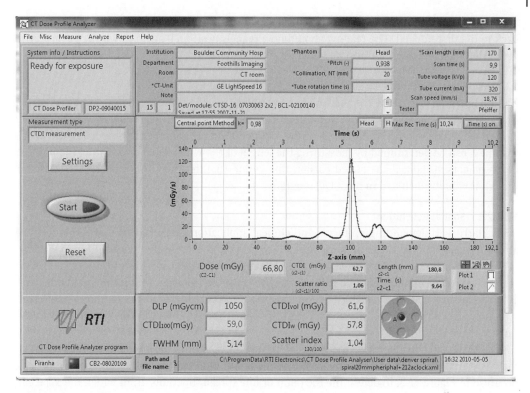

Figure 12.2 The display of one approach to electronic determination of beam width by electronic means. With this device, dosimetry information is also provided. *Source:* RTI Electronics.

12.2.2.2 Scan Localization and Scout Prescription Accuracy

It is essential that the scanner places the radiation only in the region defined by the radiologic technologist. Most often, the planning of the scan is done off of the scout (scanogram, plan scan, etc.) view. It is therefore necessary to verify that the scanned region agrees with the prescribed region. While the alignment light is generally only used for gross positioning of the patient, it is also used to ensure that the patient is properly centered in the scanner. More importantly, on systems used for biopsies, it may be used for precise needle placement. For these reasons, it is important to verify that the alignment light is accurate to ±2 mm.

To accomplish these verifications, a phantom with radiopaque fiducial markers must be scanned. The series should be planned off of the scout image, taking care to center the first slice on the fiducial marker. At the same time, verify that the laser alignment light is centered on the fiducial marker. Scan the series as prescribed.

On the resultant images, find the image containing the fiducial marker. This should be the "0" position image, ±2 mm. Assuming that the alignment light also correctly indicated the position of the fiducial marker at the "0" position, this also is the offset of the alignment light, which also should be correct to within ±2 mm.

12.2.2.3 Table Travel Accuracy

For this evaluation, a phantom with two fiducial markers separated by a known distance must be available. Position the phantom so that the alignment light marks the first fiducial; set this is position 0. Translate the table to the second fiducial and note the reading. This value should be correct to within ±2 mm of the known value. Translate the table the extent of its calibrated distance and back to the first fiducial. The reading should now read as position 0 again to within ±2 mm. Also verify that the table has not translated laterally during this test.

12.2.2.4 Image Thickness

The thickness of the reconstructed image has implications both on the noise properties of the image and the z-dimension spatial resolution. Phantoms incorporate beads, bars, or thin wires set at a known angle relative to the z-axis of the scanner. Using trigonometric properties, the image thickness can be determined by measuring the length of the wire visible or counting the number beads or bars visualized. As stated earlier, this is not a failure mode on modern CT scanners, though it remains included in most QC programs.

12.2.2.5 Spatial Resolution

Particularly with demanding protocols and clinical applications, exquisite spatial resolution, the ability to visualize small structures, is extremely important. Most frequently, resolution in the axial (x-y plane) is determined. Measurements are made most often with bar patterns (Figure 12.3), with the observer determining the highest frequency that can be resolved. Minimum standards, typically 6–7 lp cm^{-1}, have been established, but the performance is highly dependent upon the reconstruction algorithm selected. Focal spot size has some impact, but it is small compared to the impact of the algorithm.

It is also possible to determine the modulation transfer function (MTF) of the system. The MTF may be estimated using bar patterns [13] or with small, high contrast beads in a uniform field, observed in Figure 12.3, to determine the point or line spread functions, from which the MTF can be determined. The advantage of the bead method is that the MTF in any plane can be determined, not just the axial plane.

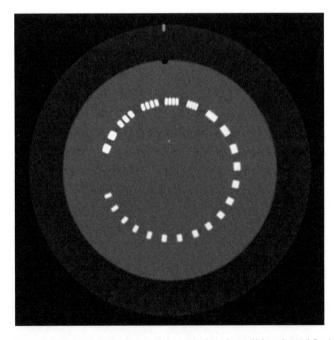

Figure 12.3 Bar pattern used for determining spatial resolution. A small bead used for MTF determination is also visible just superior of isocenter.

Experience has shown that this is not a common failure mode for CT scanners, but measurement is important for understanding the impact of the various reconstruction algorithms on images.

12.2.2.6 Low Contrast Performance

Low contrast visibility is determined by the noise in the image. For a target to be visible, the contrast (signal difference from the background) must exceed the noise by a significant amount. The signal different to noise ratio (SDNR) required for visualization typically follows the Rose model [14, 15]. It is important to note, however, that a simple SDNR measurement will not provide results that can be compared to Rose model performance. This would require normalization to the number of pixels included in the ROI. While the quantum mottle in an image is determined by the dose used, which is also a factor of image thickness, the visibility of the noise is again highly subject to the specific reconstruction algorithm used. Low contrast performance is therefore not truly a system performance measurement, but a protocol test. It allows the determination of whether the dose and reconstruction algorithm are appropriate for the diagnostic challenge.

Two methods are typically employed for low contrast performance evaluation. Most often, targets of known contrast and decreasing size are placed in the x–y plane. This volume is imaged using the protocol in question and the visibility of targets versus target size and contrast is determined (Figure 12.4). It is also possible to measure the signal and noise in a target and in the immediate background, allowing one to calculate the SDNR (Figure 12.5).

The challenge is how these measures compare to clinical needs, as phantoms rarely reflect patient attenuation, making the visual test questionable, and SDNR does not have a good clinical correlate for determining acceptance criteria.

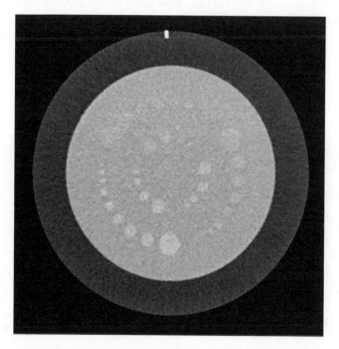

Figure 12.4 Low contrast test objects. Note the presence of targets of both decreasing size and decreasing contrast, allowing determination of a contrast-detail curve if desired.

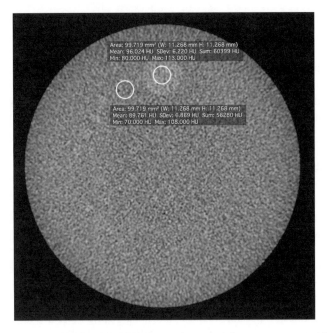

Figure 12.5 Determination of SDNR using ROI measurements in a low contrast test object image.

12.2.2.7 Artifact Analysis

Artifact analysis is arguably the most important quality control measurement that a medical physicist makes on a CT scanner. Artifacts are the most likely deficiency to be observed and have the greatest likelihood for interfering with the appropriate interpretation of the CT image.

Analysis is performed simply by searching a uniform image for non-uniformities. Except for rare cases, artifacts will most likely be either rings or streaks [16]. All observed artifacts should be noted. Those that are likely to interfere with interpretation must be addressed immediately (Figure 12.6).

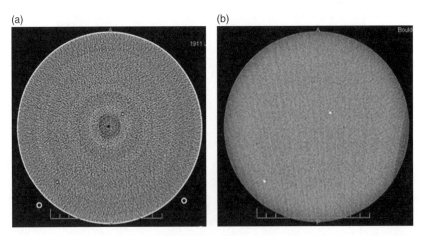

Figure 12.6 Typical artifacts found in CT imaging. (a) demonstrates ring artifacts typically caused by detector miscalibration. (b) demonstrates streak artifacts, often caused by foreign material in the beam path.

12.2.2.8   Display Monitor Evaluation

While the display monitors on CT acquisition stations are not used for primary diagnosis, they must provide adequate image quality for technologists to properly position the scans and evaluate the resultant images. Further, technologists are often called upon to make decisions regarding further scans or contacting the radiologist based on the anatomy and pathology they see. Therefore, some level of quality control for acquisition station monitors is essential.

Regular QC must involve evaluation of a TG18-QC or similar test image. It must be verified that the 0%/5% and 95%/100% patches are visible and that the gray scale is adequately displayed. The image must be free of geometric and brightness non-uniformities. Spatial resolution capabilities must be verified through the bar patterns provided.

Along with these visual evaluations, the medical physicist must make photometric measurements to verify that the minimum and maximum brightness meet standards and that brightness uniformity is acceptable. LCD monitors are prone to brightness fade over time. It may therefore be necessary for the medical physicist to make adjustments to the monitor brightness and contrast settings to maintain adequate performance.

12.2.3   Radiometry

As stated earlier, dosimetry in CT has always been problematic. Yet determination of dose in CT is extremely important due to the relatively large exposures used.

The earliest definition of dose in CT was the multiple slice average dose (MSAD), which accounted for the non-rectangular radiation dose profile and scatter contributing to the dose in a given slice [17]. However, early scanners were too slow for effective measurement of MSAD. It was determined that MSAD could be estimated from a single scan [5], the estimate being called the computed tomography dose index (CTDI). Note that this is termed an index, not dose. Misuse of the CTDI over the years has led to much confusion. The CTDI has developed into its current common form of $CTDI_{vol}$.

Modern scanners can easily support MSAD measurement, but CTDI is well entrenched in testing protocols and reporting. It has been demonstrated that modern wide beam scanners break the assumptions of CTDI, and the actual dose index is significantly under-reported [7, 9]. Efforts have been made to establish a protocol for such scanners [18]. Task Group 111 of the American Association of Physicists in Medicine, "The Future of CT Dosimetry," redefined CT dosimetry for modern scanners, but a method for practical implementation of this new formalism has not been developed.

Of practical importance in all methodologies at this time is that they are based on standardized dosimetry phantoms: acrylic cylinders, typically 15 cm in length, with diameter of either 16 or 32 cm. Few humans are accurately represented by the attenuation of either one of these phantoms. To help correct for this deficiency, the size-specific dose estimate (SSDE) was developed [19]. While useful for better understanding and monitoring patient dose, no clear guidelines are available for what appropriate SSDE values are [20].

Another problem with $CTDI_{vol}$ is that it does not account for the length of a scan. Clearly, a scan that covers twice the length of a patient, other factors held constant, will deposit twice the radiation energy into the patient. However, $CTDI_{vol}$ have the same value regardless of the length scanned. This is useful for comparing scans to each other, but not for knowing what patient dose might be. Therefore, the dose-length product (DLP) was developed. The DLP simply multiplies the $CTDI_{vol}$ for a scan by the length of the scan. This is a better estimate of patient exposure, but it does not use the SSDE correction and is of limited utility for patient dose calculation.

An important dose-saving feature of modern scanners is the ability to automatically modulate the tube current based on the actual patient attenuation. This can be modulated in the x–y plane, the z-axis, or both. The benefit to patients is clear, but it is not clear how to report the dose index from such a scan, as each rotation could theoretically use a completely different dose from the adjacent rotations. It might seem clear that an average mA should be reported, but this loses information about what dose a particular organ within the scan may have received.

In the end, it is organ dose that is most important for any proper determination of potential risk to a patient [21–23]. Practical implementation of patient-specific organ dose calculation is still in the future. Some commercially available software packages have made great efforts to make a best estimate of patient organ doses using the available data, and such programs may provide an avenue for further development.

Even once we have patient organ doses, relating the dose to a risk factor remains problematic [24]. When patients ask what their dose was, they generally are really interested in knowing what their risk is. At best, we can only provide broad, uncertainty-limited estimates of population risk.

12.3 Testing Paradigm and Clinical Implementation

Each of the tests discussed has application in multiple environments. These various situations are discussed below.

12.3.1 Acceptance Testing and Commissioning

A newly-installed scanner must necessarily undergo more comprehensive testing than might be required under normal annual testing circumstances. All of the above tests should be performed. It is important to fully characterize the system and ensure that it is performing according to manufacturer specifications.

To this end, all performance tests contained in the operator or quality control manual should be performed, using phantoms and techniques as specified in the manual. The resulting values must be compared to the values stated in the testing document. Only after it is confirmed that the scanner meets all manufacturer or bid specifications should other tests be performed.

It is important at acceptance testing to ensure that reconstruction algorithms and other features, such as mA modulation or automated kV selection, are working as expected. This is also the time to ensure that all options agreed upon in the purchase document are installed and functioning.

Some features on a new scanner may be new to the facility. It is therefore recommended that they be tested such that their use can be understood and taught to the facility, supporting and augmenting the information provided by the applications training provided by the manufacturer.

Another evaluation that is not part of regular quality control testing, but is vital at acceptance testing, is to ensure that the radiation shielding for the room has been installed properly and is providing the necessary radiation protection. The best situation would allow for visual inspection of the shielding during construction. This allows for positive verification that the lead installed meets the design specifications and that it is installed without voids or gaps. This is often not the case, so special care must be used during the subsequent radiation protection survey.

To perform the survey, a patient-representative scatter phantom must be placed in the beam and scans made using techniques sufficient to exceed the minimum detection capabilities of the survey meter. All barriers must be evaluated. Pay particular attention to areas where penetrations were made, such as junction boxes. If it is possible to bring a radioactive source into the room, this can make it easier to detect voids and gaps, as the survey meter can be used in rate mode and a complete scan of the room can be completed.

Ideally, acceptance testing is performed prior to patient use, but should in any case be performed as early as possible after installation.

12.3.2 Quality Control

CT scanners are amazingly reliable considering the complexity of the system. Nonetheless, a regular quality control program is essential to ensure that the system is functioning properly and the images are free from artifacts. This is the responsibility of the qualified radiologic technologist. The specific requirements for regular quality control vary by accreditation program and municipality.

12.3.2.1 American College of Radiology

The ACR requires daily quality control measurements of the CT scanner performed by the radiologic technologist. These measurements must consist of CT number accuracy, CT number standard deviation consistency, and artifact analysis. Additionally, the performance of the acquisition display monitor must be checked on a monthly basis.

The requirements for medical physics testing required by the ACR are more extensive. On an annual basis, the following evaluations must be performed.

- Review of Clinical Protocols
- Scout Prescription and Alignment Light Accuracy
- Image Thickness – Axial Mode
- Table Travel Accuracy
- Radiation Beam Width
- Low-Contrast Performance
- Spatial Resolution
- CT Number Accuracy
- Artifact Evaluation
- CT Number Uniformity
- Dosimetry
- Gray Level Performance of CT Acquisition Display Monitors

The review of clinical protocols is not intended to be a comprehensive evaluation of all protocols. Instead, a subset of commonly used or dose-intensive protocols should be reviewed. Generally, these should include adult head, adult abdomen, pediatric head and abdomen (if pediatric studies are performed), high resolution chest, and brain perfusion (if performed). A total of six protocols should be reviewed, so if some of the above protocols are not performed, then common protocols for that scanner should be reviewed.

Each protocol should be inspected to verify that automatic dose reduction is being used properly. The reconstruction algorithms should be appropriate for the typical clinical use of the protocol. Image thickness should also be appropriate to the clinical task. Verify that the resultant dose is as low as diagnostically appropriate, making comparisons to diagnostic reference levels when available [25–28]. If doses are not significantly less than the DRLs, then the protocols should be reviewed with the radiologist and technologist to determine what modifications are possible. On subsequent visits, it is important to verify that these protocols have not been changed since the last evaluation. If they have, a log tracking those changes with their justification should be available.

Since low contrast performance is more of a protocol test than a scanner test, it should be performed for the four main clinical protocols: adult head and abdomen and pediatric head and abdomen. Absolute performance criteria are difficult to define for this evaluation. Verify first that the values have not changed significantly from previous measurements. Also compare the values to the standards in the ACR CTAP. If the measured values do not meet the ACR CTAP standards, then verify that the clinical image quality is adequate for the clinical task by consulting with the radiologist.

CT number accuracy should meet manufacturer specifications or the standards given in the ACR CT QC Manual if the ACR Accreditation Phantom are used:

Material	CT Number Range
Water	−7 – +7 HU
Air	−970 – −1005 HU
Teflon (bone)	850 – +970 HU
Polyethylene	−97 – −84 HU
Acrylic	+110 – +135 HU

Note that these limits are not appropriate for some scanner models due to specifics of image reconstruction, beam hardening corrections, and the CT # correction factor implemented by the manufacturer. In such a case, verify that the scanner meets manufacturer specifications and then establish action limits appropriate to the scanner.

The dosimetry evaluation has several aspects to it in the ACR program. First, dose indexes should be determined for all four standard protocols and compared to the reference levels provided. Specifically, they should not exceed the reference levels values in the table below and must not exceed the pass/fail criteria.

Examination	Reference Levels	Pass/Fail Criteria
Adult Head	75 mGy	80 mGy
Adult Abdomen	25 mGy	30 mGy
Pediatric Head	35 mGy	40 mGy
Pediatric Abdomen	15 mGy	20 mGy

Further, it is important to verify that the displayed dose values are acceptably accurate, as these are being used with increased regularity, at times by regulatory mandate, for reporting along with the interpretation of the images. The reported values should be within 30% of the measured values.

12.3.2.2 RadSite

The RadSite accreditation program does not have any specific requirements for a technologist quality control program. The annual medical physics testing must include the following elements.

- CT number accuracy
- Slice thickness verification

- CT number uniformity
- CT noise measurement
- High contrast spatial resolution
- Low contrast detectability
- Review of the site's CT quality assurance program.
- Patient radiation dose for clinically utilized scans

The requirements for these tests are largely the same as for the ACR CTAP, with a few exceptions. CT number accuracy has standards specified for a number of different phantoms, and no modification of these limits is allowed. Low contrast performance is based on a visual analysis. Again, specific requirements are specified using the site adult and pediatric head and abdomen protocols.

12.3.2.3 The Joint Commission

Similar to the RadSite accreditation program, no technologist QC tests have been defined. While TJC has established requirements for the performance of annual medical physics testing, no specifics or action limits have been provided. The required tests are listed below.

- Image uniformity
- Slice thickness accuracy
- Slice position accuracy (when prescribed from a scout image)
- Alignment light accuracy
- Table travel accuracy
- Radiation beam width
- High-contrast resolution
- Low-contrast resolution
- Geometric or distance accuracy
- CT number accuracy and uniformity
- Artifact evaluation

The physicist should establish action limits appropriate to the scanner and in accord with the standards of other nationally or internationally recognized programs.

12.3.3 Manufacturer QC

Some manufactures have provided automated quality control functions into their scanners. These applications can provide an advantage when performing regular quality control procedures. They often allow automated analysis and comparison to manufacturer specifications. This can save time for the operator and helps to avoid confusion when a deficiency is detected. It must be noted that artifact analysis is always a visual analysis that must be performed manually by the technologist.

Additionally, some manufacturers recommend periodic tuning or calibration to help ensure optimal performance of their scanners. Regardless of the requirements of a particular accreditation program, these calibration functions should be performed.

12.3.4 Optimization of Use

CT scanners are increasingly complicated devices with great capabilities. With this increased capability comes also the possibility of increased risk to the patient or inferior image quality if not used properly.

Therefore, facilities should establish a program of reviewing every protocol to ensure that it is optimized, properly utilizing the capabilities of the scanner to provide clinically necessary image quality at the lowest diagnostically appropriate dose.

To achieve this, the establishment of a protocol review committee is recommended. This committee should include, at a minimum, a radiologist, a technologist, and the medical physicist. It should programmatically consider each protocol, considering aspects of image quality, dose, and clinical implementation. Each protocol should be optimized and then locked in. The protocol editing function should be password protected. Thereafter, no modifications should be made to the protocols without approval by the committee and records should be kept of each change and the reasons for that change.

12.3.5   Accreditation and Compliance-Related Matters

The requirements for each accreditation program have been briefly reviewed above. Each program has the goal of ensuring adequate image quality at an appropriate radiation dose. However, accreditation bodies are not the only authorities involved in this effort. State regulations are increasingly incorporating quality control requirements.

Some of these are very specific in regulation or guidance, similar to the accreditation programs.[1] Others are more general and leave the QC program up the facility, as stated above. Regardless of any accreditation requirements a facility has, regulatory requirements must be fulfilled.

12.3.6   Training

As stated earlier, modern CT scanners are extremely complex with many advanced features. Because of this, substantial training on the scanner and its capabilities is necessary.

Technologists regularly are provided with applications training at the purchase of a new scanner. However, as technologists leave and new ones come in, that initial training may be lost or diluted. Facilities must make efforts to ensure that all technologists are appropriately trained in the specifics of each scanner at the facility. Included in this training must be the quality control procedures, including those required by the manufacturer, required by regulation, and by the applicable accreditation program. Often it is the medical physicist who is best equipped to provide the quality control training.

The largest challenge often is for the medical physicist to become properly familiar with the scanner at the facility. In order to be able to provide guidance regarding protocol optimization, they must know what the capabilities of the scanner are. However, most often medical physicists are not included in applications training. It is therefore incumbent upon the medical physicist to make the effort required to understand the system. Operator and technical manual may be the best source of information. It might be necessary to contact a physicist or engineer with the manufacturer to learn the details. Professional societies and colleagues can also be valuable resources.

12.4   CT 1.5 – the Shifting Landscape

As is true with all diagnostic modalities, a shift in the concept of medical physics support for computed tomography must shift from being as equipment focused as it has historically been to more facility focused. This is particularly true in the realm of protocol evaluation and

---

1 NJ, NY regulations.

development. The complexity and capability of modern scanners require multiple areas of expertise to properly implement: radiologist, technologist and medical physicist.

More and more, for various reasons, patients are asking more questions about the dose of the scans they are getting and what the risks might be. The medical physicist is best equipped to provide the information needed to answer such questions. In many cases, the physicist might be the best person to speak to the patient.

This mandates a shift in the typical relationship that many medical physicists currently have with facilities.

Recognizing that most CT scanners are supported by non-employee consultant medical physicists, the typical model is for the physicist to arrive at a facility and test the scanner in as little time as possible so as to have minimal impact on patient flow. Often this is after normal business hours. In such a situation, it is very possible that the physicist may see no one but the technologist and perhaps the administrator. Radiologists are busy with their interpretation and are loath to sacrifice valuable, productive time to what might be viewed as unproductive conversation. Physicists, also being busy, might also be loath to spend time that could otherwise be used testing equipment.

Many technologists have forgotten much of their physics and do not see speaking with the medical physicist as beneficial time. Many medical physicists are not facile at speaking in a manner understood by technologists. This limits the ability to establish a relationship required for such a truly consultative role in the facility.

Further, it is reasonable for the physicist to expect to be compensated for the additional time required. Facility managers may not see the value in the additional consultative support.

Along with these shifts, the equipment also needs to be tested in ways not mandated by accreditation programs or regulations. Automatic mA modulation features play a role for CT that automatic exposure control systems play for radiographic equipment. Just as adequate testing of an x-ray room includes automatic exposure control (AEC) performance evaluation, so should complete testing of a CT scanner include dose modulation function evaluation.

Testing of automatic dose modulation functions is accomplished by placing phantoms of varying diameter on the cradle. These need to be butted up against each other to minimize any air gap at the transition. The specific phantoms used are not as important as the consistency in which they are positioned, as one wishes to verify that the modulation remains acceptably consistent over time.

Perform a scout or planning scan of the phantom and plan a series covering the extent of the phantom. Some systems will allow you to view and document the planned tube current prior to the scan; for other systems, this information may only be available after the scan has been completed. In either case, record the mA specified for each segment of the phantom (Figure 12.7). At this time no standards are available for establishing action limits; it is, however, not unreasonable to expect no more than 20% variation scan-to-scan. If this level of performance is not met, the physicist should consult with the manufacturer's service engineer or applications specialist.

Some systems also provide automated kV selection based on patient size. As with automated dose modulation features, this function should also be annually evaluated to ensure consistent performance. While a simple phantom of uniform diameter may be used for this testing, it is recommended to use a more complicated phantom, such as that described above for the mA modulation evaluation, to stress the system in a more clinically representative manner. One would expect the same kV to be selected for a given configuration every time. Again, if this is not the case, the physicist should consult with the manufacturer's service engineer or applications specialist.

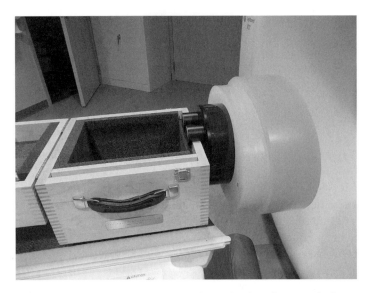

Figure 12.7 A phantom configuration that can be used for evaluation of automatic dose modulation. The changes in effective diameter should drive the mA in a consistent manner from measurement to measurement. If the scanner has automatic kV selection, the resultant kV should also remain constant.

It should also be noted that automatic exposure controls in CT are not simply on or off. Manufacturers implement these functions in different ways, and much adjustment by facilities is often available, and may be necessary. For example, on General Electric scanners, the mA is controlled by a Noise Index, which is approximately equal to the standard deviation in the central region of the image when a patient-equivalent uniform phantom is scanned and reconstructed using the standard reconstruction algorithm [29]. Several researchers have reported that it is necessary to modify the Noise Index based on patient size, using a lower index for smaller or pediatric patients and a higher index for larger patients. If this is not done, smaller patient images may be unacceptably noisy and large patients may receive more dose than is necessary.

Another caveat with the use of automated dose modulation is that the patient must be very well centered in the gantry. While the magnitude of the effect varies scanner model to scanner model, all exhibit it to some degree. Medical physicists must work with facilities to help them understand the importance of proper patient positioning in CT.

In 2010, the National Electrical Manufacturers Association published standard XR 25, Computed Tomography Dose Check [30]. This standard introduced a system by which CT scanners will prospectively compare the dose from a single series and from multiple scans on the same patient to limits set in the scanner. If any of the limits will be exceeded, a warning message is displayed that must be acknowledged by the facility. While every manufacturer incorporates Dose Check into its systems, not every facility is using this feature, as many are not comfortable with establishing values to be entered as limits. The medical physicist can play a vital role in helping facilities to use Dose Check properly.

Other recent developments include multiple x-ray tubes and detector arrays in the gantry and more advanced iterative reconstruction models. Such developments necessitate deeper involvement by the medical physicist in clinical operations. Often, such options come with a spectrum of implementation options. The medical physicist must characterize the system to be able to help guide the facility, along with the applications specialist, in applying the features to clinical scans. If this is not done carefully, it is very easy to mis-apply the options, resulting in inferior image quality or excessive dose due to repeated studies.

12.5 Conclusion

Most testing currently performed on CT scanners is driven by accreditation programs and some regulatory bodies. These mandates are often based on testing protocols developed for scanners that were much simpler than modern scanners, with failure modes very different from what is commonly observed now. As is true throughout diagnostic imaging, advances in scanner performance and capability are driving changes in medical physics support.

Each accreditation program and jurisdiction has its own requirements, and the medical physicist must be knowledgeable regarding those applicable to a given scanner. Further, modern developments are pressing medical physicist to consider additional tests and more involvement with facilities than may have been necessary in the past. This situation is not without its challenges, as modern scanners may demand more time for appropriate medical physics support, and there will be a cost associated with support.

References

1 Lin, P., Beck, T., Borras, C. et al. (1993). AAPM Report No. 39 – Specification and acceptance testing of computed tomography scanners:101.

2 Editors Goldman, L.W. and Fowlkes, J.B. (1995). *Medical CT and Ultrasound: Current Technology and Applications*. Advanced Medical Publishing.

3 American College of Radiology (2011). CT Accreditation Program Requirements. Revised 1/26/2011.

4 American College of Radiology (2015). CT Accreditation Program Requirements.

5 Cody, D., Pfeiffer, D. et al. (2012). *Computed Tomography Quality Control Manual*. American College of Radiology.

6 https://www.cms.gov/Medicare/Provider-Enrollment-and-Certification/ SurveyCertificationGenInfo/Accreditation-of-Advanced-Diagnostic-Imaging-Suppliers.html (accessed 29 November 2019).

7 Shope, T., Gagne, R., and Johnson, G. (1981). A method for describing the doses delivered by transmission x-ray computed tomography. *Medical Physics* 8: 488–495.

8 Leitz, W., Axelson, B., and Szendro, G. (1995). Computed tomography dose assessment – a practical approach. *Radiation Protection Dosimetry* 57: 377–380.

9 McCollough, C.H., Brenner, D.J., and Orton, C.G. (2006). It is time to retire the computed tomography dose index (CTDI) for CT quality assurance and dose optimization. *Medical Physics* 33 (5): 1189–1191.

10 Dixon, R.L. and Boone, J.M. (2013). Dose equations for tube current modulation in CT scanning and the interpretation of the associated CTDIvol. *Medical Physics* 40 (11): 1119–1120.

11 Boone, J.M. (2007). The trouble with CTD100. *Medical Physics* 34 (4): 1364–1371.

12 TJC standards effective 7/1/2015

13 Droege, R.T. and Morin, R.L. (1982). A practical method to measure the MTF of CT scanners. *Medical Physics* 9 (5): 758–760.

14 Verdun, F.R., Lepori, D., Monnin, P. et al. (2004). Management of patient dose and image noise in routine pediatric CT abdominal examinations. *European Radiology* 14 (5): 835–841.

15 Burgess, A.E. (1999). The rose model, revisited. *Journal of the Optical Society of America* 16: 633–646.

16 Cody, D.D., Stevens, D.M., and Ginsberg, L.E. (2005). Multi-detector row CT artifacts that mimic disease. *Radiology* 236 (3): 756–761.

17 Rothenberg, L.N. and Pentlow, K.S. (1992). Radiation dose in CT. *Radiographics: A Review Publication of the Radiological Society of North America, Inc.* 12 (6): 1225–1243.

18 Geleijns, J., Salvadó Artells, M., de Bruin, P.W. et al. (2009). Computed tomography dose assessment for a 160 mm wide, 320 detector row, cone beam CT scanner. *Physics in Medicine and Biology* 54 (10): 3141–3159.

19 Christner, J.A., Braun, N.N., Jacobsen, M.C. et al. (2012). Size-specific dose estimates for adult patients at CT of the torso. *Radiology* 265 (3): 841–847.

20 Brink, J.A. and Morin, R.L. (2012). Size-specific dose estimation for CT: how should it be used and what does it mean? *Radiology* 265 (3): 666–668.

21 Mcdermott, A., White, R.A., Mc-Nitt-Gray, M. et al. (2009). Pediatric organ dose measurements in axial and helical multislice CT. *Medical Physics* 36 (5): 1494–1499.

22 Fearon, T., Xie, H., Cheng, J.Y. et al. (2011). Patient-specific CT dosimetry calculation: a feasibility study. *Journal of Applied Clinical Medical Physics / American College of Medical Physics* 12 (4): 3589.

23 Kamei, O., Ojima, M., Yoshitake, T. et al. (2015). Calculating patient-specific organ doses from adult body CT scans by Monte Carlo analysis using male-individual voxel phantoms. *Health Physics* 108 (1): 44–52.

24 Hendee, W.R. and O'Connor, M.K. (2012). Radiation risks of medical imaging: separating fact from fantasy. *Radiology* 264 (2): 312–321. https://doi.org/10.1148/radiol.12112678.

25 Verdun, F.R., Gutierrez, D., Vader, J.P. et al. (2008). CT radiation dose in children: a survey to establish age-based diagnostic reference levels in Switzerland. *European Radiology* 18 (9): 1980–1986.

26 ICRU (2001). ICRU Diagnostic Reference Levels (March 4): 1–12.

27 McCollough, C., Branham, T., Herlihy, V. et al. (2011). Diagnostic reference levels from the ACR CT accreditation program. *Journal of the American College of Radiology: JACR* 8 (11): 795–803.

28 Aldrich, J.E., Bilawich, A.-M.M., and Mayo, J.R. (2006). Radiation doses to patients receiving computed tomography examinations in British Columbia. *Canadian Association of Radiologists Journal = Journal l'Association Canadienne Des Radiologistes* 57 (2): 79–85.

29 General Electric. AutomA-SmartmA Theory. http://www3.gehealthcare.cl/sitecore%20modules/web/~/media/documents/us-global/education/education/product-education-clinical/tip-app-library/gehealthcare-education-tip-app-library_ct-automa-smartma-theory.pdf (accessed 18 February 2015).

30 NEMA (2010). Standards Publication XR 25–2010 Edition 1, Computed Tomography Dose Check. National Electrical Manufacturers Association, Arlington, VA, October 2010.

13

Clinical CT Physics: Emerging Practice

Ehsan Samei[1] and Joshua Wilson[2]

[1] Departments of Radiology, Medical Physics, Physics, Biomedical Engineering, and Electrical and Computer Engineering, Duke University Medical Center, Durham, NC, USA
[2] Clinical Imaging Physics Group, Duke University, Durham, NC, USA

13.1 Philosophy and Significance

The role of imaging physics in medical imaging is well established. The foundation of the technology, its initial realization, and its continuous development have all been enabled by the broad field of imaging physics, as exercised by imaging physicists within multiple professional disciplines (engineering, mathematics, computer science, etc.). This role has continued and will continue for the foreseeable future, begetting innovation, superior design features, and superior intrinsic performance.

The role of physicists in clinical practice likewise has been well established, where the performance of computed tomography (CT) devices is ascertained by clinical physicists. In this process, the goal is to ensure that the CT systems are in compliance with, and their features and characteristics meet, vendor specifications, regulations, professional guidelines, or accreditation standards. This provides assurance about the quality and consistency of the intrinsic quality of CT systems and their technical compliance with certain minimum technical criteria. The procedures toward that goal are well detailed in Chapter 12.

While compliance and assurance of technical performance are essential, one can argue that they are not enough. The purpose of diagnostic techniques in general, and medical imaging in particular, is to supply meaningful information for the management of the patient. That is the only purpose for which medical images are acquired. As such, technical performance and compliance are relevant to the extent that they relate to medical information. Technical specification assurance alone fails to fully assure clinical performance. It further does not provide much provision about optimized use of the system, nor consistency of the quality of the images that it produces. Added to those limitations, technical compliance as regulatory expectations, by their existential necessity, are out of phase with the latest technological offerings, and thus not most relevant to latest technologies.

In the era of value-based care, a technological advancement or specification should be ascertained and optimized toward the value that it provides in the explicit context of patient-care. In the case of CT, the value is the safe rendition of high resolution details of patient and disease anatomy and function. This requires the deployment of clinical metrics: physics-based metrics and metrology that can be related to clinical quality. This clinically-informed characterization, while reflective of the attributes of the technology being used, is a hallmark of the Medical Physics 3.0 practice. Further, these clinical surrogates of quality can and should be optimized for the clinical task at hand and monitored over time. Finally, to ensure that the desired targeted performance is achieved, metrics of quality and safety based on patient data should be retrospectively collected and analyzed to ascertain and inform the *actual* (as opposed to presumed) outcome of the image acquisition process. Within the enterprise of clinical practice, medical physics can provide the needed expertise to enable these aims, leading to improved patient care.

13.2 Metrics and Analytics

13.2.1 Intrinsic Performance

Intrinsic characteristics of CT systems are foundational to their performance. For example, the accuracy of kV calibration of a system has implications on the resulting imaging and safety performance of the system. A CT system should thus be fully inspected and qualified in term of its intrinsic attributes. Most of these attributes and their testing methods are detailed in Chapter 12. Most of the quantities listed there are those that are related to conventional CT systems, those that are *easier* to ascertain, and those that are claimed and reported by the manufacturers, enforced by manufacturing and regulatory standards. However, there are many additional intrinsic attributes that are rarely evaluated but have strong implications on the quality of the image outcome. For example, the x-ray spectra (measured through half-value layer) can have a marked effect on dose, the size of the focal spot impacts image resolution in a way that can be kV and mA dependent, and system alignment affects its geometrical accuracy. Such attributes are not commonly evaluated during the acceptance testing or commissioning of CT systems, but should and may be considered by a seasoned medical physicist depending on the anticipated use of the technology.

13.2.2 Qualimetry

As in any imaging modality, the purpose of CT imaging is to capture images. Image quality thus is an existential requirement of CT imaging and a cornerstone of its qualification. Conventionally, physics techniques have focused primarily on intrinsic attributes of the system. Image quality is also characterized, but at its most basic level that may not be as readily extrapolatable to clinical quality. However, such evaluations can be "upgraded" toward higher degrees of clinical relevance and applicability.

The key attributes of image quality in any imaging system are the following, each of which is conventionally evaluated in a contrived manner but can support a more relevant metrology:

1) Detail rendition reflects how well an imaging system can produce the spatial features of interest. Most closely reflected in terms of spatial resolution, line pair patterns are a conventional method to measure CT resolution via visual evaluation. This method, however, only reflects the limiting resolution in terms of a subjective characterization. Resolution can be more completely characterized in terms of the modulation transfer function (MTF), which reflects the ability of a system to render any spatial frequency of a feature of interest (Figure 13.1). The American Association of Physicists in Medicine (AAPM) Task Group 233 offers specific methods to ascertain the MTF or its counterpart, the task transfer function (TTF) which reflects the contrast and noise dependency of the MTF

[1]. The detail rendition also applies to temporal details, which may be characterized in terms of a temporal MTF, but this has not been formalized or clinically implemented.

2) Detail contamination reflects unwanted signal in the image that interferes with the rendition of detail. This takes form in either stochastic contamination (aka noise) or structured ones (aka artifacts). Noise is conventionally characterized in terms of standard deviation of fluctuations within an otherwise uniform background. This is an easily measured metric and a good quantification of noise magnitude. However, noise affects the utility of an image for its intended task via both its magnitude and its texture, as depicted in Figure 13.1. The noise power spectrum (NPS) is an analogue of the MTF in terms of noise, reflecting not only the magnitude (the area of the NPS = noise variance) but also the texture of the noise (the power of the fluctuations at a given spatial frequency). The AAPM Task Group 233 also offers specific methods to ascertain the NPS [1].

The detail contamination through non-stochastic processes are generally recognized as artifacts. In CT, such artifacts include streaks (due to the non-linear response of the CT detector elements as a function of exposure), beam hardening artifact (due to preferential absorption of lower energy photons of the spectrum as a function of cross sectional thickness), and scattering artifact (due to the contribution of varying levels of scattered radiation in the acquisition process). There are methods to qualify these artifacts in the context of simple phantoms (Figure 13.2), and further consider their relative importance depending on the location of the abnormality of interest in the image.

3) Material rendition reflects the accuracy of CT system to render the attenuation characteristics of the interest with accuracy. The methodology to quantify this performance attribute of CT is primarily based on measuring the Hounsfield Unit value of phantom inserts with known material properties and ascertaining the accuracy of the values. This method is well established and noted in many guidelines documents including AAPM TG233 and the American College of Radiology (ACR). Of importance in these quantifications is the fact that the ground truth of the methodology is defined only relatively. As CT uses a poly-energetic spectrum subject to changing kV and filtration, there is no *single* attenuation value to be ascribed to a material. CT systems use varying kV-dependent calibration methods to conform the CT numbers (particularly those of water and air) to certain predefined values independent of the imaging condition. The calibration, however,

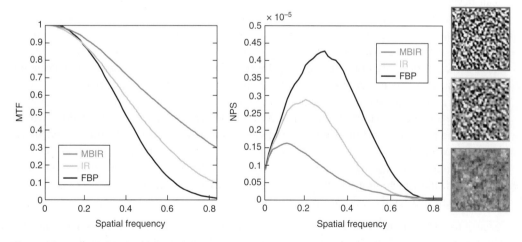

Figure 13.1 The MTF and NPS of a CT system using filtered-back projection (FBP) reconstruction, iterative reconstruction (IR), and model-based IR (MBIR).

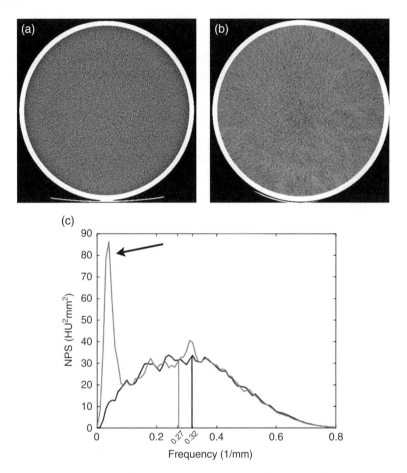

Figure 13.2 Analysis of the NPS in uniform phantom images revealing non-uniformities due to an oil leak and air bubble in the x-ray tube of a CT system.

can never be perfect given its empirical basis, necessitating characterization of system performance at multiple acquisition conditions according to the intended clinical use of the system.

4) The attributes noted above capture the foundational components of information content that a CT image is expected to deliver. In the clinical use of the image, what is most important is the task-based performance of the images, e.g. the detection or characterization of an abnormality of interest. This is commonly reflected in the concept of task-based performance. CT performance metrology should ideally include task-based characterization, the most common of which are lesion detectability and estimability of lesion volumes. The characterization involves specialized phantoms and integration of individual information transfer features listed above. The AAPM TG233 details specific methodology for characterizing the detectability and estimability of volume [1]. Task-based performance should ideally be extended to other forms of image characterization including radiomics [2, 3] so that physics evaluation can be more directly related to the expected specific output of CT images.

Each of the attributes noted above is highly influenced by the object within and through which the quantity is measured. Of note, these measurements are highly influenced by the size of the phantom and patients as well as how a CT system adapts to variation in the size of the imaged body part.

Table 13.1 Standardized protocols for testing of CT systems according to AAPM TG233.

Nomenclature[a]	CTDI (mGy)(32 cm phantom)	Tube potential (kV)	Tube current (mA)	Mode, Pitch	Reconstruction
TG233-F1	0.75	120	Fixed mA to achieve target CTDI ±10%	Helical, ~1	FBP, IR at medium strength, higher than medium strength, and maximum strength settings
TG233-F2	1.5				
TG233-F3	3.0				
TG233-F4	6.0				
TG233-F5	12.0				
TG233-F6	24.0				"standard" kernel
TG233-F3LK	3.0	70 (or 80)		Helical, ~1, unless a lower pitch is needed to achieve the CTDI	~0.6 and 5 mm image thickness
TG233-F3MK	3.0	100			
TG233-F3HK	3.0	150 (or 140)			
TG233-M2	1.5	120	TCM setting to achieve target CTDI ±10%	Helical, ~1	
TG233-M3	3.0				
TG233-M4	6.0				
TG233-M3-A	3.0	120	Same as above	Axial	

[a] F refers to fixed mA, M to TCM, one to six to dose setting, and LK, MK, HK to low, medium, and high kV settings, respectively.

A measurement made with an imaging technique on a particular size phantom cannot readily be predictive of a different size patient and different technique. As such, the technique used for the evaluation should be reflective of the techniques intended for the clinical use of the system. Alternatively, a set of preset techniques can be used to offer benchmarking across multiple evaluations (Table 13.1).

In terms of phantoms, the results are also dependent on the characteristics and size of the phantom. Multiple phantoms have been used for these evaluations. Among them, the Mercury Phantom provides a comprehensive platform for multiplicity of features and attributes of CT performance including the MTF, the NPS, artifacts, Hounsfield unit (HU) values, and task-based performance (Figure 13.3). Of note, the phantom not only offers multiple sizes, enabling measurements relevant to ranges of patient sizes from pediatric to bariatric, but also offers that within a single habitus, thus enabling testing of the adaptive component of the CT system (e.g. the tube current modulation system that adjusts the x-ray flux as a function of patient thickness). This enables evaluation of the CT system not in an idealized fixed mA but also variable mA condition, thus providing more confidence that the measurements made on a phantom are more predictive of clinical performance, an explicit objective of any physics evaluation.

The four attributes noted above can also be measured in the context of clinical images, a topic that we discuss below.

13.2.3 Radiometry

In CT imaging, radiation dose is a major concern. This is due to the fact that CT requires more exposure than alternative x-ray imaging methods, as it provides information with three (and sometimes four)-dimensional discrimination. Further, its utility and effectiveness has fueled its

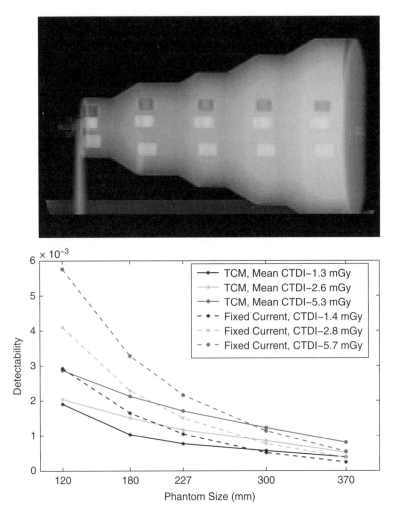

Figure 13.3 Measured detectability index as a function of size using the Mercury Phantom (top) with fixed mA and modulated mA set to output specific CTDI values.

increased use. So, both individual and population dose need to be quantified and managed. As noted in Chapter 12, CT output-based metrics (such as computed tomography dose index (CTDI) and dose length product (DLP)) have been the primary quantities of use in CT. But, as in the case of quality metrics, a quantity for radiometry is most relevant if it is related to or informed by the specifics of the patient and the examination. Between the two, DLP is more the patient-relevant metric (as opposed to technology) as it is closer to the total radiation burden of the patient during a CT examination. But DLP still does not go far enough to be a truly patient-relevant quantity.

One way to make the CTDI and DLP more relevant to the patient is through the concept of Size-Specific Dose Estimate (SSDE) [4]. SSDE is a metric derived from the CTDI with the inclusion of a size-specific adjustment factor. This makes the dose estimate size-dependent, as in the application of the Mercury Phantom above, and thus the metric more reflective of dose absorption in a patient of corresponding size. SSDE can also be extended to include the length of the scan (akin to DLP). The concept has not been endorsed by the AAPM TG which devised the concept, however, one can argue

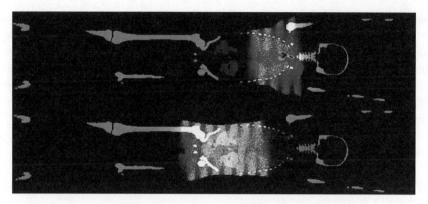

Figure 13.4 Pattern of energy deposition in a patient following chest (top) and abdomin-pelvis (bottom) CT scans. The differentials in the pattern and their geometry are largely ignored by CTDI, SSDE, and their extracts. Imparted energy integrates this total absorbed energy while effective dose and risk index account for relative radiosensitivity of the tissue.

that SSDE, if not extended to include the total radiation burden of the patient, does not go far enough to be of most relevant utility to CT radiometry [5].

Both DLP and SSDE-DLP are surrogates of Imparted Energy (IE), which can be more directly quantified as a metric of total energy deposited in the patient during the CT exam. The metric can be ascertained by an estimate of the patient body contour and the impinging radiation field of the CT exam [6]. DLP, SSDE-DLP, and IE reflect total radiation deposited in the body, not accounting for variation in radiosensitivity across human tissues (Figure 13.4), as not all tissues are equal in terms of radiosensitivity. For example, a quantity of deposited energy within an extremity has far less potential effect than that of the same quantity to the heart. In order to potentially account for this effect, it is important to estimate energy imparted to organs in terms of organ doses. Multiple prior efforts have been made to quantify CT irradiation in terms of organ doses [7, 8]. While methods vary, the ones that most closely account for the exact geometry and condition of the CT radiation including tube current modulation tend to be more accurate. With the knowledge of organ doses, the radiation burden to the patient can be quantified in terms of a number of possible scalar values including effective dose (ED) and Risk Index (RI) [9].

The metrics of CT radiometry follow a continuum from those specifying the average irradiation field in terms of dose deposited in a standardized-size object (i.e. CTDI) to patient-specific estimated risk associated with the exposure (i.e. RI). Along this continuum, the metrics have varying degrees of patient specificity from least to most. The ones that are more patient-specific tend to be more relevant but involve more assumptions, the validity of which is subject to scrutiny. Further, each has different degrees of uncertainty. For example, CTDI is a much more robust metric than SSDE, as the latter requires an addition adjustment factor that subjects the metric to an additional level of variability [10]. For a given application and need, a seasoned physicist should be aware of these tradeoffs and make sensible choices in balancing uncertainty and relevance of the metric to be applied for CT radiometry.

13.3 Testing Implication of New Technologies

CT systems are continuously evolving, with new technologies being introduced to the market every year. These new technologies have implications for clinical medical physics and how a physicist might evaluate these technologies. The developments have changed the needed physics support, as they offer features that are not targeted by traditional physics testing methods or metrics. In such conditions, it is paramount to determine the quality of the feature being offered, not to just characterize the system, but to provide key information to better implement the system in the clinic. Highlighted below are some of these implications. Maintaining a focus on the clinical relevance of the medical physics evaluation, the technology itself is not discussed in detail, rather the focus is mostly on the medical physics implications.

13.3.1 Hardware

New systems are frequently introduced with new and updated hardware including tubes, bowtie filters, anti-scatter provisions, and detectors.

Relevant evaluation of x-ray tubes should be in terms of allowable maximum mA as a function of kV and the impact of high kV and mA settings on the focal spot size. The focal spot blooming at high kV and mA settings has a direct impact on system resolution and thus the MTF, while kV-mA ranges can limit the size of the patients that can be effectively imaged on the scanner to have sufficient signal to noise ratio at reasonable scanning speed.

New models of CT systems often involve changes to beam shaping and scatter reduction: from the source-side active beam limitation of dynamic collimation, filter material, and filter shape (i.e. bowtie matched to patient habitus), to the post-patient anti-scatter grid. All of these naturally influence the magnitude of primary and scatter signal being detected. The scatter, as well as similar effects due to beam hardening and the choice of bowtie filter and field of view is corrected by the system. However, the adequacy of this correction in terms of HU accuracy and image uniformity should be verified as a function of kV and patient size.

In terms of detectors, an evaluation of the noise or signal-to-noise performance of the hardware using the detector quantum efficiency (DQE) is what makes the most sense. The metric should ideally be estimated across the exposure range to ascertain detector linearity and the potential influence of that in image quality as a function of signal level.

The hardware characterizations noted above can be done in terms of physics metrics such as uniformity, DQE, or MTF, but as in all physics evaluations, those metrics should ideally be extended to TTF and NPS as well as related to task-based performance such as detectability or estimability so that the measures can be made more relevant to clinical performance and explainable to other healthcare providers.

13.3.2 Acquisition Methods

In addition to, and in conjunction with, new hardware features of CT systems, the systems deploy a host of acquisition conditions and processes that influence the resulting images. A physics evaluation of the CT system will be incomplete if the influence of such features is not evaluated.

Scanning mode has a direct influence on CT image quality and dose. Among those features of modern CT systems is the choice of axial versus helical scanning of varying pitch including high-pitch mode for improved temporal resolution, choice of cone angle, mA modulation as a function of patient thickness with additional provision for organ-sparing angular modulations (to reduce dose to the eyes and female breasts), and kV modulation. Each of these features should be evaluated by tests that target the very specific outcome that the feature claims. For example, a breast dose reduction modulation should evaluate the changes in the anterior portion of the imaged patient/phantom with the features turned on and off to ascertain the effect on dose and image quality, and ascertain the potential influence on patient imaging. Likewise, the choice of increased pitch and cone angle trades azimuthal resolution for potential improvement in the scanning speed and thus improved temporal resolution. A phantom with an actuating apparatus can quantify the tradeoffs. A seasoned physicist may design such tests for each of the aforementioned features targeting the exact claims of the feature and influence on patient dose and task-based image quality. The specific use of the system can then be ordained by the results.

Modern CT systems are also equipped with a host of advanced scanning modes for cardiac, contrast enhanced, and perfusion imaging. These modes, likewise have their own operating features, claims, and processes. Ascertaining the quality and effectiveness of these features through simplified phantoms is challenging. But again, a seasoned physicist should be creative to devise methods that assess the operation of the system in a representative way with those features to make reasonable predictions of the clinical performance based on their physics evaluations.

13.3.3 Image Processing and Analysis

Recently, CT has seen significant progress in terms of image reconstruction and processing. Images can be rendered in a multiplicity of ways, not only by changes in the reconstruction slice thickness, but in the applied reconstruction kernel, a host of iterative and statistical reconstruction algorithms, and machine-learning-based (so called deep-learning) reconstruction techniques. Beyond reconstruction, some systems deploy post-processing methods (similar to those of radiography and mammography) which further influence the rendition of the image data. These topics, by and large, have remained outside the purview of medical physics. However, if the medical physicist is responsible for the quality of the medical images, the profound influence of reconstruction and processing should be fully embraced by physics oversight.

The influence of image rendition on image quality can be readily characterized by reconstructing a set of images (either phantom or patient images) under multiple acquisition techniques. The results can then be evaluated in quantitative terms using image quality metrology detailed above. In that process, the inherent non-linearity and non-stationarity of the image rendition methods should be taken into consideration. For example, iterative reconstructions typically reduce noise in the images, but the reduction is mostly in relatively uniform areas of the image. They further create a noise texture that has more power at lower spatial frequencies than those of more conventional filtered-back-projection (FBP) reconstructions. These effects, if deemed undesirable, can be somewhat tempered by mixing the iterative reconstructed images with FBP images through user-selectable desired weightings. The results influence task-based performance. The AAPM TG233 offers a set of reconstruction conditions to sample the reconstructions and kernels of the system with task-based evaluations [1]. A seasoned physicist can devise a strategy based on the TG233 blueprint to assess the image quality across a variety of clinically-representative image rendition conditions so that the results are reasonable surrogates to decide on the best rendition for a given type of exam.

13.3.4 New System-Wide Technologies

Some new CT systems deploy technologies for specific clinical needs. Among those are cone-beam systems for extremities, interventional, and dental applications as well as spectral images for material differentiation.

Many of the fan-beam CT metrologies cannot be readily extended to cone-beam CT. For example, cylindrical phantoms deploying cylindrical inserts designed for fan-beam CT do not well represent the image quality conditions of cone-beam images. The same can be said about dosimetry methods; cone-beam geometry violates some of the assumptions of CTDI measurements. A standardized set of methods to evaluate cone-beam CT in such a way that is reflective of dose and image quality in patient exams is currently lacking. Drawing from the primary principles of clinical representation, a seasoned clinical physicists, however, can adapt existing phantoms and measurements to ascertain reasonable surrogates of image quality and safety. Examples include phantoms with three-dimensional inserts for HU and resolution measures, 3D noise estimation methods, and dose measurement methods that better account for the scatter dose from wide beams.

Spectral imaging through dual-energy dual-scans, split filter, detector dual binning, or dual gantry presents yet another system-wide technology in need of tactful engagement of physicists. While different systems deploy different methods, they all aim for material differentiation. Evaluation should thus ascertain that outcome in terms of the quality of that differentiation. Example metrics include minimum detectable concentration of iodine or calcium, the signal-to-noise ratio in differentiation of two material (e.g. iodine and calcium, fat and soft tissue) as a function of dose. These values can be reflected into task-based performance metrics of detectability and estimability noted earlier. The spectral imaging technologies also offer unique image rendition capabilities such as mono-energetic and virtual non-contrast images. These renditions can likewise be tested in terms of their claims, in terms of accuracy of mono-energetic representation and iodine elimination, for example.

13.4   Clinical Integration and Implementation

Medical physics is most relevant when engaged and practiced in the context of a clinical operation. All medical physicists are naturally expected to have a strong understanding of the physical properties and performance of clinical systems, and clinical medical physicists have always worked *around* the clinical environment. However, only a minority have had the opportunity to fully integrate the fruits of their work *in* the clinic by engaging with clinicians and administrators. This is best illustrated by the fact that most clinicians and administrators are either unaware of our profession or are unable to explain what it is that we do. For the select few who can offer a description, it likely begins and ends with an explanation of meeting regulatory compliance, shielding calculations, radiation dose estimates, and routine equipment testing. These are all important tasks that are fundamental duties of a medical physicist, but they are only a foundation; these bedrocks of our profession are more characteristic of technicians and compliance officers than highly trained, skilled problem solvers.

One side effect of the 1.0 paradigm has been the ability to work, largely autonomously, around the clinic instead of being integrated into it: "I work around patients," "I work around radiologists and technologists," and "I do my testing around the clinical schedule." Not all physicists work this way, but those who are viewed as an integral part of the care delivery team are the exception rather than the rule.

A second side effect of the traditional, routine clinical responsibilities is a difference in vocabulary and base knowledge. Just as physicists have machine-oriented, technical jargon, clinicians speak in medical terms: procedures, indications, and pathologies. Those in the hospital administration have an entirely different vocabulary of finance, accounting, acronyms, and idioms. Physicists can get by with not knowing the difference between KPIs, PIKs, and IPKs (key performance indicator, payment in kind, and intractable plantar keratosis, respectively), but then they are also at risk of being left out of conversations establishing hospital quality metrics or optimization of the weight-bearing radiography scan parameters.

A third side effect, and arguably the most concerning, is the difference in quality and rigor of physics and non-physics needs and the overall effect on the patient care. A thoroughly tested CT scanner can easily be misused; an optimized protocol can be misapplied. If a medical physicist adopts a "not my job" attitude and does not engage with clinical colleagues on the implementation of imaging technology, then the physicist runs the risk of being complicit in providing lower quality healthcare and doing a disservice to patients.

13.4.1 Training and Communication

A key skill necessary for medical physicists to effectively integrate into the clinical environment is communication. In many instances in a clinic, the physicist will have the best fundamental understanding of the underlying imaging technologies and image formation processes. However, if this knowledge cannot be relayed in an interpretable way to a patient, clinician, or administrator, the physicist's audience will turn to a more understandable source. Professionalism has become an educational requirement for graduate and residency programs, but training in effective communication may be missed. Thus, enhancing beyond the 1.0 paradigm of having an in-depth understanding of the technologies in use and generating dense reports of measurements and calculations, we need to be a conductor and coordinator in the clinic, to bring that knowledge to the clinic, and to work with the radiologist and technologist to optimize the use the system.

13.4.2 Optimization

Classically, imaging techniques and workflow have been optimized using a combination of educated guessing, trial-and-error, phantom measurements, simulation analyses, and some luck. It is plausible that with enough time some techniques and workflows would be optimized in a hypothetical situation: a specific patient population imaged on a specific piece of equipment as positioned by a few technologists and interpreted by a small practice of radiologists. And that multi-variable "optimization" ignores the potential for converging on some locally optimized solution and missing the global optimization. It is only with patient-centered and patient-relatable metrologies of qualimetry and radiometry detailed earlier that the variables of optimization can be quantified. Once the key attributes of image quality are quantifiable, then robust, systematic, and repeatable optimization practices can proceed.

What happens when the patient population changes because a completely new pediatric imaging program is introduced? What happens when a scanner that is several years old is upgraded to a new model with different detectors, reconstruction algorithms, and kernels? What if the contracted radiologist practice changes? Each of these will necessitate a new optimization project, which a seasoned physicist should be fully capable, entrusted, and empowered to undertake. Without it, the outcome will be *ad hoc* and far from optimized, a dis-service to the patient entrusted to our care.

Protocol is a space where there can be significant variability in the clinical practice, particularly where multiple makes and models of CT scanners are used. Optimization, meaning providing the needed clinical information at the lowest dose, should be quantified with patient-centered metrics, as noted above. Ideally, the optimized protocols will also be consistent, meaning equivalency of image quality attributes across systems of different makes and models for the same exam type, across different systems.

As an example of the difficulty in optimizing protocols consistently, consider the scenario of an established radiology department in a hospital with five CT systems, from 3–10 years old, from two

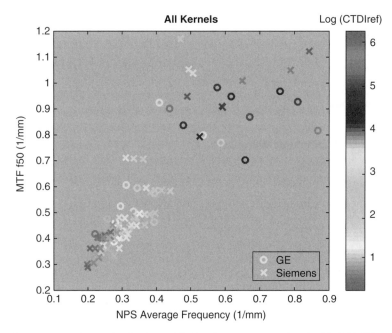

Figure 13.5 Output resolution and noise (quantified as frequency associated with 0.5 MTF and average NPS frequency) across two CT systems and their reconstruction kernel settings, enabling identifying kernels that deliver closest match in resolution and noise. Color (rendered here in grayscale) notes the dose factor necessary to deliver consistent noise magnitude.

different vendors. The department has purchased and installed the state-of-the-art CT system from one of those vendors. How does the medical physicist commission this new technology into a clinical ecosystem? Inevitably there will be new dose reduction options, workflow automation features, reconstruction flavors, and other specific applications such as dual-energy or bolus tracking. First, if the classic techniques of intrinsic performance assessment are used, then none of these new features would be evaluated. The characterization of this expensive new piece of equipment could look substantially different to the decade-old system. Second, how are imaging protocols and workflows to be adapted? If the department likes the look of the historical images and tailors protocols to match, then the new features are not being utilized. If the department simply adopts what the vendor's application specialist installs as recommended protocols, then the consistency of image quality or dose cannot be assured. If the department starts with some baseline protocols having the expectation that tweaks will be made over the coming weeks and months as patients are imaged, then the patients are being used as test subjects.

How can the multitude of questions above be addressed? This can be achieved by first quantifying attributes of image quality across systems and protocols, and use those that provide the closest matched performance across systems [11] (Figure 13.5). Then integrating new technology would be considerably more streamlined and methodical.

13.4.3 Meaningful QC

Quality assurance (QA) and quality control (QC) procedures are critical to ensuring a reliable CT operation and patient safety over time. However, QA and QC monitoring programs must be thoughtfully established both in terms of frequency and criteria. If every time QC was performed it failed, then QC is not being performed frequently enough. If QC has never failed, then a specific procedure may be inappropriate or unnecessary. Even for a well-targeted QA and QC monitoring program, the majority of the time the system will be found to be functioning as expected. This makes it easy for people who conduct QA and QC to become complacent, especially in a busy clinical environment. Because these tests are relatively easy and routine to perform but are time-consuming, the person can operate on "auto-pilot."

Increasingly, vendor software applications, the ubiquity of computers in the clinic, and the trend of going paperless have meant that many QC procedures, from set-up to analysis, have become push-button and automated. This automation improves clinical efficiency and multitasking: the technologist can press a button at the start of the shift, or better yet the scanner runs a scheduled task before anyone shows up, and then goes about making other preparations for the clinical day. Additionally, these automated QC procedures minimize user variability and can provide a wealth of data. Whereas a technologist or physicist might have been limited to reviewing a few phantom image slices, drawing some regions of interest (ROIs), and recording a few values, automated analyses can perform extensive measurements, calculations, and data-basing with ease. Automated QC has enabled opportunities that are largely still untapped potential.

For the simple phantom and flat field QC, most QC tests use rudimentary image analysis that yield a pass-fail assessment on a specific date using generic threshold criteria. This will probably flag a system that should not be used due to loss of functionality, if the thresholds have not been set so permissively so as to minimize false positives. However, this will not provide a warning that the system's performance is progressively degrading or performing sub-optimally. It is expected that x-ray tube and detector performance will drift over time and require recalibration, so an automated QC algorithm that offers trend analysis and warns of impending issues or failures *before* they manifest in patient images or require taking a scanner out of clinical service for repair is clearly preferable.

Another untapped potential of automated QC is the ease of implementing existing, and as yet to be defined, qualimetry and radiometry metrologies that were detailed earlier. Training users to measure MTF and NPS would be challenging, but automation is comparatively simple. Figure 13.6 demonstrates an example of how a QC program in terms of detectability can establish that inter- and intra-system consistency across CT systems (Figure 13.6). Metrologies such as these have already been shown to flag QC artifacts on phantom images that have passed the system's QC tests and other basic ROI measurements (Figure 13.2) [12].

13.4.4 Automated Analysis and Data Management

Considering the overall mandate of a 3.0 physicist to provide comprehensive oversight of the quality and safety across the imaging operation, in the context of this chapter CT imaging operation, it is tremendously helpful to provide that oversight through automated systems that incorporate not only phantom QC, but also all physics evaluations, CT protocols, reported issues, and equipment reports. Such a system, as a singular system, does not currently exist, but there have been attempts to take on these tasks in piecewise fashion. These have been in-house programs and limited commercial offerings that are only expected to increase over time. These empower medical physics support on a more system-wide (as opposed to equipment-focused) scale.

Paramount to the oversight of quality and safety is a mechanism to do so not only in the context of phantom data but actual clinical data. Recent advances have shown how patient radiation dose

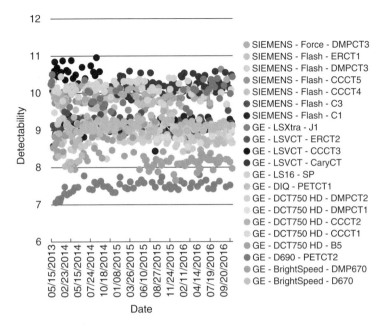

Figure 13.6 Performance of various CT systems in terms of detectability index as a function of time.

and image quality can be ascertained in a patient-specific manner from the CT exam data [10, 13, 14]. Assessments have included the measurements of noise, contrast, and resolution in patient images, extraction of detectability from the data, and matching the image geometry to computational models to compute organ doses [15]. The results have proven to be robust and offer reasonably accurate outcomes correlated to clinical measures of image quality and patient dose (Figures 13.7 and 13.8). In terms of radiation dose, an area that is a bit more advanced, these methods can further offer benchmarking against peer data [16]. These methods are expected to take more of a center stage in the future as a strong companion to the work of the physicist and their aim to advance consistency, quality, and safety of CT imaging [17–22].

13.4.5 Effective Practice

Clinical physics is expected to provide a crucial value to patient care. It then follows that the work should be a net value-add to the system by strong practices of stewardship and effective practice. The physics support should be properly resourced toward that goal.

Current clinical physics support is largely based on the 1.0 practice model focused on regulatory compliance, which is essential but not enough. In the same way, we do not wish a surgeon to just focus on following pre-ordained minimal tasks that do not fully represent what the patient needs. Practice based on the 3.0 paradigm as outlined in this chapter takes more effort. This extra effort requires strong justification (based on the added service and value to patient care), targeted regulation and accreditation guidelines, automation tools, and intentionally-designed models of efficient practice. Testing must be as efficient as possible to allow for an effective clinical role to take primacy. Through these advances, it is expected that clinical medical physics can transform from an equipment focus to a patient focus.

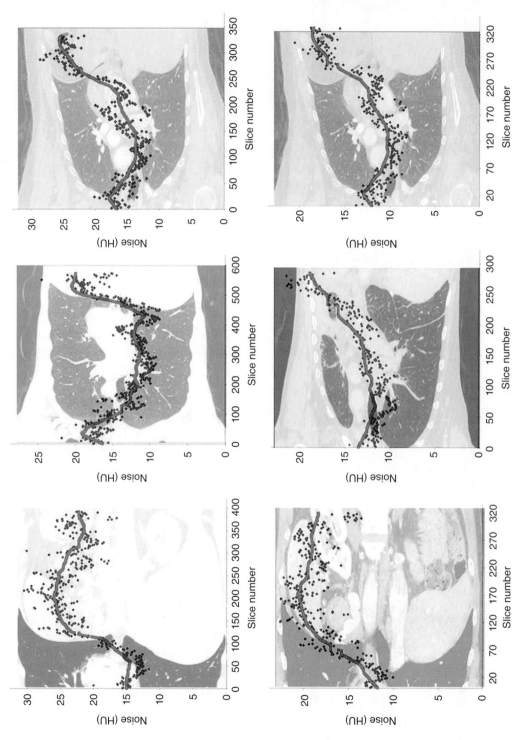

Figure 13.7 Measured noise values along the axial slices of CT scans.

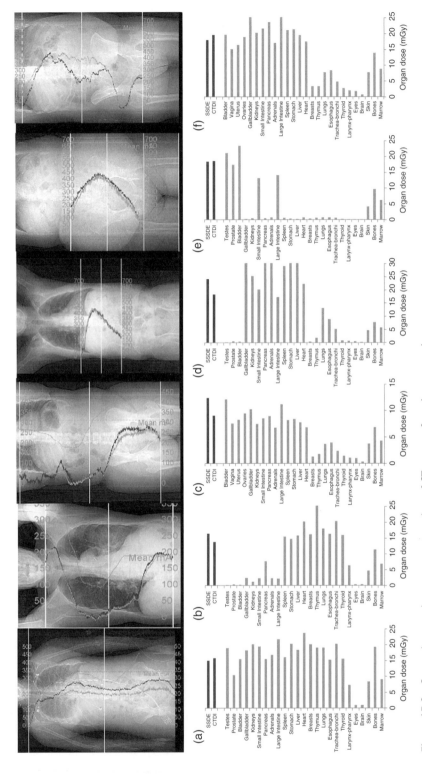

Figure 13.8 Organ doses estimates across a variety of CT exams of varying protocols.

References

1 Samei, E., Bakalyar, D., Boedeker, K.L. et al. (2019). Performance Evaluation of Computed Tomography Systems, Report of the American Association of Physicists in Medicine (AAPM) Task Group 233, *American Association of Physicists in Medicine*, Alexandria, VA.

2 Hoye, J., Solomon, J., Sauer, T.J. et al. (2019). Systematic analysis of bias and variability of morphologic features for lung lesions in computed tomography. *Journal of Medical Imaging* 6 (1), https://doi.org/10.1117/1.JMI.6.1.013504).

3 Robins, M., Solomon, J., Hoye, J. et al. (2019). Systematic analysis of bias and variability of texture measurements in computed tomography. *Journal of Medical Imaging* 6 (3): 033503.

4 Boone, J., Cody, D., McCollough, C. et al. (2011). Size-Specific Dose Estimates (SSDE) in Pediatric and Adult Body CT Examinations, AAPM TG 204, *American Association of Physicists in Medicine*, Alexandria, VA.

5 Samei, E., Christianson, O., and Zhang, Y. (2015). Comment on "comparison of patient specific dose metrics between chest radiography, tomosynthesis, and CT for adult patients of wide ranging body habitus". *Medical Physics* 42 (4): 02094–02095.

6 Sanders, J., Tian, X., Segars, W.P. et al. (2017). Automated, patient-specific estimation of regional imparted energy and dose from TCM CT exams across 13 protocols. *Journal of Medical Imaging* 4 (1): 013503–013503.

7 Li, X., Samei, E., Segars, W. et al. (2011). Monte Carlo method for estimating patient-specific radiation dose and cancer risk in CT: application to patients. *Medical Physics* 38 (1): 408–419.

8 Zhang, Y., Li, X., Segars, W.P., and Samei, E. (2012). Organ dose, effective dose, and risk index in adult CT: comparison of four types of reference phantoms across different protocols. *Medical Physics* 39 (6): 3404–3423.

9 Ria, F., Fu, W., Zhang, Y. et al. (2018). Characterization of radiation risk across a clinical CT patient population: comparison across 12 risks metrics. Proceedings of the Scientific Assembly and Annual Meeting of the Radiological Society of North America, Chicago, IL, Nov. 2018, *RSNA'18 Proc*.

10 Samei, E. and Christianson, O. (2014). Dose index analytics – more than a low number. *Journal of the American College of Radiology* 11 (8): 832–834.

11 Winslow, J., Zhang, Y., and Samei, E. (2017). A method for characterizing and matching CT image quality across CT scanners from different manufacturers. *Medical Physics* 44 (11): 5705–5717.

12 Jaffe, T.A., Winslow, J., Zhang, Y. et al. (2019). Automated early identification of an excessive air-in-oil x-ray tube artifact that mimics acute cerebral infarct. *Journal of Computer Assisted Tomography* 43 (1): 18–21.

13 Abadi, E., Sanders, J., and Samei, E. (2017). Patient-specific quantification of image quality: an automated technique for measuring the distribution of organ Hounsfield units in clinical chest CT images. *Medical Physics* 44 (9): 4736–4746.

14 Sanders, J., Hurwitz, L., and Samei, E. (2016). Patient-specific quantification of image quality: an automated method for measuring spatial resolution in clinical CT images. *Medical Physics* 43 (10): 5330–5338.

15 Tian, X., Segars, W.P., Dixon, R.L., and Samei, E. (2016). Convolution-based estimation of organ dose in tube current modulated CT. *Physics in Medicine and Biology* 61 (10): 3935–3954.

16 Kanal, K.M., Butler, P.F., Sengupta, D. et al. (2017). U.S. Diagnostic reference levels and achievable doses for 10 adult CT examinations. *Radiology* 284 (1): 120–133.

17 Christianson, O., Winslow, J., Frush, D.P., and Samei, E. (2015). Automated technique to measure noise in clinical CT examinations. *AJR* 205: W93–W99.

18 Jaffe, T.A., Tian, X., Bashir, M.R. et al. (2018). Clinically acceptable optimized dose reduction in computed tomographic imaging of necrotizing pancreatitis using a noise addition software tool. *Journal of Computer Assisted Tomography* 42 (2): 197–203.

19 Cheng, Y., Smith, T.B., Jensen, C.T. et al. (2019). Correlation of algorithmic and visual assessment of lesion detection in clinical images. *Academic Radiology* https://doi.org/10.1016/j.acra.2019.07.015.

20 Ria, F., Wilson, J., Zhang, Y., and Samei, E. (2017). Image noise and dose performance across a clinical population: patient size adaptation as a metric of CT performance. *Medical Physics* 44 (6): 2141–2147.

21 Ria, F., Davis, J.T., Solomon, J.B. et al. (2019). Expanding the concept of diagnostic reference levels to noise and dose reference levels in CT. *AJR* 213 (4): 889–894.

22 Cheng, Y., Abadi, E., Smith, T.B. et al. (2019). Validation of algorithmic CT image quality metrics with preferences of radiologists. *Medical Physics* 46 (11): 4837–4846.

Part V

Nuclear Imaging

14

Clinical Nuclear Imaging Physics: Perspective

Douglas E. Pfeiffer

Boulder Community Health, Boulder, CO, USA

14.1 Historical Perspective

The roots of nuclear imaging reach back as far as some of the origins of modern physics. In 1896, Henri Becquerel reported to the French Academy of Science his discovery of what was later to be known as radioactivity [1] through his film darkening experiments with uranium. His discovery led Marie and Pierre Curie to conduct further research, discovering the elements radium and polonium. Ernest Rutherford started his work to better understand the atom and discovered alpha and beta particles. In the early 1900s, Rutherford paired up with Frederick Soddy and worked out the process of radioactive decay as the source of the radiations being detected [2, 3]. In the 1920s, George de Hevesy established the radioactive tracer principle [4]. In 1934 Irène Curie and Jean Frédéric Joliot discovered that radioactivity could be induced when a lighter element, such as boron or aluminum, was bombarded with alpha particles. This discovery eventually led Ernest Lawrence to invent the cyclotron, which made it possible to create radioactive isotopes in greater quantities.

E. Lawrence's brother, John Lawrence, realized the possible applications of the cyclotron for medicine, proposing that radioactive compounds could be used to treat cancer. His first trials were in 1935 when he injected mice having leukemia with ^{32}P. He also did early work on the biological effects of neutrons, determining them to be five times more harmful than x-rays. This work lead to the development of the first radiation safety regulations. In 1939 he performed the first radioisotope therapy treatment in a human, using ^{32}P to successfully treat a patient with polycythemia vera.

A major achievement came in 1946 when Sam Seidlin found that ^{131}I could halt the growth of thyroid cancer. The use of ^{131}I expanded from treating thyroid cancer to include imaging the thyroid gland, determining thyroid function, and treating hypothyroidism.

Imaging of the thyroid was achieved through the use of a rectilinear scanner developed by Benedict Cassen. This was a relatively crude device consisting of a NaI crystal approximately 1.3 cm in diameter and 5 cm thick coupled to a photomultiplier tube (PMT). A mechanical printer followed the boustrophedon pattern of the scanner, placing dots on the paper as gamma rays were detected. This technique was very slow with poor spatial resolution. It did, however, usher in a new era of *in vivo* imaging of the human body, with a fundamental difference from other modalities in

Clinical Imaging Physics: Current and Emerging Practice, First Edition. Edited by Ehsan Samei and Douglas E. Pfeiffer.
© 2020 John Wiley & Sons, Inc. Published 2020 by John Wiley & Sons, Inc.

that it was effectively imaging function – in the case of the thyroid, metabolic uptake – rather than anatomy. In spite of its limitations, the rectilinear scanner developed and was in use up to the 1970s.

Hal Anger worked to overcome the limitations of the rectilinear scanner and introduced the first scintillation camera in 1957. This device became regularly known as the Anger camera. As with the rectilinear scanner, a NaI crystal is coupled to PMTs. However, Anger used a much larger crystal and a hexagonal array of PMTs. He also placed a parallel hole collimator in front of the crystal to improve spatial resolution. The output of the PMTs was fed to position logic circuits that enabled the system to determine the location of the scintillation event in the crystal. The *x* and *y* coordinates of the event were sent to a cathode ray tube (CRT) along with the pulse height (Figure 14.1). The image was then viewed on the CRT. The images could be recorded using a Polaroid camera or a matrix camera for transparency film. While the technology has certainly developed since the 1950s, the basics of the Anger camera are still prevalent in modern nuclear imaging cameras. Of primary importance is that fact that this device allowed, for the first time, imaging of an entire organ without any movement of the device.

Nuclear imaging expanded dramatically after the realization that the properties of ^{99m}Tc made it an excellent imaging agent. The 140 keV gamma is easily detectable by scintillation cameras. It is a relatively pure gamma emitter (just under 88%), helping to minimize patient dose. Finally, the six-hour half-life allows for an adequate short-distance distribution and imaging time without large decay corrections or extended radioactivity. The development of ^{99}Mo generators in 1958 greatly increased the availability of ^{99m}Tc, and the 66-hour half-life of ^{99}Mo made the distribution of generators over large distances feasible.

The metastable isotope of technetium was discovered in 1938, but remained unexploited until the 1950s when Powell Richards began to understand its potential. The first publication including

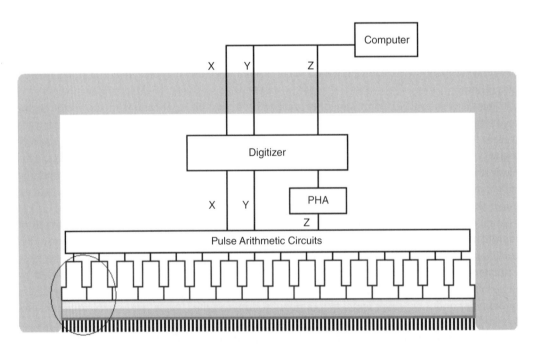

Figure 14.1 Illustration of the Anger scintillation camera. *Source:* Fizzy at en.wikipedia [GFDL (http://www. gnu.org/copyleft/fdl.html) or CC-BY-SA-3.0 (http://creativecommons.org/licenses/by-sa/3.0)], from Wikimedia Commons.

the use of ^{99m}Tc scanning was in August 1963 [5]. It remains the most widely used imaging isotope to date. The development of radiopharmaceutical tracers continued until it was possible to image processes in almost every major organ, plus bones.

In 1962, David Kuhl and Roy Edwards published their first work in tomographic imaging with radioisotopes [6]. Using a scintillation detector, they scanned patients in a boustrophedon pattern from multiple angles (Figure 14.2), using back-projection techniques to reconstruct images in a plane. Other researchers, such as John Mallard with University of Aberdeen and J. Brill and his colleagues continued to develop this method of using scintillation detectors for tomographic imaging.

The use of the Anger camera for tomographic imaging was first investigated by Paul Harper and his colleagues at the University of Chicago. In early systems, patients sat on a chair that was rotated in front of the camera (Figure 14.3). 1976 saw the introduction of gantry-mounted cameras at the Annual Meeting of the Society of Nuclear Medicine (SNM). One of these was called the Humongotron SPECT (single photon emission computed tomography) scanner (Figure 14.4), developed by John Keyes. In the late 1970s a dual head scanner was investigated and produced. This early system had corrections for attenuation and scatter and was also capable of acquiring body contour information and gated cardiac data.

Nuclear cardiac imaging began in the 1950s with potassium and rubidium and has been central to the practice since the 1960s. Early cardiac imaging was performed with ^{131}Cs and planar views. In 1973 ^{43}K was used, with ^{201}Tl coming on the scene in 1975 [7]. ^{99m}Tc, now a mainstay of cardiac imaging, was introduced in 1985. It has several advantages over ^{201}Tl. First, the 140 keV photon energy is better suited to gamma camera imaging than the 68–80 keV of ^{201}Tl. The much shorter half-life of ^{99m}Tc (6 hours) compared to ^{201}Tl (73 hours) results in much better dosimetry, allowing a higher dose, which allows for higher quality images in shorter scan times. This also allows for cardiac gating, so that both myocardial perfusion and left ventricular function can be evaluated.

Positron Emission Tomography (PET) imaging is often considered to be a relatively late development in nuclear imaging. However, Sweet [8] and Wrenn et al. [9], both published independently

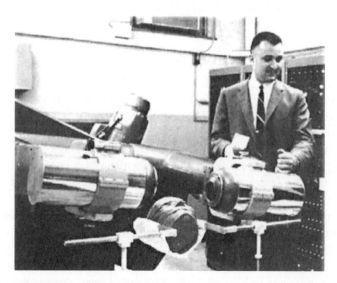

Figure 14.2 David Kuhl and his rectilinear scanner, called the Mark II. *Source:* Image © Institute of Physics and Engineering in Medicine Reproduced by permission of IOP Publishing. All rights reserved. Phys. Med. Biol. 51 (2006) R99–R115. doi:10.1088/0031-9155/51/13/R07.

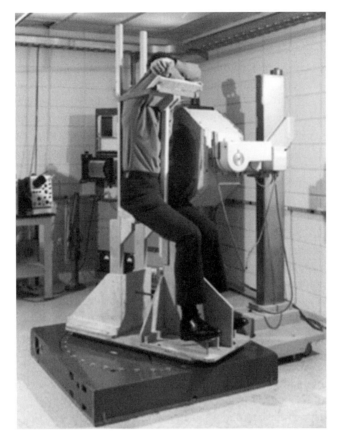

Figure 14.3 Rotating chair system used for cardiac imaging. *Source:* Image © Institute of Physics and Engineering in Medicine Reproduced by permission of IOP Publishing. All rights reserved. Phys. Med. Biol. 51 (2006) R99–R115. doi:10.1088/0031-9155/51/13/R07.

on positron imaging of the brain in 1951. Several groups continued to develop PET imaging techniques and instrumentation, but it wasn't until 1974 that the first human PET image using filtered back-projection reconstruction was produced [10, 11]. These early scanners were constructed using NaI(Tl) detectors in hexagonal arrays, typically up to 48 individual detectors. Early development was hindered due to the fact that most positron emitters have quite short half-lives, making it necessary to have a cyclotron on site for production of the isotope.

Because PET imaging depends on the detection of coincident photons, the decay time of the detector crystal is very important for accurate determination of coincidence events. Additionally, since the photons have high energy (511 keV), the stopping power of the crystal is also important. NaI(Tl) crystals were used because they were readily available. They also had good light output, so the signal received per photon was relatively high. However, NaI(Tl) has a relatively low density and effective atomic number, so its linear attenuation coefficient at 511 keV is low. In 1975, BGO (bismuth germanate) was developed. This material has higher density and effective atomic number than NaI(Tl) and so it is much more effective at stopping 511 keV photons. Its decay time is somewhat longer than NaI(Tl), and its light output is significantly lower. Overall, this was found to be a better crystal for PET imaging than NaI(Tl). Around 1990 a new crystal was developed, lutetium oxyorthosilicate (LSO) [12]. As seen in Table 14.1, its linear attenuation coefficient is similar to BGO, but with a much shorter decay time and better light output, making it a much better scintillator for

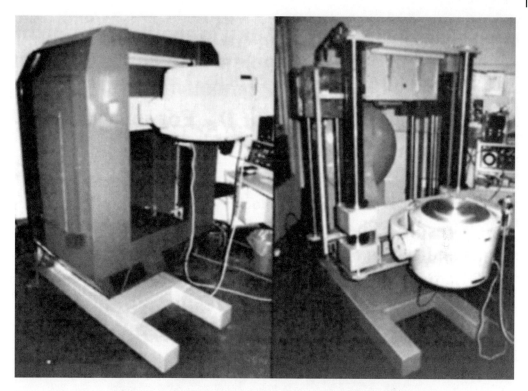

Figure 14.4 The Humongotron SPECT scanner by John Keyes, introduced at the 1976 Annual Meeting of the Society of Nuclear Medicine. *Source:* Image © Institute of Physics and Engineering in Medicine Reproduced by permission of IOP Publishing. All rights reserved. Phys. Med. Biol. 51 (2006) R99–R115. doi:10.1088/0031-9155/51/13/R07.

Table 14.1 Scintillation crystal comparison.

	NaI(Tl)	BGO	LSO	BaF$_2$	GSO
Effective atomic number	51	75	66	54	59
Linear attenuation coefficient (at 511 keV)	0.34	0.92	0.87	0.44	0.62
Decay constant (nS)	230	300	40	0.8	56
Relative light output [% NaI(Tl)] (at 511 keV)	100	15	75	0.8	41

PET imaging than either NaI(Tl) or BGO. Table 14.1 also includes characteristics of two other potential scintillators, barium fluoride (BaF$_2$) and germanium oxyorthosilicate (GSO). Research into other scintillators continues.

Early PET imaging was performed using ^{11}C-glucose, ^{15}O-water, ^{13}N-ammonia, ^{15}O-oxygen, and ^{18}F-fluoride. In 1978, FDG (^{18}F-deoxyglucose) was developed by Brookhaven [13]. This compound was approved by the Food and Drug Administration (FDA) in 1999 and remains the mainstay of PET imaging. ^{82}Rb-chloride was first used for cardiac imaging in 1979, approved by FDA in 1989. As stated earlier, the short half-lives of these isotopes limit the facilities at which they can be used. This is one of the reasons that ^{18}F with its 110 minute half-life, is so popular as an agent, as it can be produced outside of the facility and transported without too high of a decay penalty. Small ^{82}Rb generators were produced commercially around 2000 making its use for general cardiac imaging more popular.

As with all imaging, improved spatial resolution in PET is achieved by using a larger number of smaller detectors. In 1984, the block detector was developed. With this detector, a two-dimensional array of scintillator crystals is coupled to a set of four PMTs via a light guide. By taking ratios of the signals in the four PMTs, the location of the scintillator causing the light can be determined. This approach greatly increased the number of scintillators that could be used and allowed them to be much smaller, leading to substantially improved spatial resolution. The first blocks contained an array of 32 crystals over 4 PMTs. This rapidly increased to more than 144 crystals per PMT in 1998 [14].

14.2   Current and Upcoming Technologies

As with other imaging modalities, nuclear imaging technology has continued to advance. Most SPECT systems still use NaI(Tl) as the scintillator, but field sizes have continued to increase. Moderns systems cite 40 cm × 50 cm fields of view for general purpose and have reconstruction matrices up to 512 × 512 (Figure 14.5). Such capabilities come at a price, one of which is system

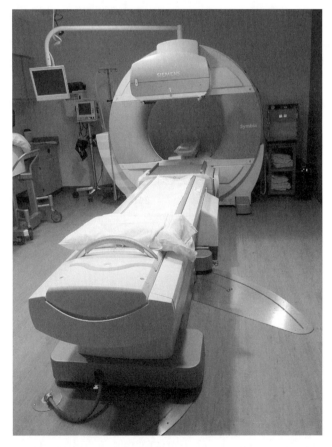

Figure 14.5   A modern SPECT system incorporating advanced technology NaI/PMT detectors, a 44.5 × 59.1 cm field of view, and integrated quality control radioactive sources for automated quality control (QC).

weight: it is not uncommon for these systems to have gantry weight more than 2000 kg. The NaI scintillator detectors have become more sensitive with less energy dependence. Rotations are now automatically contoured to the anatomy for more optimized SPECT studies. Systems are incorporating automated quality control functions, including flood images and center of rotation (Figure 14.6).

All of these advances led to better image quality, lower patient doses, and shorter scan times. Technologist handling of radioactive materials is reduced, as is the time that must be devoted to quality control efforts.

Scintillators also continue to be developed. Manufacturers are starting to use solid state detectors. Both CdTe and CdZnTe are being used as single detectors or segmented monolithic detectors. Solid state detectors offer many advantages over NaI, along with limitations [15]. The atomic numbers of the components are relatively high, yielding excellent quantum efficiency and linear attenuation, so detectors can be thinner. Since the absorbed photon is directly converted to signal, their energy resolution is much better than NaI, so suppression of Compton scatter is improved, leading to improved contrast. Each detector element can be much smaller, so spatial resolution is greatly improved. However, charge collection is not ideal, so the thickness is limited. Field of view is limited due to the cost of these detectors.

The cost is less of an issue for smaller detector sizes, so solid state is finding inroads in specialty cameras, particularly for cardiac and breast imaging. Some systems use pixelated detectors that look otherwise similar to conventional NaI detectors. One cardiac system uses a series of small, independently-addressed solid state detectors that rotate individually within a housing (Figure 14.5). Sophisticated reconstruction algorithms allow creation of a SPECT series from these acquisitions.

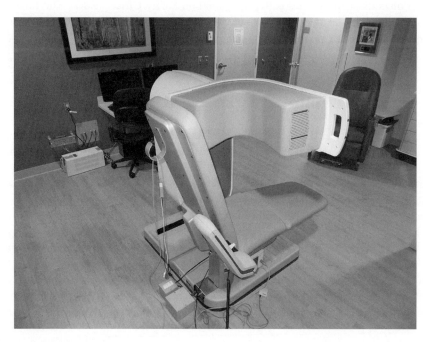

Figure 14.6 SPECT system dedicated to cardiac imaging. Note the housing, which contains an array of solid state detectors and is conformal to the torso. Both the housing and the patient remain stationary during SPECT acquisition.

While the early imaging was done using filtered back-projection algorithms, much modern imaging is done with iterative or more advanced algorithms. These, too, are continually being developed and improved for shorter reconstruction times and better image quality. Additionally, the focus is increasingly moving toward the functional aspects. Indeed, even the name of the specialty is changing from nuclear imaging, focusing on the creation of the image, to molecular imaging, focusing on the purpose of the image.

It is becoming increasingly difficult to purchase a general-purpose nuclear imaging system that is not a hybrid with another modality, particularly computed tomography (CT). In fact, no manufacturer currently markets a PET scanner on its own; all are sold as PET-CT systems. CT yields vital attenuation correction information and provides anatomical information that is not present in nuclear studies. SPECT systems may be sold with a very limited CT capabilities used only for attenuation correction, or they may be full diagnostic CT scanners for fully fused SPECT and CT images. Work is progressing to develop hybrids with magnetic resonance imaging scanners as well.

Finally, the imaging agents themselves continue to develop. Especially in PET imaging where much of the focus has been on oncologic imaging, efforts are being made to improve cardiac imaging and branch into other diagnostic areas.

14.3 The Movement from 1.0 to 3.0

Much of the regular quality control work in nuclear imaging is performed by the technologist. Medical physicists, as in other modalities, may only be present for an annual test of the camera. However, nuclear imaging presents multiple needs that are well addressed by medical physicists (Table 14.2).

The most obvious of these roles is that of Radiation Safety Officer (RSO). The RSO may be a medical physicist, a physician, or a technologist as long as regulatory requirements for training and education are met. Nuclear medicine is perhaps the most highly regulated modality in medical imaging, and few individuals are as intimately familiar with regulations as a medical physicist.

Table 14.2 Comparison of Medical Physics 1.0 and 3.0 paradigms.

Nuclear Medicine	1.0	3.0
Focus of medical physicist' (MP) attention	Equipment, radiation safety	Radiation safety, equipment
Image quality evaluation	Visual, subjective	Mathematical, quantitative
MP "tools of the trade" for image quality evaluation	Spheres, rods in phantom; uniform flood images	Advanced uniformity, noise component analysis
Ongoing QC	Individual subjective evaluation of image quality, manufacturer-specified tests	Automated, remote analysis of advanced image quality metrics
Patient dosimetry	MIRD	Advanced radiation transport, humanoid phantoms
Radiation risk estimation	MIRD	Advanced radiation transport, humanoid phantoms
Commonly used imaging technologies	NaI, PMT	Solid state, direct conversion

Further, medical physicists are often called upon to perform periodic audits of the compliance program for the facility. This level of interaction is helpful as the profession transitions from machine-based support to facility-based, patient-centric support.

The guidelines for testing nuclear cameras have not changed substantially over time. The prevailing document, NEMA NU-1 was originally published in 1980 [16]. Except for the inclusion of SPECT testing, the 2012 version of the document [17] is remarkably similar. The National Electrical Manufacturers Association (NEMA) standard for PET imaging, NU-2, was first published in 1994 [18]. Its 2001 update [19] made significant changes and improvements, but it has not been substantially changed since then. Note also that these publications are equipment-centric. No link to clinical performance is evident. As capabilities and technology of the equipment has advanced, it is necessary to modify test protocols to address clinically relevant issues. Current testing paradigms are not even applicable to some of the new cardiac imaging systems.

Many physicists supporting nuclear imaging facilities are devoted solely to nuclear imaging. While this allows for truly excellent support for those facilities, the prevalence of hybrid imaging systems is necessitating the addition of knowledge and skills in the associated modalities. As with the nuclear imaging, support in the hybrid modality must be clinically focused rather than equipment focused. Issues of dose, clinically relevant image quality metrics, and patient care must be the focus.

As in all imaging modalities, patient dose is receiving increasing attention. Especially for pediatric patients, doses should be scaled by body weight [20]. The Society of Nuclear Medicine and Molecular Imaging also notes that doses should be optimized for all patients [21]. Medical physicists should have the knowledge and experience to assist in this optimization.

The transition to Medical Physics 3.0 should be somewhat easier in nuclear imaging facilities, as physicists supporting them are familiar with involvement beyond just equipment evaluations. It will be necessary to address practice patterns to be more focused on patient care rather than just regulatory compliance. This is a level clinical involvement that may be unfamiliar to some medical physicists.

References

1 Becquerel, H. (1896). Sur les radiations invisible émises par les corps phosphorescent. *Comp. Rend. Acad. Sci.* 122: 501–503.

2 Rutherford, E. and Soddy, F.L.X.I.V. (1902). The cause and nature of radioactivity. – Part I. *Philos. Mag.* 4 (21): 370–396.

3 Rutherford, E. and Soddy, F.L.X.I.V. (1902). The cause and nature of radioactivity. – Part II. *Philos. Mag.* 4 (23): 569–585.

4 de Hevesy, G. (1962). Adventures in Radioisotope Research, The collected papers of George Hevesy. New York: Pergamon Press.

5 Sorensen, L. and Archambault, M. (1963). Visualization of the liver by scanning with Mo99 (molybdate) as tracer. *J. Lab. Clin. Med.* 62: 330–340.

6 Kuhl, D. and Edwards, R. (Apr 1963). Image separation radioisotope scanning. *Radiology* 80: 653–662.

7 Strauss, H.W., Harrison, K., Langan, J.K. et al. (1975). Thallium-201 for myocardial imaging. Relation of thallium-201 to regional myocardial perfusion. *Circulation* 51: 641–645. https://doi.org/10.1161/01.CIR.51.4.641.

8 Sweet, W.H. (1951). The use of nuclear disintegration in diagnosis and treatment of brain tumors. *N. Engl. J. Med.* 245: 875–878.

9 Wrenn, F.R. Jr., Good, M.L., and Handler, P. (1951). The use of positron emitting radioisotopes for localization of brain tumors. *Science* 113: 525–527.

10 Phelps, M.E., Hoffman, E., Mullani, N. et al. (1976). Design considerations for a positron emission transaxial tomograph (PET III). I.E.E.E. Trans. Biomed. Eng. NS-23:516–522.

11 Hoffman, E., Phelps, M., Mullani, N. et al. (1976). Design and performance characteristics of a whole-body transaxial tomograph. *J. Nucl. Med.* 17: 493–503.

12 Melcher, C.L. (1991). Lutetium orthosilicate single crystal scintillator detector. US Patent 5,025,151, June 18.

13 Ido, T., Wan, C.N., Casella, J.S. et al. (1978). Labeled 2-dexoy-D-glucose analogs: 18F labeled 2-deoxy-2-fluoro-D-glucose, 2-deoxy-2-fluoro-D-mannose and 14C-2-deoxy-2-fluoro-D-glucose. *J. Label. Compd. Radiopharm.* 14: 175–183.

14 Schmand, M., Dahlbom, M., and Eriksson, L. (1998). Performance of a LSO/NaI(Tl) phoswitch detector for a combined pet/spect imaging system. *J. Nucl. Med.* 39: 9P.

15 Darambara, D.G. and Todd-Pokropek, A. (2002). Solid state detectors in nuclear medicine. *Q. J. Nucl. Med.* 46 (1): 3–7.

16 National Electrical Manufacturers Association (1980). NEMA Standards Publication NU 1–1980 Performance measurements of scintillation cameras.

17 National Electrical Manufacturers Association (2012). NEMA Standards Publication NU 1–2012 Performance measurements of scintillation cameras.

18 National Electrical Manufacturers Association (1994). NEMA Standards Publication NU 2–1994: Performance Measurements of Positron Emission Tomographs.

19 National Electrical Manufacturers Association (2001). NEMA Standards Publication NU 2–2001: Performance Measurements of Positron Emission Tomographs.

20 Gelfand, M.J., Parisi, M.T., and Treves, S.T. (2011). Pediatric radiopharmaceutical administered doses: 2010 north American consensus guidelines. *J. Nucl. Med.* 52 (2): 318–322.

21 Society of Nuclear Medicine and Molecular Imaging SNMMI Position Statement on Dose Optimization for Nuclear Medicine and Molecular Imaging Procedures. June 2012. http://snmmi.files.cms-plus.com/docs/SNM_Position_Statement_on_Dose_Optimization_FINAL_June_2012.pdf (accessed 20 March 2015).

15

Clinical Nuclear Imaging Physics: Current and Emerging Practice

Jeffrey Nelson and Steven Mann

Clinical Imaging Physics Group, Duke University, Durham, NC, USA

15.1 Introduction

The evolution of new evaluation methodologies in the field of clinical nuclear medicine physics has recently become relatively stagnant, despite the availability of several new commercial offerings of nuclear imaging technologies and features in clinical practice. Additionally, improved access to acquired data and to computer processing now allows more advanced image interrogation not possible in years past. An updated approach to practicing medical physics in nuclear medicine is necessary.

As the landscape of healthcare moves toward precision medicine, where outcome focused results are mandatory in the eyes of hospital administration, nuclear medicine physicists must learn to shift from the traditional focus on equipment performance and more into actual clinical outcomes. The medical physicist must demonstrate value as an integral part of the clinical operation as a whole to remain a vital fixture within the nuclear medicine landscape.

This chapter is intended to provide ideas for advancing the practice of medical physics in nuclear medicine through updated methodologies of equipment evaluation, dose monitoring, and process improvements. The end goal is to move the practice of nuclear medicine physics toward more relevant objectives that demonstrate the value provided by diagnostic medical physicists to the clinical operation.

15.2 Philosophy and Significance

15.2.1 Compliance Assurance

Traditionally, the presence and the scope of a medical physicist within the clinical domain are mostly driven by regulation. For the x-ray modalities, facilities are required by regulation to ensure that equipment performance meets some minimum established compliance or potentially face financial penalty and possible revoked usage rights. Therefore, facilities often utilize a medical physicist to oversee equipment performance. However, in the nuclear medicine setting, Federal, and State regulatory requirements focus largely on the safe handling and accountability of radioactive material (RAM) [1], requiring the utilization of individuals with a health physics background. There is also a

Clinical Imaging Physics: Current and Emerging Practice, First Edition. Edited by Ehsan Samei and Douglas E. Pfeiffer.
© 2020 John Wiley & Sons, Inc. Published 2020 by John Wiley & Sons, Inc.

historic precedence (past regulations) of detailed requirements pertaining to ancillary equipment, such as the dose calibrator, survey meter, and well counter. However, there are currently no regulatory requirements in the United States pertaining to the nuclear imaging equipment's performance or use; the component without which the administration of RAM would be useless in most cases. Unfortunately, without a regulatory mandate in place, it becomes challenging for medical physicists to justify or expand their role within the clinic.

On the equipment evaluation front, professional organizations have published recommendations pertaining to gamma camera quality control (QC) and performance evaluations [2–7]. For a facility, following these recommendations is optional; they are viewed as good practice, but not required except by some accreditation bodies. While it is likely that many nuclear medicine facilities do abide by these recommendations as good internal practice, relying on recommendations alone may be insufficient justification for many medical physicists to expand their operational scope into the nuclear imaging realm.

Nuclear medicine imaging equipment manufactures also publish equipment performance results based on the testing strategies published by the National Electrical Manufacturers Association (NEMA) [4]. By following these detailed testing and analysis procedures, it allows the consumer the ability to directly compare various camera manufactures' systems "apples-to-apples." While these NEMA testing strategies have essentially become the standard for equipment performance evaluations in nuclear imaging, without the backing of being a regulatory requirement, facilities may choose whether to utilize a medical physicist to assess these performance measures.

More recently, the American College of Radiology (ACR) has developed a required set of annual imaging equipment evaluations, which must be carried out by a qualified medical physicist, in order for the imaging center to achieve accreditation status [8]. ACR also defines routine equipment QC evaluations and testing frequencies. Although not a regulatory requirement, currently stand-alone imaging facilities are required to meet and maintain accreditation in all applicable imaging modalities by a designated accrediting organization (such as ACR) to receive full monitory reimbursement from Medicare [9]. Although a step in the right direction for nuclear imaging facilities, these ACR equipment evaluations and QC standards are not groundbreaking, as they are almost identical to the recommended publications referenced above [2, 3, 6] which have been accepted as good practice for decades. Relying on published standards or regulations to gain a foothold into the clinic is advantageous, but relying on them as a best practice is impractical as they are not updated as frequently as new technology is introduced. For instance, the current ACR annual testing requirements, while applicable to the majority of systems, do not currently include guidance on evaluating and monitoring the performance of non-traditional systems which are becoming more prevalent in the clinical practice.

15.2.2 Relevancy of Performance Evaluations

Though developed decades ago, the generally accepted routine QC tests required by the ACR [8] and other accreditation bodies are still largely relevant today, and will likely lead to the identification of a majority of major equipment performance issues prior to imaging patients in the clinic. Most of the basic and most important equipment performance characteristics are monitored: uniformity, linearity and resolution, and single-photon emission computed tomography (SPECT) performance. However, the methods of analysis are largely subjective, or they rely on metrics developed almost 50 years prior [10]. As technology continues to improve and evolve, physicists must reevaluate the current testing methodologies and consider the potential benefits gained with updated or newly developed methods. Updating techniques or metrics may provide improved sensitivity in detecting performance issues that may be missed with current methodologies [11]. Indeed, as alluded to earlier, the current rubric of testing is not even applicable to some modern devices.

Accreditation bodies must have a solid rubric of requirements for sites to follow in order to ensure a minimum level of quality is maintained. Because these requirements must be followed by a wide variety of practice settings, the requirements are typically very basic. It is often difficult for accreditation bodies to update their requirements for fear that some sites may not have the means for compliance. Some facilities may take their own initiative to modify QC strategies, analysis methods, or testing frequencies in order to improve identification of an issue or to optimize clinical efficiency. These modifications would naturally lead to facilities replacing a less reliable test in favor of an updated testing strategy. An unintended consequence of perhaps antiquated accreditation requirements is, in order to become accredited, these sites are now forced to revert back to the required traditional methods which were determined superfluous. It may unintentionally stall the development of testing methodologies by penalizing efforts to improve upon inferior techniques.

Accreditation bodies also typically define medical physics equipment evaluation requirements (Table 15.1). The types of evaluations as defined in the ACR standards are relevant and relatively good indicators of basic equipment performance characteristics of the traditional gamma camera. They assess basic image formation and processing characteristics applicable to clinical use of these systems.

While uniformity, spatial resolution, sensitivity, and energy resolution are all important performance indicators, some of the current standard evaluation techniques and analysis processes are outdated; many of them are still purely subjective. While assessing the spatial resolution subjectively using a four-quadrant bar phantom (Figure 15.1) may be convenient, it does not provide the most meaningful and comprehensive description of the system's resolution performance. Additionally, at the time many of the current standards were developed, the landscape of computer processing was significantly more limited than today. It was difficult for most physicists to harvest the acquired images for off-line analysis, and many of the camera workstations were limited to pixel value-based analysis.

Table 15.1 List of the technologist required quality control tests as required by the American College of Radiology for accredited gamma camera systems [8]. The required frequency and purpose are also noted.

NM Technologist QC Test	Frequency	Purpose
Intrinsic or System Uniformity	Each day of use	To verify components are properly functioning and provide a uniform image in response to a uniform flux of radiation
Intrinsic or System Spatial Resolution	Weekly	To verify detector spatial resolution is satisfactory for clinical imaging
Center-of-Rotation (SPECT systems)	Monthly	To maintain ability to resolve details in clinical SPECT studies
High-Count Floods For Uniformity Correction	As recommended by a qualified medical physicist	To correct for residual detector and collimator non-uniformity and to minimize the production for artifacts in clinical studies
Overall System Performance for SPECT Systems	Semiannually required, quarterly recommended	To qualitatively verify system has maintained its capabilities with respect to tomographic uniformity, contrast, and spatial resolution that maximize the benefits in clinical studies

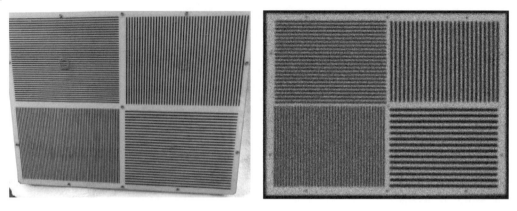

Figure 15.1 Left: Photograph of a typical four-quadrant bar phantom. Right: Extrinsic acquisition of the bar phantom using Co-57 sheet source for seven-million counts.

In order for equipment evaluation strategies to remain relevant, they must follow the growth and evolution of the modality as advancements in technology occur. One recent and significant growth in the nuclear imaging field has been the widespread adaptation of hybrid SPECT/computed tomography (CT) imaging. Current SPECT/CT units typically employ either a fully diagnostic or a low-output CT component for providing anatomical information and attenuation correction for the SPECT emission data. Some SPECT/CT systems are also capable of being used as a stand-alone clinical diagnostic-quality CT unit. Although clinical CT equipment evaluations and QC procedures are well established, with the wide variety in the utilization of the CT component in the nuclear imaging setting, modification to the standard evaluations may be necessary.

Whenever a new component is introduced into the clinical field, such as the addition of CT to SPECT, the medical imaging physicist is the expert within the clinic with the knowledge and training to define appropriate physics evaluations and QC procedures. Facilities will utilize these new technologies differently, specific to the needs of their particular clinic, making it necessary for the medical imaging physicist to interact with the clinical staff to help decide appropriate methods of performance evaluation and monitoring. These interactions are necessary in order for the medical physicist to become fully integrated into the clinical setting.

Most of the current nuclear medicine performance testing has been designed around the predominant Anger-style gamma camera. However, an increasing number of non-traditional systems are being introduced which replace the traditional sodium iodide (NaI) scintillation crystal/photomultiplier tube (PMT) configuration. New detector technologies, such as solid-state detectors, and systems employing non-traditional imaging configurations have entered the clinical practice [12–15]. Testing methodologies must be adapted to thoroughly and appropriately evaluate these non-traditional additions.

Solid state detectors are comprised of individual pixelated detectors that function as direct detectors, converting gamma rays directly into charge for collection. The individual detector elements alleviate the need for positioning circuitry which was a source of resolution degradation in traditional camera systems. Cross-talk between detector elements is also reduced, resulting in resolution being largely dominated by detector geometry and pixel size [16, 17]. The traditional evaluation of spatial linearity, imaging the four-quadrant bar phantom, is no longer necessary. However, other routine tests may be necessary to ensure the proper functioning of solid state detectors. For example, the energy resolution of cadmium zinc telluride (CZT) detectors is typically superior to traditional NaI systems due to the improved photon-to-signal conversion efficiency [18]. However, both imperfections in CZT material and the operating electronics can lead to degraded energy resolution in the form of both incomplete charge collection ("tailing") and non-uniform performance across detector pixels [16, 17]. These new considerations may require more sophisticated evaluations beyond the measurements of a single full width at half maximum (FWHM) of the photopeak. Such evaluations may necessitate the need for access to list mode data, and, if so, the medical physicist community must stress the importance of that data to vendors. Likewise, solid state detectors often utilize collimators with matched holes-to-pixels to maximize sensitivity and resolution. Because mismatch between the collimator holes and detector pixels can reduce the performance of solid state detectors, it may be prudent to evaluate the impact of the system sensitivity and resolution when accepting a system or deploying a new collimator.

Even with these substantial changes to our imaging systems, the common performance characteristics do remain similar to those of the Anger-style systems. Ideally, our traditional testing methods should be modified to better characterize and evaluate these new technologies. In the case of uniformity testing, artifacts will manifest differently; from PMT artifacts in the Anger-style systems, to pixel-based artifacts [19] in the solid state systems. Traditional strategies for objectively evaluating uniformity images may need to be reevaluated to ensure sensitivity to the presence of these new type of artifacts. It is also likely some of the staple evaluations that are commonly performed on the Anger-style systems will not be needed with the new solid state based systems. For instance, planar spatial linearity is a very important evaluation in traditional scintillation systems. The scintillation light is collected non-uniformly across the face of the PMT. This requires a specific linearity correction in order to calibrate the X–Y spatial locations across the field of view (FOV). However, since the solid state detectors are pixelated, there will be no need to evaluate this characteristic.

The current traditional equipment evaluation strategies may not only be lagging behind due to the new technological advancements in the modality. There are technologies introduced many years ago which are now completely integrated into the clinical workflow that still need standard testing strategies defined. For instance, continuous whole body imaging is quite common in the clinical nuclear medicine setting, yet typically no evaluations are performed on the whole body mode of the system. The timing of the electronic collimators opening and closing accurately, as well as scan speed accuracy are both vital for the uniformity of clinical whole-body scans, yet are typically not part of a medical physicist's evaluations. This can be evaluated simply by performing a clinical bone scan acquisition with a Co-57 sheet source lying on the detector. Visual analysis of the image uniformity and image profile plot as well as a quantitative uniformity analysis would be appropriate for analyzing the image (Figure 15.2). Cardiac gating is another example of a commonly used mode in the clinic which has not yet found its way into the medical physicist's equipment report. The proper binning of acquisition data acquired according to the patient's cardiac rhythm is critical in the dictation of both myocardial perfusion imaging and MUGA studies. Evaluating this feature would require an ECG simulator, which is a common tool found in a hospital Biomedical Department. For example, a point source of activity could be imaged while simulating a constant rhythm and analyzing the time activity curve.

15.2.3 Clinical Focus

Perhaps more importantly, medical physicists must expand their responsibilities beyond a solely equipment-focused mindset to providing a more hands-on approach to improving the clinical operation. There is importance in ensuring the imaging equipment is operating appropriately by performing quality assurance evaluations, but it is equally important to ensure the imaging machine is being used appropriately. One area the medical physicist can provide great benefit to

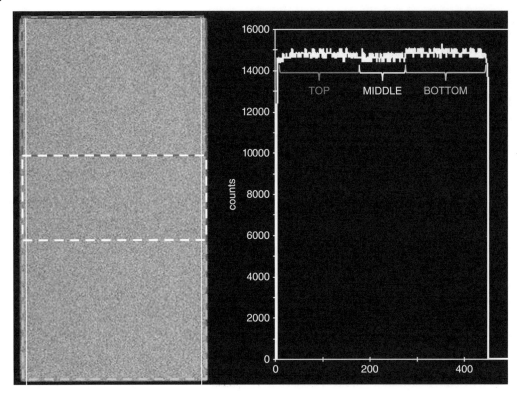

Figure 15.2 A 100 cm acquisition and profile analysis of a Co-57 sheet source using a continuous whole body acquisition mode. In this example the top, middle, and bottom areas of the image show similar counts on the profile, indicating adequate timing of the electronic collimators and table motion.

the clinic is in the area of protocol development. Having knowledge in the intricacies of each machine within the fleet, and knowing how each machine is different from the adjacent room, protocol definitions may be transformed from blanket "one size fits all" into patient/equipment specific protocols in order to deliver high quality personalized imaging.

Medical physicists must seek out opportunities where their physics knowledge and unique perspective may be used to greatly impact the clinical operation. Within the clinical operation, there are tasks which the medical physicist may help to streamline, helping the clinic save time and energy. For example, the daily technologist uniformity test contains several steps including acquiring, analyzing, issue reporting, and archiving the uniformity image. Perhaps for the acquisition task, the medical physicist may look to adjust the parameters to better optimize the acquisition time/artifact detection trade-off. The medical physicist may develop improved metrics for the task of identifying relevant clinical artifacts, or adjust the thresholds to better flag potential problems, ensuring clinical studies will not be suboptimal. Working hand-in-hand with the clinical staff, the medical physicist may help develop a strategy to streamline the workflow to not only improve efficiency, but also improve the task of detecting and expediting repair of artifacts.

Another important clinical focus for the medical physicist is how to communicate testing results to their consumer, the clinic, in a meaningful way. As data is interrogated from equipment performance and QC evaluations, the medical physicist should focus on how those results are directly related to clinical imaging performance. Rephrase testing results from reporting just numbers into terms of how they affect clinical use; make the results more meaningful or clinically relevant to the clinical users. Instead of only reporting a simple value for percent-difference, add wording as to how this number will impact clinical acquisition or task detection.

Physicists should also be more engaging with end users, the interpreting physicians. Routinely ask for their input on clinical quality improvement projects; they have a good understanding on which projects would be most beneficial to the clinical operation. Be more direct with inquiring about physician needs in the clinic in order to identify current situations which result in suboptimal image quality or operational inefficiencies. Also, providing education to technologists, physicians, even patients is a vital part of the medical physicist's responsibilities.

In addition to staying clinically and operationally engaged, medical physicist must make time for professional development as well. Take the time to review recent scientific publications in order to bring new ideas into the practice and to keep up to date on what is going on in the field. Understand the benefits and risks of emerging technologies that may become a clinical option in the near future. Perhaps there is a new option on the market which will fulfill a current clinical need or help solve an inefficiency within the clinic. These are the types of topics many hospital administrators will want to discuss with their medical imaging physicist for input with purchasing decisions.

Hospital administrations are also paying increasingly close attention and devoting many resources to ensuring hospital accreditation requirements are being followed. This area is an opportunity for medical physicists to demonstrate to the hospital administrators the value they bring beyond equipment performance evaluations. Many of the accreditation-required processes lend themselves nicely for medical physicist involvement or even becoming project lead. Physicists must go one step beyond the traditional equipment-focused mindset and put their worth into the context of improving the overall clinical practice.

15.3 Metrics and Analytics

Over the past few years, medical physicists have benefited from the advances in digital image transfer and storage. This has lead to easier access to acquired image data; both clinical images and QC data. Along with greater image processing power and improved methods, the opportunity now presents for better analysis in the areas of physics equipment evaluations as well as clinical image quality evaluations. In years past, analysis methods were limited to relatively first-order methods, based mostly on pixel values. Some evaluations are even purely subjective. Unfortunately, most of these rudimentary techniques are still in use today. There is great opportunity for the medical physicist to develop better evaluation strategies.

15.3.1 Intrinsic Performance

One of the most important performance characteristics of a nuclear medicine imaging system is the uniformity of the image across the FOV. The traditional Anger-style gamma camera is considered relatively unstable within the realm of clinical medical imaging equipment. Each individual dynode within each PMT requires a precise voltage to achieve uniformity across the entire FOV. Additionally, there are inherent structural differences in the scintillation crystal itself, as well as numerous electronics including amplifiers, positioning circuits, analog to digital converters, and power supplies, which may be a source of non-uniformities. As a result, each day, prior to patient imaging, it is traditionally required that a uniformity test be performed. After acquiring an image from a uniform flux of radiation, the image is analyzed, typically by subjective visual assessment. It is also common to perform an

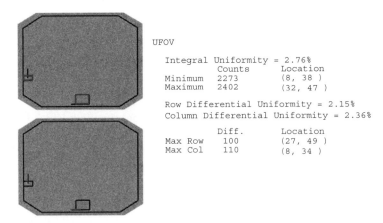

```
UFOV

Integral Uniformity = 2.76%
                Counts        Location
Minimum     2273          (8, 38 )
Maximum     2402          (32, 47 )

Row Differential Uniformity = 2.15%
Column Differential Uniformity = 2.36%

                Diff.         Location
Max Row     100           (27, 49 )
Max Col     110           (8, 34 )
```

Figure 15.3 Image analysis using the Integral and Differential uniformity calculations. Top image highlights (in red) the areas used for Integral Uniformity calculation, bottom image highlights the areas used for Differential Uniformity calculation.

Integral and Differential uniformity calculation (Figure 15.3). One criticism of this uniformity calculation is it sometimes fails to detect instances of visually apparent subtle non-uniform structure within the image (Figure 15.4). While these non-uniformities may be subtle, they are nonetheless important to identify as they indicate an emerging issue with the imaging system. Medical physicists now have the capability to develop and utilize more sophisticated analysis methods to better identify imaging system problems.

One method commonly used in image analysis in medical imaging modalities is the Noise Power Spectrum (NPS) which analyzes the frequency component of the image to infer the texture of the image [20–22]. This method has proven beneficial when extended to nuclear medicine for analysis of uniformity images [11, 23, 24]. Integrating this technique into a uniformity analysis metric, any non-uniform structure (i.e. non-stochastic) would be identified as a spike in the frequency spectrum compared against the expected stochastic properties of a completely uniform image (Figure 15.5). This technique could allow for a better description of the image instead of only using the Integral Uniformity which describes the variance in pixel values across the smoothed image to indicate if a non-uniformity is present or not.

Another important performance aspect of nuclear medicine imaging systems is the linearity. Because of the inherent non-uniform collection of scintillation light across the surface of PMTs (Figure 15.6), the imaging system requires a linearity correction file which maps the physical X–Y location of known calibration points throughout the FOV to create a linear image. As is the case with uniformity, as the voltage of the PMT drifts, the linearity of the image may be affected and should be evaluated on a regular frequency (weekly per current ACR requirements). The linearity performance evaluation traditionally involves the imaging of a phantom consisting of horizontal and vertical lead bars of varying widths (bar phantom) (Figure 15.2) and subjective visual inspection of the resulting image. As with most subjective evaluations, the quality of this assessment is dependent on the analysis time and quality of observer, which may change from week to week. This type of subjective analysis is not ideal for a QC evaluation which requires consistency from week to week. A better alternative for analyzing the images would be designing an objective analysis program, perhaps utilizing mutual information algorithms. This could be achieved by acquiring an x-ray image of the phantom used in order to create the template. An algorithm could then detect differences between the acquired image

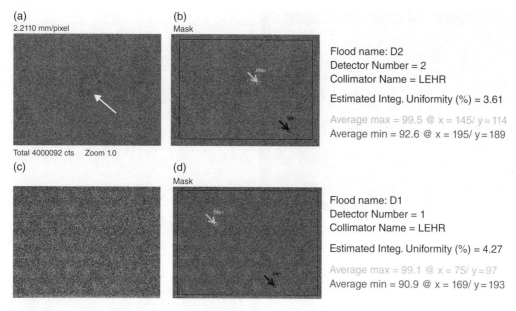

Figure 15.4 Examples of two flood field images with visually apparent artifacts and their Integral Uniformity calculation results. Top flood field image (a) and (b) contains a single PMT artifact in center of image (white arrow), bottom image (c) and (d) contains several PMT artifacts throughout the image, most visible in the lower left quadrant. The reported Integral Uniformity values are within acceptable limits (<5.0%).

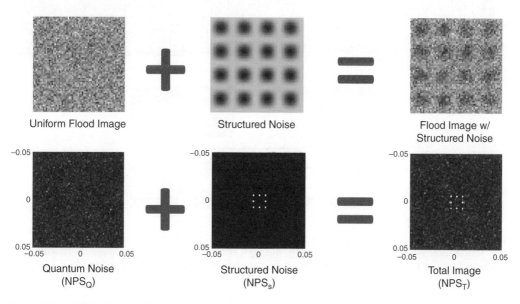

Figure 15.5 Example of how the 2D-NPS changes when structured noise is added to a uniform flood image. The top left image represents a uniform flood image with its corresponding NPS in the bottom left. The center top image represents structured noise from photomultiplier tubes and its corresponding NPS shown center bottom. The right top image represents the structured noise added to the uniform flood image with the corresponding NPS shown bottom right demonstrating the presence of spikes in the NPS at the corresponding frequencies. Quantification of these spikes may be used to design a uniformity analysis metric [11].

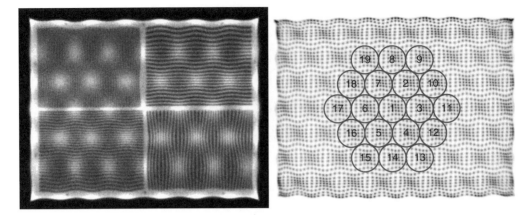

Figure 15.6 Left: Bar phantom imaged with no linearity correction. Right: Solid lead sheet with evenly spaced holes imaged with no linearity correction. The approximate location of the PMTs is shown.

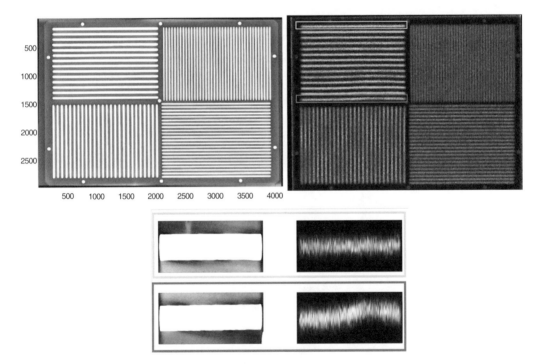

Figure 15.7 Left: X-ray template of a bar phantom. Middle: Overlay of NM bar phantom acquisition on X-ray image with two example bars highlighted with light and dark boxes. Right: Example of linearity analysis on the light and dark boxed bars showing a linearity defect along the bottom blue bar.

and the template (Figure 15.7). A scoring rubric would also be created to track performance from week-to-week and a threshold established for flagging outliers. This analysis method would save time, be objective and reproducible, be able to quantify the phantom results that can then be tracked over time.

A third common performance specification in nuclear medicine is spatial resolution. Traditionally, gamma camera resolution is evaluated by imaging line sources filled with radiotracer and measuring the FWHM and maybe the full width at tenth maximum (FWTM) of the line spread function (LSF). It is a quite simple way to quantify the resolution of the system, but several assumptions also come along with using this method. The FWHM only represents the center of the peak, so it is possible for several differently shaped peaks to measure the same FWHM value. This analysis method makes assumptions that the peaks are symmetrical, and the distribution is Gaussian. A more complete assessment would be to measure the modulation transfer function (MTF) across the detector to characterize the system performance of spatial resolution in the frequency domain. Edge or radial MTFs could be measured from square or circular objects (such as petri dish) at several locations across the FOV (Figure 15.8). The MTF could also be determined from images of a line source, however, to obtain MTF information at multiple locations across the detector would require the placement of multiple sources in various orientations [25].

15.3.2 Qualimetry

Describing the system's resolution performance in the frequency domain via the MTF and the system's uniformity characteristics in the frequency domain via the NPS are useful measures independently as described in the previous section. An additional use of these frequency descriptions

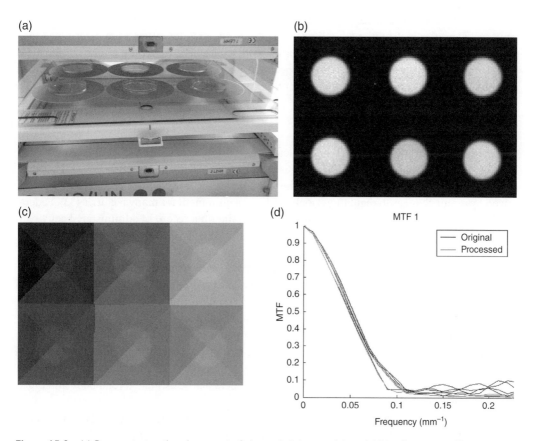

Figure 15.8 (a) Demonstrates the placement of six petri dishes positioned 10 cm from top collimator surface. (b) Acquired image of the six petri dishes. (c) Demonstrates the four radial MTF measurements which can be made from each petri dish. (d) Resulting MTF curves from one of the petri dishes. This method can be used to characterize the MTF at multiple locations across the detector.

of imaging system characteristics would be to combine these into a single performance metric called the detectability index [26–29]. The detectability index quantifies the likelihood of the imaging system detecting a particular object, as defined by a task function. The task function may model a tumor, defining the contrast, size, shape, and edge profile. By utilizing actual system characteristics, such as noise (NPS) and resolution (MTF), and taking into account human visual frequency filters which include viewing distance and display size, the detectability index equation can provide an estimate of detectability of the object. For a detectability index to be applied in the context of nuclear medicine, consideration would need to be made for the distance-dependent resolution of the detector. This metric may be useful for many clinical situations including comparison of different imaging systems, in protocol development, and determining the impact of QC results in clinically applicable terms.

When QC results are near or exceed defined failure thresholds, it is the responsibility of the clinical imaging physicists to determine how and to what degree this result will affect the clinical performance of the system. Currently, using traditional means, the impact is nearly impossible to quantify. However, by measuring an MTF and NPS from the failing system, and incorporating these into the detectability index, one would be able to confidently provide a meaningful answer in the context of the clinical needs. This would allow for a more informed decision about using the system for clinical diagnosis.

Another use of the detectability index in nuclear medicine would be as an aid in developing system specific protocols. Traditionally, clinical studies are acquired for either a pre-determined time or number of counts, regardless of the imaging system. Being able to utilize the resolution and noise properties of the system would allow for protocols tailored specific for each system, especially those with significantly different imaging components such as the crystal thickness, or PMT vintage.

15.3.3 Radiometry

There are several specific areas where nuclear medicine as a modality is lagging behind other imaging modalities; patient dose monitoring is one example. The idea of monitoring patient radiation dose, or some surrogate [30–32], for the CT modality is now becoming common practice, driven by recent changes to regulations making this a requirement for many facilities [33]. Federal regulations do require nuclear medicine facilities to maintain a record of administered activity to patients; however, it is not common practice to take this one step further and employ any type of patient dose calculation/monitoring in the clinical setting.

In the United States, the approval process for a radiopharmaceutical includes submission of radiometric data including estimated absorbed radiation dose conversion factors [34]. Separate tables specific to age groups or gender are also common. With this wealth of information easily assessable to the medical physicist, taking the next step to calculate and database patient dose estimates should be a low hanging fruit. After the patient administration record is harvested for the nuclear medicine (NM) database (most facilities have converted to electronic records), the medical physicist may find a way to combine the data with look-up-tables of conversion factors, based on radiopharmaceutical, and patient age and gender, to calculate the estimated total body and organ dose for each patient.

There are many uses for calculating patient dose data in nuclear medicine. Having patient values represented in effective dose equivalent (millisievert) rather than administered activity (millicurie) will allow us to compare and better understand the true magnitude of any outliers. Just as five millicuries of two different radiopharmaceuticals may have orders of magnitude differences in effective dose equivalent, five millicuries of the same radiopharmaceutical will have

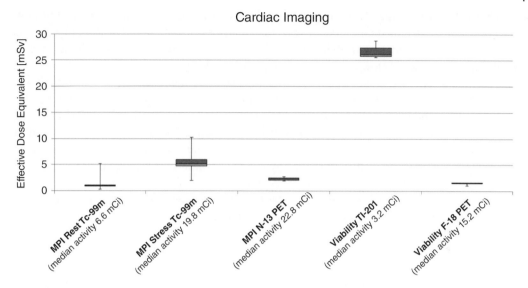

Figure 15.9 Example of how a nuclear medicine dose monitoring program can be used for comparing the effective dose equivalent from five different cardiac imaging studies. The median injected activity for each study is also noted in parentheses. This example nicely illustrates that the injected activity would not be a useful metric for comparing various clinical imaging studies.

a different effective dose equivalent across genders and age. Hence, describing outliers in reference to the effective dose would be more informative than by administered activity. We may also use this patient dose data to aid in protocol optimization; balancing imagine quality with demographic specific risk. The data may also be useful when comparing two nuclear imaging studies using different radiopharmaceuticals, or to demonstrate the result of a changed protocol (Figure 15.9). Finally, calculating, and recording the dose data may be useful for comparing dose across different modalities and creating a facility-wide dose record for the patient.

15.4 Testing Implication of New Technologies

As new technologies continue to enter into the clinical setting, it presents a challenge to the medical physicist of how to properly evaluate a new feature or new imaging technique. Additionally, the clinical operation is challenged with how to best utilize these advancements, ensure it is performing as intended, and quantify the benefit it provides. These are all important aspects to determine, and are best answered with guidance from the medical physicist. This is not an easy task; the physics community must come together to develop new testing strategies for these systems and share knowledge gained from performance evaluations. Publishing testing methods, participating in listservs, and presenting at conferences are all opportunities to help the physics community in this realm.

15.4.1 Hardware

One of the more recent hardware advancements in the nuclear medicine modality is the addition of CT to nuclear medicine SPECT systems. When first introduced in the commercial clinical scene, circa 1999, the x-ray component was typically comprised of a low-power x-ray generator which slowly rotated around the patient (typically 20 seconds/rotation) [35]. The image quality from these CT series was limited due to the low mA (maximum 2.5 mA) produced by the x-ray tube. As a result, their use was limited to attenuation correction and localization purposes. Physics evaluations from these relatively low-risk tubes were typically limited to a SPECT-to-CT registration test, and perhaps a few basic image quality evaluations using the manufacturer supplied phantom. However, as time passed the technology improved, and the majority of current SPECT/CT systems now include the option of a fully functional, diagnostic quality, multi-slice CT system. This not only leads to questions about who is qualified to operate these units, but also how they should be evaluated by the medical physicist. The medical physicist should design the QC and annual testing based on how the system is being used clinically. If the CT is used solely for attenuation correction and localization of nuclear medicine studies, it would be acceptable to perform only limited testing – perhaps evaluation of co-registration, basic CT performance, and modified image quality aspects would be adequate. However, if the system is used for full diagnostic CT studies, a complete comprehensive CT evaluation is warranted.

For all systems utilizing CT for NM attenuation correction, the medical physicist should assess the NM-CT co-registration, and perform a comprehensive interrogation of the HU accuracy. These are important aspects to evaluate as the attenuation correction is derived directly from the CT data. The CT numbers should be evaluated for the clinically used kVp settings as the HU-kVp dependence is not typically stable [36, 37]. An expanded test could be deployed to assess the kVp and depth (attenuation) dependence of HU. The Mercury phantom [22] would be a logical choice for this new evaluation as it contains multiple rods of a wide range of HU materials embedded within cylinders of varying diameters. The results from this evaluation would also aid with protocol definitions for determining the lowest appropriate mA one may use for low-dose attenuation only studies while still ensuring the fidelity of HU values as well as minimal image quality attributes.

After the fidelity of the HU is determined, the next step would be to evaluate if the system is properly calculating the attenuation. If the system attenuation map is available to the user, reviewing the attenuation coefficients used for reconstruction would be an ideal approach. If the correction map is not viewable, one could assess this by imaging identical concentrations of radiotracer through varying amounts of attenuating material and reconstructing using attenuation correction software. To provide a clinically-meaningful assessment, it will be important to use scanner and attenuation conditions similar to those encountered in clinical study conditions.

The QC requirements for these SPECT/CT will also depend on the clinical use of the system. If the system is used for performing any diagnostic-quality CT exams, the full gamut of the CT department QC program should be followed. Unfortunately, because these scanners are often in a different hospital department than the stand-alone diagnostic CT scanners, and typically under different management, they are often not thought of in the same context and may be overlooked. If the CT component is not used in a full diagnostic-quality capacity, the medical physicist should design a QC program focused around the extent of its clinical use.

New collimator designs for gamma cameras are also becoming more common in the clinical arena. Until recently, the vast majority of collimators in clinical use have been traditional parallel-hole collimators (with the exception of the pinhole collimator commonly used for thyroid imaging studies). The properties of these collimators are relatively straight forward and our traditional testing strategies are designed around these designs. Understanding the performance characteristics of parallel-hole collimators has become second nature; the resolution degrades with increasing distance while sensitivity remains relatively constant [16]. Recently, as manufacturers continue to strive for the upper hand in the nuclear medicine market, alternative collimator designs, each specifically designed for an imaging task, are being utilized more frequently. For instance, for the task of cardiac imaging, vendors are introducing a variety of converging and multi-pinhole designs (and camera rotation orbits) in an attempt to improve the resolution and sensitivity of the cardiac FOV [38, 39]. Performing a physics evaluation of resolution, sensitivity, count rate, and SPECT performance will not follow traditional testing strategies. Medical physicists must take the time and effort to work directly with the manufacturer to develop and publish appropriate testing strategies specific to the technology.

New detector technology is also entering into the clinical realm. Replacing the traditional NaI scintillation crystals paired with PMTs, solid state detectors made from CdTe or CZT are increasingly entering the market. The availability of solid state detector designs is due in large part to improvements in the fabrication of solid state materials. Detectors made from CdTe or CdZnTe (CZT) are pixelated and, in the case of parallel-hole collimators, are combined with hole-matched collimators. Combining the design with the elimination of the inefficiencies of light spreading and PMT collection in traditional scintillators yields significant improvements in spatial resolution. Direct detection also results in significantly lower variability in the signal generated by an absorbed photon, yielding excellent energy resolution (2–5%) compared with traditional NaI detectors (~10%) [16–18].

For these solid state systems, the spatial resolution of the pixelated system at the detector surface will primarily be determined by the pixel pitch of the detector elements. Current standard spatial resolution tests may not be useful for this solid-state technology. The traditional method of measuring line profiles from capillary tubes filed with radiotracer could still be useful for this technology. It could be used in characterizing the spatial resolution degradation as the source to detector increases, and to compare imaging system performance with other systems in your fleet to aid in protocol optimization tasks. Care must be taken in the positioning of the line sources for pixelated detectors; instances where the source is aligned with the pixel rows would yield a better result than when the source is spread across multiple rows. Therefore, the average of multiple measurements as the source is slightly displaced across the detector would be important in order to return a more accurate measurement result [4]. For a more complete measurement, a pre-sampled MTF measurement could be accomplished using the capillary tube measurements or a petri dish filled with a shallow radioactive solution. Similar to radiography, this measurement would provide information about the detector characteristics across a range of spatial frequencies and be less influenced by the relative positioning of the source to the detector pixels. Unlike the NaI detector, where resolution and linearity can be highly dependent on the position on the detector face, the MTF of a solid state unit should be largely independent of location.

Another characteristic in which solid-state detectors differ from our traditional Anger-style gamma cameras is the analysis of count rate performance. Some solid-state systems may not demonstrate the same dead-time behavior as measured in traditional NaI systems (Figure 15.10). Measuring the count rate on the typical Anger-style clinical systems demonstrates the text-book paralyzable dead-time curve. The solid-state detector designs allows for independent signal readout and processing for each detector element within the detector, allowing for linear count rate response at even very high count rates [40]. It is imperative that the medical physicist understand the operational parameters of the unit to know the impact of both photons absorbed during dead-time and system-specific acquisition thresholds.

There may also be aspects of a traditional performance test where only slight modification may be required. With the improved energy resolution solid-state technology brings, the current energy resolution testing of reporting a peak energy and the FWHM percentage may not be sufficient to fully characterize or assess the performance of these systems. Incomplete charge collection in solid state detectors can significantly impact energy resolution due to a broadening of the lower-energy

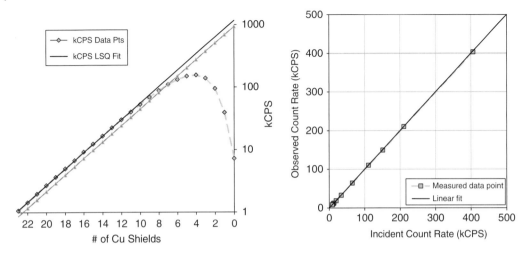

Figure 15.10 Count Rate Performance Evaluation measured for (LEFT) a traditional NaI scintillation gamma camera (GE Discovery 630) and (RIGHT) a solid state CZT dedicated cardiac camera (GE Discovery 530c).

side of the photopeak. The non-Gaussian response of the detector may require more sophisticated measures of energy resolution than a system-reported FWHM; it may be necessary to require vendors to give medical physicists access to full-spectra or list mode data to assess the impact of incomplete charge collection across the entire detector. Additionally, with the improvement in energy resolution, clinical tasks may begin to routinely include imaging studies using multiple isotopes. Simultaneous Technetium-99 m and Iodine-123 dual-radionuclide imaging has clinical promise in myocardial, parathyroid, and brain imaging [41–44]. With new clinical tasks in mind, a possible strategy to modify current energy resolution performance evaluations would be performing the test using a mixed-isotope source. This dual-isotope analysis may also be beneficial to assess uniformity and sensitivity.

15.4.2 Acquisition Methods

Nuclear imaging systems having non-traditional imaging geometries are also becoming more common in the clinical realm. Many of these systems are designed for cardiac-specific imaging applications. For instance, to take advantage of the magnification properties provided by pinhole collimators, one system is employing multiple pinhole collimators coupled with solid-state pixelated detectors [13, 45], with each detector-collimator pair precisely angled to provide a complete coverage of the heart. This allows for stationary acquisition protocols. Another cardiac-specific system is designed using rotating detector arrays to properly sample the heart [14, 19]. These non-traditional alignments present some interesting challenges when trying to carry out performance testing using traditional evaluation strategies. The traditional SPECT phantoms, designed to evaluate a large FOV system, will not work in all situations. Developing new phantom designs, ideally which more closely relate to the clinical task at hand, are needed to properly evaluate these new novel imaging systems.

Properly evaluating the sensitivity of these non-traditional imaging geometries may also be a challenge. In traditional systems, because of the corrections applied, the sensitivity is relatively uniform across the FOV [16]. However, for systems specifically designed to fully sample only a targeted region, it will require new evaluation strategies. The geometry of the source used for the evaluation will be important, as well as placement of the source within the FOV. One strategy for mapping out the sensitivity of these unique systems is imaging a point source at several locations throughout the FOV [45] to better characterize the system sensitivity. These results will be useful for optimizing the clinical imaging operation including patient positioning.

The need for updated testing strategies is not limited to new technologies; some of the acquisition methods commonly employed in the clinical setting for several years or decades are still not included in the traditional evaluation scheme. One example is dynamic mode imaging which is common in the clinical setting, used to capture the initial flow of a radiopharmaceutical as it is enters the body or evaluate the physiological movement over a defined time. This mode is often used for quantitative imaging studies, in which the precision and accuracy of each acquired frame is important. Evaluation of this imaging mode may be performed by intrinsically imaging a point source for a set time (perhaps 30 seconds) with both a static acquisition and a dynamic acquisition using the shortest frame time available with the number of frames to match the total time of the static acquisition [6]. Use a stopwatch to physically time each image acquisition. Record the counts for the static image and each frame of the dynamic images. The physical time, static image time, and sum or the apparent frame times should vary by no more than 5%. Also, perform a chi-square analysis for the counts of the dynamic frames using a 95% confidence limit. Excessive variation in apparent frame times may indicate an issue in the camera-computer interface, or issues with the camera such as a drifting pulse height analyzer window.

Likewise, gated mode acquisitions are common in the clinical setting, especially for performing cardiac imaging studies. When acquiring cardiac studies in this mode, the acquisition data is binned based on ECG cycle allowing for assessment of cardiac wall motion. With high precision needed for accurate quantification, and the clinical importance of this procedure, it is vital to ensure all aspects of the cardiac gating is functioning properly. Designing an evaluation scheme for the gated acquisition mode may require additional hardware, such as an ECG simulator (which can often be borrowed from a hospital biomedical department), but the reward of identifying an issue or verifying proper working order upon installation into the clinic would make it worthwhile. One strategy to evaluate gated acquisition mode is to image a point source using typical exam settings and a normal ECG signal. The resulting time-activity curve of the point source should form a horizontal line with a suggested variation limit of three times the standard deviation of the random counting error (square root of the mean) [6].

15.4.3 Imaging Processing and Analysis

SPECT imaging has become a vital part of the current clinical nuclear medicine setting. When first introduced, clinical reconstruction of the projection images was performed using simple back-projection methods employing a ramp filter to remove the $1/r$ blurring, along with a post-process filter to smooth the image in order to make it more palatable [16]. There were only a few settings to change, mostly adjusting the post-processing filter to tweak the smoothness of the image. As computing power grows, it is becoming increasingly common for vendors to provide some iterative reconstruction filter options. Iterative filters are typically more sophisticated than filtered back projection (FBP) as they can account for particular aspects of the imaging system, including resolution and noise properties, as well as attenuation and scattering properties. Such sophisticated reconstruction methods allow for more dramatic changes to the image with the intent of improving the image quality. With these filters there are often several user options to set, including the number of iterations and subsets as well as the processing filter levels as with the FBP.

Many vendors are offering iterative reconstruction processing techniques as additional software processing packages for purchase. The advertising claims for many of these packages are allowing for less injected activity, shorter acquisition times, and providing superior image quality [46, 47]. However, consumers may be skeptical of this win-win-win situation which defies the traditional balance between injected activity and acquisition time. The medical physicist plays an important role in evaluating these claims, as well as helping to ensure that the reconstruction is properly setup and utilized appropriately in the clinic. It is not uncommon for vendors to provide a 30-day trial of new processing software programs, allowing the medical physicist time to interrogate the product and inform the clinic of any limitations within their clinical operation. Suggestions made by the medical physicist will directly impact the purchasing decision process, potentially giving the clinic improved leverage in negotiations. Additionally, publishing these trial results will help educate others in the imaging community. The unbiased data will be especially helpful to those facilities unable to include a medical physicist in the decision-making process.

15.4.4 New System-Wide Technologies

With the recent commercialization of new detection technologies, including solid state and pixelated systems, as well as the evolution of iterative reconstruction methods, there are many opportunities for medical physics to play a key role in the adaptation and utilization of these technologies in the clinical setting. Aside from developing new evaluation and characterization strategies, the adaptation of these technologies in the clinical setting requires modification of the current traditional imaging protocols. Currently, solid state detectors are emerging in organ-specific scanners, such as dedicated cardiac systems. Designing specific application systems allows manufacturers the opportunity to significantly deviate from traditional imaging geometries in order to gain advantages in certain performance aspects, such as sensitivity or resolution. As a result, clinics may have the option of altering their typical imaging protocols, including decreasing the administered activity or acquisition time, without sacrificing image quality. Medical physicists have the opportunity to become involved in helping to determine the best way to optimize the new protocols to take advantage of the changes in technology.

As a part of protocol optimization, the medical physicist must also educate the clinic on the findings from their thorough evaluations and understanding of the new technology's capabilities. For instance, it is possible that some systems are designed with non-uniform sensitivity across the FOV in order to achieve the greatest sensitivity in the typical organ location. This is vastly different from the traditional parallel-hole collimator scintillation camera which has roughly the same sensitivity across the central FOV. Utilizing the measured sensitivity data from the physics evaluation, the medical physicists must educate the clinic on this particular characteristic of the system so they may better understand these differences and prevent a poor clinical quality scan.

Proper assessment of this new technology will also likely require redesigning or developing new phantoms. Ideally phantom designs should mimic the unit's clinical utility in both size and geometry, and measure the traditional system characteristics of resolution, sensitivity, and uniformity. Data from these phantoms will be instrumental in defining new protocols and image processing settings for the clinical implementation of this technology. The new phantoms may also be designed to represent clinically-relevant anatomy, such as the already existing cardiac phantom with interchangeable stenosis inserts [48] which would be extremely beneficial for comparing new technology against the traditional systems and evaluating protocol changes.

15.5 Clinical Integration and Implementation

It is important that practicing clinical medical physicists be an integral part of the clinical operation. The medical physicist brings additional knowledge to the table which the other clinical staff (technologists, radiologists, radiopharmacists, service engineers, etc.) will not have. It is also important for the medical physicist to recognize the contributions and knowledge that other clinical staff members bring to the clinic outside of the physicist's expertise. A symbiotic relationship must exist between medical physics and the clinic.

15.5.1 Training and Communication

Within the clinical setting, the addition of new equipment and technological offerings can become very disruptive. When new equipment is installed, it will take the technologists and radiologists time to become comfortable operating, processing, and viewing images from the new equipment. Additionally there may be new acquisition or processing features they will need to learn. It is often difficult for clinical staff to afford the time to become an expert on all aspects of new offerings. This is an area where the medical physicist may provide great benefit to the clinical environment. Medical Physicists have the skills to understand the workings of these technologies to help guide its deployment into an already established clinical setting. After deployment, the medical physicist can provide ongoing support by providing educational staff in-service sessions and through discussions with the radiologists to help optimize protocols and workflows.

Ongoing professional development, especially in the context of continuing education, is an important component of a Medical Physicist's job requirements and should never be overlooked. Staying up to date on the latest technological offerings will not only help with educating others and answering questions, but will become invaluable during the equipment purchasing process. Medical physicists are uniquely positioned to look past the sales pitch and identify meaningful differences in technology between the vendors. From a practical clinical sense, the medical physicist should know which features are important for the facility. If multiple vendors are considered, the medical physicist should provide a comprehensive comparison of the features and usability of each system, including how each may advance or possibly deter the clinical operation. Occasionally vendors may inaccurately portray the features of their system and the medical physicist should be a clinical advocate to question or clarify claims. The physicist can explain and reiterate the needs of the clinic and the benefits new technology may provide to ensure everyone involved understands how this new purchase or feature may change the landscape of the clinical environment.

Communication and interaction with the clinic also helps drive quality improvement projects. By communicating with the radiologists and technologists, a medical physicist can better understand what is working well and what may need attention in the clinic. Perhaps a tool already exists within the medical physics tool box to quickly help improve a clinical problem. If a tool does not exist, the medical physicist must make a decision on how and to what extent to intervene. Depending on the severity of the problem, or the amount of clinical improvement solving the problem may provide, the medical physicist must be mindful about the amount of resources used to help resolve an issue. Developing a strategy to help resolve the problem, including a timeline, is a good way to keep a project on track.

Another effective method of communication between medical physics and the clinic would be to host regular meetings to discuss the current landscape of physics, the recent accomplishments, and develop a road map of the future [49]. Having the entire clinical team, including physicians, technologists, engineers, administration, and medical physicists, gathered in one location is a tremendous opportunity to better understand the needs of the clinic and get buy-in on proposed projects. Also, use these meetings as a platform for demonstrating the great value provided by medical physics, and the importance of including the medical physicist as a part of the clinical team. Scheduling these meetings in advance and on recurring intervals, perhaps quarterly or with higher frequency depending on the clinical needs, usually helps ensure maximum participation.

One of the challenges medical physicists often face is in communicating test results to other members of the clinical team. Medical physicists often communicate test results in a way only fellow physicists can comprehend. Within an issued report, most of the results are reported in numbers and percentages. Medical physicists should find a way to translate these cryptic results into clinical relevance to bring meaning for the intended report consumer. For instance, if the measured energy resolution in FWHM is 14.5% instead of the aim value of 9.0%, the medical physicist should communicate the impact this change will have on the patient images being sent for interpretation. Physicists must strive to make test results translatable back to the clinical task to provide maximum clinical impact.

15.5.2 Optimization

By shifting beyond the traditional equipment evaluation mantra into more of a clinical operation focused mindset, the medical physicist may discover the opportunity to provide valuable input on imaging protocols. Hospitals should consider the formation of a protocol review team to review and justify changes to imaging protocols in nuclear medicine. The review team should consist of at least a radiologist, technologist, and medical physicist. This effort emphasizes the importance of involving every part of the imaging team in the protocol landscape.

Within the protocol landscape, the scrutiny of a protocol review remains somewhat undefined. Reviewing an imaging protocol to look for gross errors or outdated methods is very different than reviewing with the intent of optimization. Within nuclear medicine there is a balance between the activity of injected radiopharmaceutical (patient radiation dose) and the acquisition time of an image. Additionally, patient-specific factors, such as body mass index (BMI) and age must be considered. Patients with higher BMI will generally attenuate the injected radiopharmaceutical more, leading to a lower photon flux to the detector, requiring longer imaging times. As for age, one must consider the difficulty for pediatric patients to remain motionless during long acquisitions. Since motion will lead to decreased spatial resolution in the image, it is not always optimal to only consider the radiation dose to the pediatric patient. The post-injection wait time is also an important consideration of the protocol; it may be possible in some cases to estimate the metabolism of the radiopharmaceutical within patient and adjust the wait times to better maximize the target to background ratio.

The specific characteristics of each imaging system must also be considered. The increased sensitivity offered by many of the solid state system designs and iterative reconstruction options typically allows for faster imaging times, resulting in greater patient throughput. Alternatively, this increased sensitivity can allow for decreasing activity of radiotracer injected to reduce the radiation burden to the patient. Medical physicists provide the expertise needed to evaluate and help optimize this injected activity-acquisition time balance in the clinical practice.

Advancements in the traditional Anger-style scintillation systems have also led to improvements in sensitivity and resolution properties, however the facility protocols often remain static. The medical physicist must lead the task of translating these equipment improvements into the protocol space and tailor protocols to the actual performance of the specific imaging system. Using input from the radiologists and technologists, the medical physicist can identify which systems are producing the best image quality and use that as a starting point for improving the fleet to bring both consistency and improvements to the image quality across the operation.

Also, while diving into protocol optimization, the physicist should invest time to discover why the radiologist has identified a particular image as superior over another. As scientists, medical physicists should develop ways to quantify these aspects and create new metrics which may be used as a retrospective image analysis quality assurance tool. This will allow for an objective comparison of the image quality across the entire imaging fleet.

Medical physicists also play a valuable role in troubleshooting issues. Traditionally the clinical staff are used to reporting to the engineer whenever a problem arises. If the problem stems from equipment malfunction, such as a power supply or corrupt correction file, then the engineer may be the correct person to turn to. However, in instances where the problem may be related to the image protocol or processing, the clinical staff must become accustomed to notifying the medical physicist as a first response. The engineer may not have the expertise to aid in some issues, or will only verify the system is operating properly and not identify the true problem, and therefore the issue never becomes resolved. Even in instances when the engineer is notified for an equipment repair issue, the medical physicist should also be made aware in case follow-up action is required to verify the baseline performance of the system has not changed. Also, with the advancements in automated camera corrections, it becomes easier to unintentionally mask a problem instead of identifying and correcting the root cause (Figure 15.11).

15.5.3 Automated Analysis and Data Management

The medical physicist also serves a vital role in the equipment QC program. The traditional QC evaluations, which may be required by accreditation bodies, may not always be the most useful in their traditional capacities. Many of the tests rely solely on subjective analysis, making it difficult to meaningfully track results as QC operators may change from week-to-week.

As discussed previously, there is a need for the development of new metrics in nuclear medicine, especially to help remove or at least supplement the subjectivity and become an asset in QC programs. For example, a template-based bar phantom image analysis, discussed earlier in Section 15.3.1, would serve well in a QC program and could be incorporated with little or no

Figure 15.11 An example of how a uniformity correction file can cover up a photomultiplier tube (PMT) which is decoupled from the scintillation crystal. (LEFT) An intrinsic Tc-99 m uniformity image (six million counts) showing a slight non-uniformity in the center of the image caused by a decoupled PMT. (CENTER) The source of the non-uniformity is evident when reviewing the correction file (120 million counts). The correction file shows a previous attempt to mask the decoupling PMT problem that has since progressed in severity. (RIGHT) The intrinsic Tc-99 m uniformity image (60 million counts) acquired shortly afterwards demonstrating the correction file is substantially masking the PMT issue. However, because the underlying problem was not corrected, the artifact continued to progress and until the proper, time-intensive repair was completed.

additional effort asked of the clinical technologists. Implementing such an analysis program would not only serve as a secondary review, but would also quantify the likelihood of a non-linearity being present. This would allow the tracking of more in-depth system performance which will improve the quality of the operation by flagging gradual degradation in system performance more quickly.

One possible way to integrate new metrics into the QC program with little or no extra effort from the clinical technologists would be to setup a DICOM repository within the facility network where images can be sent, received, and processed using these new advanced analysis metrics. At the completion of the QC acquisition, the technologist would send the QC image to this location, where automated programs could analyze and write results into a QC database. The program could automatically send email alerts to physics and clinical staff if predefined thresholds are exceeded. Such a program would not only help in tracking system performance, but would also promote communication between clinical and physics staff to help expedite the repair process. Through the automation of new improved analysis metrics, physics can provide meaningful results at the cost of only minimal, or no added effort by the clinical staff. In the long run, implementing automated analysis programs may lessen the technologist workload by reducing or even eliminating the time needed to subjectively analyzing the images and charting the results.

Protocol development is one opportunity previously mentioned for medical physicist engagement. Automated image data extraction also allows for tracking to ensure consistency with new or recently changed protocols. The medical physicist may be the facilitator to develop a protocol monitoring strategy where the acquisition data from all images is pulled from the DICOM header and placed in a database. Some of the useful elements to track in nuclear medicine images would be acquisition date and time, camera name, study description, operator's name, patient demographics, counts accumulated, acquisition duration, matrix size, acquisition zoom, and photon energy range acquired. Programs can then be developed which comb through the data and identify any discrepancies from the current physician approved protocol. Reviewing the collected data may also help identify instances when a protocol is routinely changed on the fly by the user, perhaps indicating the protocol itself may need to be adjusted. This will help ensure consistency across the operation.

Beyond capturing and databasing image attributes, calculating, and recording the patient radiation dose in nuclear medicine based on administered activity, as discussed earlier, may also lead to several clinical benefits. Since most facilities utilize radiopharmacy management software packages designed to record administered activity for compliance purposes, it provides a convenient avenue for the medical physicist to access and retrieve the patient administration records. Typically, for the feature of populating patient demographics, the software is already connected into the hospital computer network, and may allow for the automated flow of data directly to the medical physicist data base. This lends itself to building an automated nuclear medicine patient dose monitoring program. Some of the benefits of having the dose monitoring program as an automated system instead of a quarterly or monthly manual data dump is the option of setting up automated alerts. Also, if other modalities within the facility have real-time patient dose monitoring, then at any time, a user can obtain the current dose history of a patient.

Oftentimes one of the major challenges within an imaging environment is the sheer size of the operation. It is often difficult to maintain daily in-person interactions between physicians, technologists, imaging managers, and medical physicists. This not only leads to challenges when a radiologist has a question for the technologist about the patient history, but also when the radiologist has an issue with the image quality of a clinical image, or when the technologist has a question about the appropriateness of a technique. The hurdles are compounded when considering large, multi-facility health systems, each with their own clinical staff, but supported by the same physicist(s). An efficient and high quality operation must have an uncomplicated method to streamline the communication between these parties for important issues. Many hospital IT or clinical engineering departments have a third-party, ticket-based tracking system for problem reporting, but similar systems for communication of image quality issues are relatively rare. Using email to report and track these issues may be an option, but much too often inboxes become cluttered and emails overlooked or forgotten. Another, more comprehensive option would be to design a simple in-house program for this purpose. It should be designed to not only help organize and catalog reported issues, but also create accountability to ensure a task is followed through to completion (closed ticket). An essential feature for this program would be the ability to enter work notes for tracking progress through resolution, as some issues may take an extended time to resolve. Having this work note option will allow the issue reporter to keep informed on the status and progress of resolving the concern they raised.

15.5.4 Meaningful QC

The work of the medical physicist may not always be about developing new analysis metrics or processes. One important task is to evaluate what is currently being performed to ensure it is meaningful. Oftentimes QC tests originate from a common problem or a peculiarity of a device. The test may continue to be performed years later without anyone investigating if it is still relevant and if the frequency is still appropriate. In nuclear medicine, the routine QC tests performed on the imaging equipment [2] are likely still relevant. Even though the dependability and reliability of the PMTs and electronics within the imaging systems have improved, the daily uniformity evaluations are still justified. Clinically significant artifacts continue to be identified routinely with this relatively simple QC procedure.

After determining that current tests remain meaningful and appropriate, the medical physicist should also evaluate if the analysis methods used are still appropriate. Some QC procedures originated as a subjective test but are now also analyzed using a complimentary objective metric [9]. While objective methods provide a consistent evaluation metric, the role of any objective test in the overall QC procedure must be well understood. It is likely multiple analysis methods complement each other instead of replacing. For example, for daily uniformity, a subjective critical analysis should be the gold standard. Other useful analysis metrics, such as Integral and Differential Uniformity, were developed to complement the critical visual inspection. While this metric definitely adds value to the analysis, too often too much weight is given to the objective metric score that the value of the subjective visual assessment has become lost. This metric is not designed to assess the visual uniformity of the image and may not identify images with subtle structural artifacts which may be clinically relevant [11]. Additionally, the medical physicist must assess if the pass/fail criteria are clinically relevant. Perhaps the limit is too sensitive where non-clinically relevant artifacts are consistently being flagged, or the limit not sensitive enough and may miss flagging some of the clinically relevant artifacts.

Medical physicists should be pleased with all of the progress the field has made. However, it is important to not become stagnant. Through routine performance evaluations and QC one can only infer the quality of the nuclear medicine exam will be adequate. Adding in protocol review and optimization establishes a clinical environment that will likely lead to quality images; however, the only way to truly assess if the nuclear medicine unit is producing high quality images is to analyze the actual clinical images produced. As a field, medical physicists should aim to develop methods to estimate the clinical image quality from patient images directly, which will in turn allow for the creation of analysis programs to QC the actual clinical images. We may begin this process with common established metrics such as noise, CNR, and SNR, but likely it will require some combination of more sophisticated metrics, such as NPS and MTF, to completely quantify the nuclear medicine image such as can be done in other modalities [27, 28]. This retrospective patient image analysis QC will prove useful for performing protocol optimization and driving the continued pursuit of excellence in health care.

References

1 Medical use of byproduct material (2002). 10 C.F.R. § 35.

2 American Association of Physicists in Medicine. Nuclear Medicine Committee (1982). *Computer-Aided Scintillation Camera Acceptance Testing*. New York, N.Y: Published for the American Association of Physicists in Medicine by the American Institute of Physics.

3 American Association of Physicists in Medicine. SPECT Task Group (1987). *Rotating Scintillation Camera SPECT Acceptance Testing and Quality Control*. New York, N.Y: Published for the American Association of Physicists in Medicine by the American Institute of Physics.

4 NEMA (2012). *Performance Measurements of Gamma Cameras*. Rosslyn, VA: National Electrical Manufacturers Association.

5 IEC (1984). *Characteristics and Test Conditions for Anger-Type Gamma Cameras*. Geneva: International Electrotechnical Commission.

6 IAEA (2009). *Quality Assurance for SPECT Systems*. Vienna: International Atomic Energy Agency.

7 Bolster, A. (ed.) (2003). *Quality Control of Gamma Camera Systems*. United Kingdom: Institute of Physics and Engineering in Medicine.

8 American College of Radiology. American College of Radiology nuclear medicine accreditation program requirements, revised 1/4/2019. American College of Radiology website. http://www.acraccreditation.org/modalities/nuclear-medicine-and-pet#s1 (accessed 3 August 2019).

9 Medicare improvements for patients and providers act of 2008. US Government Printing Office. Public Law 110-275, Page 112, STAT. 2494 (July 15, 2008).

10 Cox, N.J. and Diffey, B.L. (1976). Letter: a numerical index of gamma-camera uniformity. *Br. J. Radiol.* 49: 734–735.

11 Nelson, J.S., Christianson, O.I., Harkness, B.A. et al. (2014). Improved nuclear medicine uniformity assessment with noise texture analysis. *J. Nucl. Med.* 55: 169–174.

12 Gambhir, S.S., Berman, D.S., Ziffer, J. et al. (2009). A novel high-sensitivity rapid-acquisition single-photon cardiac imaging camera. *J. Nucl. Med.* 50: 635–643.

13 Esteves, F.P., Raggi, P., Folks, R.D. et al. (2009). Novel solid-state-detector dedicated cardiac camera for fast myocardial perfusion imaging; multicenter comparison with standard dual detector cameras. *J. Nucl. Cardiol.* 16: 927.

14 Erlandsson, K., Kacperski, K., van Gramberg, D. et al. (2009). Performance evaluation of D-SPECT: a novel SPECT system for nuclear cardiology. *Phys. Med. Biol.* 54: 2635.

15 O'Connor, M., Rhodes, D., and Hruska, C. (2009). Molecular breast imaging. *Expert. Rev. Anticancer. Ther.* 9 (8): 1073–1080.

16 Cherry, S.R., Sorenson, J.A., and Phelps, M.E. (2003). *Physics in Nuclear Medicine*, 3e (Chapter 10). Saunders.

17 Knoll, G.F. (2000). *Radiation Detection and Measurement*, 3e (Chapter 13). Wiley.

18 Eisen, Y., Shor, I., and Mardor, I. (1999). CsTe and CdZnTe gamma ray detectors for medical and industrial imaging systems. *Nucl. Inst. Methods Phys. Res.* 428 (1): 158–170.

19 Allie, R., Hutton, B.F., Prvulovich, E. et al. (2016). Pitfalls and artifacts using D-SPECT dedicated cardiac camera. *J. Nucl. Cardiol.* 23: 301.

20 Dobbins, J.T. 3rd, Samei, E., Ranger, N.T., and Chen, Y. (2006). Intercomparison of methods for image quality characterization. II. Noise power spectrum. *Med. Phys.* 33: 1466–1475.

21 Solomon, J.B., Christianson, O., and Samei, E. (2012). Quantitative comparison of noise texture across CT scanners from different manufacturers. *Med. Phys.* 39: 6048–6055.

22 Wilson, J.M., Christianson, O.I., Richard, S., and Samei, E. (2013). A methodology for image quality evaluation of advanced CT systems. *Med. Phys.* 40: 031908.

23 Tsui, B.M., Beck, R.N., Doi, K., and Metz, C.E. (1981). Analysis of recorded image noise in nuclear medicine. *Phys. Med. Biol.* 26: 883–902.

24 Grossman, L.W., Anderson, M.P., Jennings, R.J. et al. (1986). Noise analysis of scintillation camera images: stochastic and non-stochastic effects. *Phys. Med. Biol.* 31: 941–953.

25 Madhav, P., Bowsher, J.E., Cutler, S.J., and Tornai, M.P. (2009). Characterizing the MTF in 3D for a quantized SPECT camera having arbitrary trajectories. *IEEE Trans. Nucl. Sci.* 56 (3): 661–670.

26 International Commission on Radiation Units and Measurements (ICRU) (1996). Medical imaging – The assessment of image quality, ICRU Report No. 54 (Bethesda, MD, 1996).

27 Richard, S. and Samei, E. (2010). Quantitative breast tomosynthesis: from detectability to estimability. *Med. Phys.* 37: 6157–6165.

28 Richard, S. and Samei, E. (2010). Quantitative imaging in breast tomosynthesis and CT: comparison of detection and estimation task performance. *Med. Phys.* 37: 2627–2637.

29 Gang, G.J., Lee, J., Stayman, J.W. et al. (2011). Analysis of Fourier-domain task-based detectability index in tomosynthesis and cone-beam CT in relation to human observer performance. *Med. Phys.* 38: 1754–1768.

30 American Association of Physicists in Medicine (2011). Size-specific dose estimates (SSDE) in pediatric and adult body CT Examinations: report of AAPM Task Group 204. College Park, MD: American Association of Physicists in Medicine.

31 Wang, J., Duan, X., Christner, J.A. et al. (2012). Attenuation-based estimation of patient size for the purpose of size specific dose estimation in CT. Part I. development and validation of methods using the CT image. *Med. Phys.* 39: 6764–6771.

32 Wang, J., Christner, J.A., Duan, X. et al. (2012). Attenuation-based estimation of patient size for the purpose of size specific dose estimation in CT. Part II. Implementation on abdomen and thorax phantoms using cross sectional CT images and scanned projection radiograph images. *Med. Phys.* 39: 6772–6778.

33 Cody, D.D., Fisher, T.S., Gress, D.A. et al. (2013). AAPM medical physics practice guideline 1.a: CT protocol management and review practice guideline. *J. Appl. Clin. Med. Phys.* 14: 3–12.

34 Siegel, J.A., Thomas, S.R., Stubbs, J.B. et al. (1999). MIRD pamphlet No. 16: techniques for quantitative radiopharmaceutical biodistribution data acquisition and analysis for use in human radiation dose estimates. *J. Nucl. Med.* 40: 37S–61S.

35 Hutton, B.F. (2014). The origins of SPECT and SPECT/CT. *Eur. J. Nucl. Med. Mol. Imaging* 41: S3–S16.

36 Copp, R.J., Seslija, P., Tso, D. et al. (2013). Scanner and kVp dependence of measured CT numbers in the ACR CT phantom. *J. Appl. Clin. Med. Phys.* 14: 338–349.

37 Patton, J.A. and Turkington, T.G. (2008). SPECT/CT physical principles and attenuation correction. *J. Nucl. Med. Technol.* 36: 1–10.

38 Hawman, P. and Hsieh, J. (1994). The cardiofocal collimator: a variable-focus collimator for cardiac SPECT. *Phys. Med. Biol.* (3): 439–450.

39 Nakajima, K., Okuda, K., Momose, M. et al. (2017). IQ-SPECT technology and its clinical applications using multicenter normal databases. *Ann. Nucl. Med.* 31: 649–659.

40 Bocher, M., Blevis, I.M., Tsukerman, L. et al. (2010). A fast cardiac gamma camera with dynamic SPECT capabilities: design, system validation and future potential. *Eur. J. Nucl. Med. Mol. Imaging* 37: 1887–1902.

41 Blaire, T., Bailliez, A., Bouallegue, F.B. et al. (2018). Frist assessment of simultaneous dual isotope (123I/99mTc) cardiac SPECT on two different CZT cameras: a phantom study. *J. Nucl. Cardiol.* 25: 1692–1704.

42 Asseeva, P., Paladion, N.C., Guerin, C. et al. (2019). Value of 123I/99mTc-sestamibi parathyroid scintigraphy with subtraction SPECT/CT in primary hyperparathyroidism for directing minimally invasive parathyroidectomy. *Am. J. Surg.* 217: 108–113.

43 Imbert, L., Roch, V., Merlin, C. et al. (2018). Low-dose dual-isotope procedure planned for myocardial perfusion CZT-SPECT and assessed through a head-to-head comparison with a conventional single-isotope protocol. *J. Nucl. Cardiol.* 25: 2016–2023.

44 Takeuchi, W., Suzuki, A., Shiga, T. et al. (2016). Simultaneous Tc-99m and I-123 dual-radionuclide imaging with a solid-state detector-based brain-SPECT system and energy-based scatter correction. *Eur. J. Nucl. Med. Mol. Imaging* 3: 10.

45 Aarsvold, J.N., Galt, J.R., Nye, J.A. et al. (2012). The quality field of view of a Discovery 530c IEEE Nuclear Science Symposium and Medical Imaging Conference Record (NSS/MIC), Anaheim, CA, pp. 3551–3555.

46 Marcassa, C. and Zoccarato, O. (2017). Advances in imaging reconstruction software in nuclear cardiology: it all that glitters gold? *J. Nucl. Cardiol.* 24: 142–144.

47 Hughes, T., Scherbinin, S., and Celler, A. (2009). A multi-center phantom study comparing image resolution from three state-of-the-art SPECT-CT systems. *J. Nucl. Cardiol.* 16: 914–926.

48 Lyra, M., Ploussi, A., and Rouchota, M. (2014). Filters in 2D and 3D cardiac SPECT image processing. *Cardiol. Res. Pract.*: 963264.

49 American Association of Physicist in Medicine. State of the modality: integrated communication for better clinical care. American Association of Physicist in Medicine website. https://w3.aapm.org/medphys30/articles/stateModality.php (accessed 3 August 2019).

Part VI

Ultrasonography

16

Clinical Ultrasonography Physics: Perspective

Paul Carson[1], Nicholas J. Hangiandreou[2], and Zheng Feng Lu[3]

[1] *Department of Radiology, University of Michigan, Ann Arbor, MI, USA*
[2] *Department of Radiology, Mayo Clinic Rochester, Rochester, MN, USA*
[3] *Department of Radiology, University of Chicago, Chicago, IL, USA*

16.1 Introduction

This chapter will offer a high-level overview of ultrasound (US) imaging technology and clinical medical physics involvement, starting with a review of the history and current state of US performance testing. Established US imaging technology will be described, as will technologies that are only now becoming commercially available or are evolving rapidly. The current level of physics practice, Medical Physics 1.0, will be outlined. Finally, important considerations for a transition from current practice to a Medical Physics 3.0 practice model will be detailed.

16.2 An Historical Perspective on US Performance Testing

As in other imaging modality areas, clinical medical physicists have been involved in quality control (QC) and performance evaluation of US imaging systems for many years. The most important early successes resulting from these physics testing efforts have been the detection of numerous performance problems and some design issues which, in some cases, resulted in nearly immediate corrections once the vendor was notified. It was critical for medical physicists to perform this testing as vendor testing of system performance in the field was found to be essentially non-existent [1]. The continuous efforts of medical physicists and others to develop effective measurement methods have led to the use of these methods in national testing facilities and in national regulations. If anything, the impacts of these new developments, often resulting from work performed in the USA, are more consistently felt outside the USA. For example, the methods reported in AAPM Report No. 8 [2] were used to test every B-scan US system produced in the USSR before their introduction into service. In fact, however, QC and performance evaluation tests are not performed regularly on most US systems used in United States radiology departments. Another failure of these early physics efforts is the revelation that, even when testing reveals significant limitations of scanner functionality and this is reported, these problems may remain uncorrected for many years [3].

Clinical Imaging Physics: Current and Emerging Practice, First Edition. Edited by Ehsan Samei and Douglas E. Pfeiffer.
© 2020 John Wiley & Sons, Inc. Published 2020 by John Wiley & Sons, Inc.

Recently the American College of Radiology (ACR) has included reasonably meaningful US QC in its practice accreditation requirements [4] and medical physicists are working quickly to receive the necessary training and institute QC programs. Although this is a useful first step, evolution of these requirements to make them even more specific and effective is needed. This evolution in requirements and methods will be enabled as more medical physicists and clinical practices gain US performance testing experience. This will hopefully pave the way for other accrediting bodies to include meaningful testing requirements in their accreditation programs.

Development of simplified and more effective QC testing methods should make implementation of routine QC programs more cost effective. However, to date there has been relatively little published literature regarding US system failure rates and root causes, which has resulted in continued use of excessively time-consuming test procedures [5–7] for US systems. The five annual routine phantom tests reported in [7] are rarely performed on all transducers and do not exhibit sufficient reproducibility to detect modest, but significant changes. Studies identifying the most common types of imaging system defects in reasonably modern systems are appearing [8] and have resulted in recommendations for, and detailed exposition of, three relatively simple tests – image uniformity, distance measurement accuracy and maximum depth of penetration (MDOP) [6] that can detect the majority of common defects. MDOP is difficult to measure with sufficient reproducibility to reliably detect small degrees of change. Changes in distance measurement accuracy are of critical clinical importance, but measurement accuracy changes are very rarely encountered with modern equipment, except in measurements based on transducer motion-tracking systems. Except for systems that do involve transducer motion tracking, distance measurement accuracy and MDOP could be relegated to acceptance testing and other non-repetitive performance evaluation applications (or possibly performed infrequently as part of an ongoing QC program).

Current methods for evaluating image uniformity typically rely on phantom images. Although more fundamental evaluations of uniformity and element performance might be possible for 1-dimensional (1D) phased arrays without support from system suppliers, that is yet to be shown in practice. This direct approach to evaluation of 2D arrays will definitely require support from system suppliers, expensive equipment, or time consuming methods. Manufacturers have revealed that the second most common system problem reported by customer sites involves the scanner display. US scanner displays deserve careful attention, particularly in practices where patient images are read on a separate workstation, e.g. where picture archiving and communication system (PACS) are employed. In general, for most common US imaging equipment, requiring only more frequent tests of image uniformity on each transducer and tests of the scanner monitor (as well as a general visual inspection for mechanical defects) should reduce the personnel time required for testing and increase the yield of detected system issues, resulting in increased value to the practice and dedication to the QC program.

It should be noted that QC and performance evaluation are not the only areas of clinical medical physics contribution in US imaging practice, although historically the bulk of clinical physics effort has been expended in these areas. There has also been some work aimed toward testing of image processing applications and image quantification methods, and optimizing clinical imaging presets and measurements. Physicists have also been involved in development of new imaging systems and functions, although this often takes place in the research environment.

16.3 Established US Imaging Technology

US systems have evolved far beyond traditional fundamental grayscale imaging and now offer a wide variety of imaging modes. Spatial compound imaging and harmonic imaging modes can improve the image by speckle reduction and improved display of more specular reflectors, and by clutter reduction, respectively. However, compound imaging also has the potential to hide fine detail while harmonic imaging can limit the maximum imaging depth (penetration), so use of these features needs to be carefully adjusted to different patient imaging situations. In spite of these potential limitations, compound and harmonic imaging have become part of the standard of practice in US imaging. More recently, static and shear wave elasticity imaging modes are appearing on all high end systems. These modes provide a new source of contrast compared with traditional B-mode imaging (brightness-mode, or real-time grayscale imaging), that are directly related to the mechanical properties of tissues, e.g. Young's modulus. These capabilities are expected to become essential to many diagnostic and interventional US imaging applications.

3D US imaging has become common in obstetric imaging and echocardiography. The value of 3D imaging is more equivocal in abdominal and breast imaging practices, where flattening of aberrating tissue layers by a relatively thin, linear or curved linear array is critical to routinely achieving good image quality. (This is a lesson often missed when concentrating only on images of uniform phantoms.) 3D and 4D imaging is performed by mechanically scanning linear or curved linear arrays (Figure 16.1) or by using transducer arrays consisting of a 2D pattern of small piezoelectric elements. Current realizations of 2D transducer arrays are useful primarily in echocardiography, where speed is critical and only small acoustic windows into the body are available. Since small element dimensions (1λ and $\frac{1}{2}\lambda$) in a given plane are required, respectively, for strong focusing in that plane and for $>20°$ beam steering, large numbers of elements are required to achieve the large apertures and strong focusing expected for general and obstetrical imaging. 2D arrays for general and obstetrical imaging applications are now becoming available, but are not yet commonplace.

Highly miniaturized electronic components and increasing computing speeds make possible software beamforming (Figure 16.2), as well as small, low cost systems with excellent basic imaging performance, and reductions in the price of high end systems. Specialized applications (Figure 16.3) [9] provide opportunities for technology entrepreneurs to penetrate the challenging medical imaging system market (though a large medical imaging company introduced the device shown in Figure 16.3). Tablet and smart phone-based US imaging devices with software provided as a downloadable app are now available, and will become ubiquitous throughout medicine in developing as well as advanced societies.

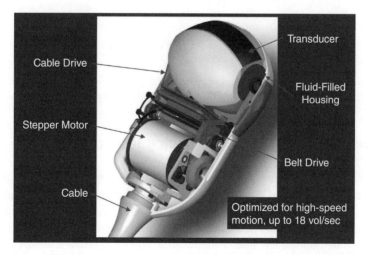

Figure 16.1 Diagram of a mechanical 3D/4D imaging probe, utilizing a curved linear array.

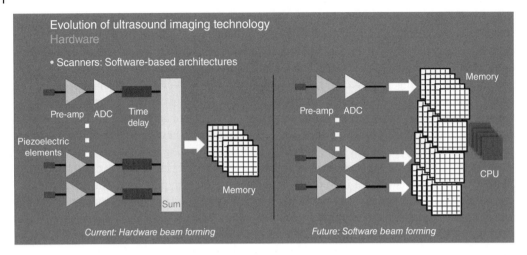

Figure 16.2 Software beamforming (right side of diagram) involves storing the full RF or base-banded RF (IQ) data to system memory so that software can provide various delays for transmit and receive focusing at each point in the image. This is in contrast with traditional hardware beamforming (left side of diagram) in which custom hardware processing pipelines perform considerable data reduction before storing results in memory.

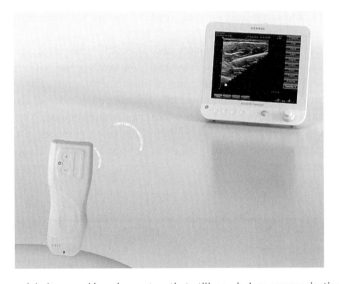

Figure 16.3 Commercial ultrasound imaging system that utilizes wireless communication of image data from the handheld transducer to a tablet-sized display. Elimination of transducer cable reduces infection risk, wrist strain, and simplifies interventional procedures.

16.4 Newer and Near Future US Imaging Technologies

Computing capabilities have advanced to the point that the phase coherent waveform to and from each piezoelectric element of a 1D transducer array can be controlled, recorded and processed in real time so that traditional transmission of many individual, focused US pulses with detection of echo trains along each individual scan line in the image (supported by hardware beamforming methods as illustrated on the left side of Figure 16.2) is no longer necessary. A few transmitted

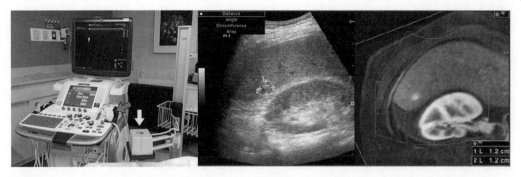

Figure 16.4 Electromagnetic tracking components, including a field generator (left panel, green arrow) and sensor clipped to a linear array transducer (left panel, red arrow), integrated with an US imaging system. This allows dynamic determination of transducer position and orientation which can be used to superimpose real time US images on treatment planning image volumes during interventional procedures, as shown in the middle and right panels [12].

waves (e.g. plane waves) covering the entire image can generate sets of echoes that may be reconstructed into an image with sharp, in-plane, focus at all depths. This approach allows ultrahigh speed imaging with remarkable consequences in most imaging modes, including color flow and elasticity imaging [10, 11]. Much more sophisticated software beamforming (right side of Figure 16.2) and reconstruction methods, using for example maximum likelihood techniques, are expected to appear on commercial systems within a few years.

Integration of ultrasound probe tracking and image fusion systems into ultrasound units has been achieved for 3D guidance of therapeutic interventions with real time imaging, registered to previous diagnostic studies (Figure 16.4). Systems for training imagers have also utilized these systems. The possibility of errors with electromagnetic tracking systems is still quite high and there is a need for development and validation of techniques, even as the systems become more accurate and robust.

Specialized breast screening US devices are now marketed, which generally allow volumetric image data to be automatically acquired and then efficiently reviewed. These systems present their own procedural and training challenges and opportunities. The relatively large number of callbacks from traditional B-mode US screening in several studies suggests that some more stringent diagnostic criterion should be applied, or that other information must be combined with the US exam. Additional types of information with potential to improve this situation include tissue bulk or elastic modulus, or attenuation coefficient (all obtainable using US methods), or vascular abnormalities evaluated with contrast-enhanced magnetic resonance imaging (MRI). Registration and fusion of B-mode US with digital breast tomosynthesis may also prove beneficial.

4D color flow contrast imaging is beginning to be implemented and is, in the opinion of the authors, the best approach for performing most contrast studies. This is especially true in practices where the diagnostician is not performing the exam. This is a very common practice model in the USA, where image acquisition is typically performed by a sonographer with images sent to a workstation for interpretation by a physician. 2D color Doppler imaging has been used for decades, but it presents procedural and thus performance issues which have contributed to a relatively limited level of clinical utilization in the radiology community in the USA, as compared with its application in cardiac imaging practices. Significant improvements in vascular US imaging and diagnosis will be provided by vector Doppler imaging modes that accurately assess 2D and eventually 3D blood flow speed and direction. Super resolution imaging methods using contrast agents as point targets also show considerable potential in this regard.

2D transducer arrays with many isotropic elements, e.g. 256×256, with true software beamforming (in which signals from all individual elements are transmitted directly to system memory) will allow imaging in 3D and 4D that is much superior to that achieved with current linear arrays. Full software beamforming and image reconstruction will enable the primary current limitations on US imaging, i.e. aberration by overlying tissues and multiple scattering, to be addressed more fully. This technology is expected to develop over the next decade, as current coaxial cables with only ~64–256 conductors significantly limit this approach.

16.5   The Movement from Medical Physics 1.0–3.0

US imaging practices are behind other radiologic modality practices in terms of utilization of basic Medical Physics 1.0 services, e.g. routine use of imaging system performance evaluation techniques and practice requirements for routine QC testing. In part his has been due to limited clinical medical physics time devoted to this modality. Thus, growth of Medical Physics 3.0 services in US, e.g. medical procedure- and clinically- focused medical physics, will be delayed unless increased physicist time is dedicated in this area. US provides high soft tissue contrast, but interacts more strongly with the tissues than would ideally be the case. Specifically, the considerable variation in tissue acoustic properties, such as attenuation and speed of sound, means that echo signals detected from one location in the body are affected strongly by overlying tissues. These basic imaging complications mean that there is considerable Medical Physics 3.0 work to be done to help optimize clinical image quality and to assure reproducible clinical imaging and measurements. Table 16.1 provides an overview of traditional, equipment-focused Medical Physics 1.0 practice in US, with a vision for Medical Physics 3.0.

For performance evaluation and routine QC, automated measurements with logging and statistical analysis of the measurement data, while well published, is only now beginning to become convenient enough to be implemented in most clinical medical physics practices. These approaches will become ubiquitous components of a Medical Physics 3.0 practice. Automated tests that include much of the overall resolution and contrast characteristics of the systems in a single measurement at each depth are desired. Spherical void phantom tests are one example (illustrated in Figure 16.5 [12]), as are direct transducer element and channel uniformity tests.

An important component of future Medical Physics 3.0 practice is much closer connection and cooperation between clinical physicists and equipment vendors. For example, when physics testing reveals substantive defects in US system hardware or software design that may have significant clinical practice impact, the equipment vendor must be contacted, whether or not the defect has been previously reported. The company should be asked to inform the physicist when a correction has been made, and if no effort to address the defect is undertaken, this situation should be pursued further, either publicly or privately. Previous (and current) US imaging systems have suffered from known functional deficiencies that have been long ignored by system vendors and accepted by the US imaging community (e.g. as reported in [3]).

Much work has been done to-date to provide acoustic exposure information to the user and to (nearly) always reduce to negligible levels the risk to the patient and fetus, except in the case of US contrast agents. Here the overall risk is likely less than that with other imaging agents, but the situation is complicated. The success of the Food and Drug Administration (FDA) 510(k) guidelines [13] in keeping acoustic exposures relatively low worldwide has actually undermined the focus of clinical users on the need to actively keep exposures as low as reasonably achievable (ALARA). Also, as the existing FDA exposure guidelines have and do limit the performance of US imaging

Table 16.1 Comparison of the current state of Medical Physics 1.0 ultrasound practice and technology, and a future vision for Medical Physics 3.0. (MP = medical physicist.)

Ultrasound Imaging and Measurement	Medical Physics 1.0	Medical Physics 3.0
Focus of MP's attention	Only a few specialists do much	Equipment, training in use of patient specific exposures and image optimization
Image quality evaluation	Visual, imaging system measurements	Automated analysis, aberration correction evaluation
MP "tools of the trade" for image quality evaluation	Visibility, dimensions, spacing of line pairs, displayed dynamic range and penetration Homogeneous phantoms	Less expensive QC and flow phantoms; Inhomogeneous, clutter, elastic, porosity, attenuation, SOS measurement phantoms
Performance evaluation Routine system QC	Done occasionally Many performance evaluation measures/metrics, rarely used	Do consistently, possibly in patients; Detection of failure occurring at highest rates
Patient exposimetry	Biophysical indices, thermal index (TI) and mechanical index (MI)	Organ, patient specific exposure estimates
Acoustic risk estimation	Comparison with 1976 levels and effects thresholds; Poor exposure estimates	Comparison with thermal and cavitational effects; Improved estimates with safety margin
Commonly used imaging technologies	Pulse echo B-mode, compounded, harmonic, color/spectral Doppler	Shear wave elasto-, visco-, and permio-graphy; Vector Doppler; Pressure, density, speed of sound, molecular, temperature, attenuation, nonlinearity, scatterer size and density
Independent element 2D arrays	Elements coupled, not capable of aberration correction	Data from independent elements with SW beamforming; Quantitative evaluation of uniformity, focus, grid ratio
Combined imaging and therapy systems	MR used to guide high-intensity focused-ultrasound therapy; Ultrasound used to guide other therapeutic modalities	High resolution thermal or surgical ultrasound therapy, with precise guidance in brain and other organs

systems, there will be efforts to raise exposure levels closer to and above bioeffects thresholds in an effort to improve image quality, especially in difficult-to-scan patients. This will increase the need for users to make more complex safety and efficacy tradeoffs while imaging patients (even as, or maybe particularly as, many of these scan parameter changes will be automated on the system). This topic of acoustic exposure and safety represents one significant area where increased and improved education provided by clinical physicists is needed in the Medical Physics 3.0 environment. Increasing the understanding of safe and effective US usage by clinical staff, as well as sales and applications representatives of companies, will continue to be a very important area of need for the foreseeable future.

Decades of research by US physicists and engineers on more quantitative imaging approaches and more accurate measurement methods is beginning to bear fruit. This work has been accelerated by the increased availability of digital RF image data from individual beam lines and, in

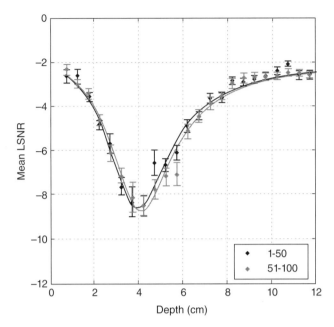

Figure 16.5 Measurements of lesion signal to noise ratio (LSNR) from automated assessment of spherical voids randomly placed in a uniform scattering material [12]. Consistency of two sets of LSNR measurements versus target depth is shown. The variability of LSNR with depth due to the variable elevational resolution clearly shows the limitations accepted with simple linear and curved linear arrays that are commonly used in current clinical ultrasound practices.

research systems and next generation clinical systems, full RF data from individual channels and transducer elements. Clinical implementation of advanced imaging capabilities will significantly increase the importance of Medical Physics 3.0 work aimed to optimize image exam protocols, image acquisition techniques and presets, data manipulation methods, and to assist development of interpretation and reporting guidelines and templates. Equipment-related, Medical Physics 1.0 work involving testing and validation of emerging imaging capabilities will continue to be important. All of this work will be facilitated by working groups organized by professional societies, such as the Quantitative Imaging Biomarker Alliance (QIBA) organized by the Radiological society of North America (RSNA). For example, the QIBA US shear wave speed profile provides benchmark data regarding measurement variance and bias that can aid clinical physicists evaluating this function on competing commercial imaging systems [14, 15]. These working groups would benefit from greater participation by clinical medical physicists in the future.

Another area that would benefit from increased involvement by medical physicists in future Medical Physics 3.0 practices involves clinical measurement data, and practice and image metadata. Improved export of image-based clinical measurement data via DICOM Structured Report functionality has great promise for improving the quality and efficiency of clinical practices, but implementation can be challenging. Efforts have only recently begun to explore opportunities and methods to leverage image and practice metadata to improve practice resource utilization and efficiency and image quality, but the potential seems significant. Increased understanding and awareness of the evolving DICOM protocol, as well as techniques for analytics data collection, analysis and presentation will be needed to maximize the benefits physicists can offer in this important developing area.

Responsibilities and opportunities for medical physicists to contribute to US practice improvement are broadened greatly by the increasingly wide distribution of medical US systems throughout the medical community. The traditional close ties of medical physicists to Radiology and Radiation Oncology practices should be expanded in the Medical Physics 3.0 environment, to provide proper guidance to practitioners in other medical disciplines on US technology and approaches for clinically- and cost-effective use of US (and other) imaging systems. Physicists specializing in US should also be very familiar with the capabilities and safety characteristics of other imaging modalities. This will allow medical physicists to advise practices on the relative technical and clinical strengths and weaknesses of various modalities, and appropriate clinical applications for these powerful tools.

We are in a time of accelerating transition to more cost effective medical services in the USA. Attacks on the assumptions of the cost effectiveness of medical imaging by competing medical disciplines, those relying almost entirely on medications and tests of extracted fluids and cells, should be met by genuine scientific objectiveness on the part of organized medical physics and medical physicists, and must be studied carefully. In the future Medical Physics 3.0 practice, this type of work will allow medical physicists to engage and contribute in valuable ways to high level discussions of best clinical practices for patient diagnosis and treatment. It will be very important for medical physicists to participate in the future to a much greater degree in persuasion and advocacy efforts organized by professional organizations such as the ACR. In particular, given the relatively low cost and significant (and expanding) capabilities in diagnosis and therapy offered by US technology, involvement by physicians and scientists who understand the technical and clinical potential of US will be especially beneficial.

References

1 Christensen, S.L. and Carson, P.L. (1977). Performance survey of ultrasound instrumentation and feasibility of routine monitoring. *Radiology* 122: 449–454.

2 Carson, P.L. and Zagzebski, J.A. (1981). Pulse echo ultrasound imaging systems: Performance tests and criteria. AAPM report #8.: Amer. Assoc. of Phys. in Medicine: pp. 73.

3 Hoyt, K., Hester, F.A., Bell, R.L. et al. (2009). Accuracy of volumetric flow rate measurements an in vitro study using modern ultrasound scanners. *J. Ultrasound Med.* 28: 1511–1518.

4 American College of Radiology (2014). Ultrasound Accreditation Program Requirements 11/7/014 [cited 6/30/2015]. https://www.acraccreditation.org/-/media/ACRAccreditation/Documents/Ultrasound/Requirements.pdf?la=en.

5 Goodsitt, M.M., Carson, P.L., Witt, S. et al. (1998). Real-time B-mode ultrasound quality control test procedures: report of AAPM Ultrasound Task Group No. 1. *Med. Phys.* 25: 1385–1406.

6 AIUM Technical Standards Committee (2014). QS, E.L. Madsen, Chair, AIUM Quality Assurance Manual for Gray Scale Ultrasound Scanners: Amer. Inst. Ultras. Med., Place Published. pp. 71.

7 AIUM Technical Standards Committee RQS (2018). Routine Quality Assurance for Diagnostic Ultrasound Equipment: Amer. Inst. Ultras. Med., Place Published. pp. 10

8 Hangiandreou, N.J., Stekel, S.F., Tradup, D.J. et al. (2011). Four-year experience with a clinical ultrasound quality control program. *Ultrasound Med. Biol.* 37: 1350–1357.

9 Acuson Freestyle ultrasound system [cited 10/18/2018]. https://usa.healthcare.siemens.com/ultrasound/ultrasound-point-of-care/acuson-freestyle-ultrasound-machine.

10 Osmanski, B.F., Martin, C., Montaldo, G. et al. (2014). Functional ultrasound imaging reveals different odor-evoked patterns of vascular activity in the main olfactory bulb and the anterior piriform cortex. *NeuroImage* 95: 176–184.

11 Provost, J., Papadacci, C., Arango, J.E. et al. (2014). 3D ultrafast ultrasound imaging in vivo. *Phys. Med. Biol.* 59: L1–L13.

12 Madsen, E.L., Song, C., and Frank, G. (2014). Low-echo sphere phantoms and methods for assessing imaging performance of medical ultrasound scanners. *Ultrasound Med. Biol.* 40: 1697–1717.

13 FDA (2008). Guidance for Industry and FDA Staff: Information for Manufacturers Seeking Marketing Clearance of Diagnostic Ultrasound Systems and Transducers, Place Published. pp. 68: http://www.fda.gov/downloads/medicaldevices/deviceregulationandguidance/ guidancedocuments/ucm070911.pdf.

14 Buckler, A.J., Bresolin, L., Dunnick, N.R. et al. (2011). Quantitative imaging test approval and biomarker qualification: interrelated but distinct activities. *Radiology* 259: 875–884.

15 Hall, T.J., Milkwoski, A., Garra, B. et al. (2013). RSNA/QIBA: Shear wave speed as a biomarker for liver fibrosis staging, in Procs. 2013 IEEE Int. Ult. Symp., Inst. Elect. Electron. Engrs., Prague.

17

Clinical Ultrasonography Physics: State of Practice

Zheng Feng Lu[1], Nicholas J. Hangiandreou[2], and Paul Carson[3]

[1] Department of Radiology, University of Chicago, Chicago, IL, USA
[2] Department of Radiology, Mayo Clinic Rochester, Rochester, MN, USA
[3] Department of Radiology, University of Michigan, Ann Arbor, MI, USA

17.1   Introduction

Diagnostic ultrasound is a rapidly evolving field. This has been especially true during the last two decades as breakthrough technologies such as tissue harmonic imaging, extended field of view, coded excitation, real time compounding, B-mode flow imaging, 4D imaging, and others have been introduced. The growing complexity of ultrasound systems makes quality assurance increasingly important, but also more challenging. The goal of an ultrasound quality assurance program is to maintain clinical ultrasound imaging equipment at an optimal and consistent level of performance. One crucial aspect of such programs is to include comprehensive quality control (QC) testing so equipment defects can be detected and corrected before they affect clinical outcomes. Of all the imaging modalities in radiology, diagnostic ultrasound is the least regulated with regards to user quality assurance programs. Some clinical sites simply employ a preventative maintenance program rather than a true quality assurance program. However, preventative maintenance programs have a different emphasis and do not include detailed and comprehensive QC testing. Some clinical ultrasound users argue that ultrasound quality assurance is not necessary because defects can be identified during clinical evaluation. While this may be true for certain severe defects, such as the one shown in Figure 17.1, gradual degradations may go un-noticed until image quality has significantly deteriorated. As shown in Figure 17.2, this old probe clearly indicates poor image quality in all of the measured QC parameters. This problem would be detected earlier if performance consistency was checked periodically using QC testing. As shown in Figure 17.3, subtle defects at early stages may not be noticed in clinical studies but can be effectively detected if careful phantom tests are done.

17.1.1   Guidelines

Simultaneously with the rapid breakthroughs in ultrasound technologies, QC testing of ultrasound equipment is also evolving. Guidelines [1–8] have been published involving visual assessments of system performance using tissue-mimicking phantoms. These published guidelines provide a

Clinical Imaging Physics: Current and Emerging Practice, First Edition. Edited by Ehsan Samei and Douglas E. Pfeiffer.
© 2020 John Wiley & Sons, Inc. Published 2020 by John Wiley & Sons, Inc.

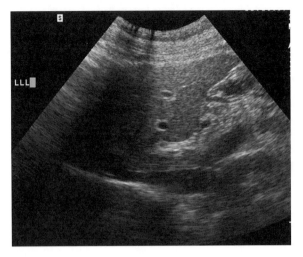

Figure 17.1 The liver image was produced by a damaged transducer that had been dropped accidentally. The defect was obvious.

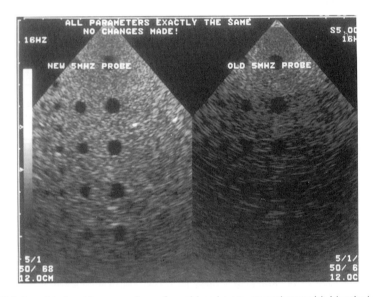

Figure 17.2 This is a side-by-side comparison of an old and a new transducer with identical system settings. The gradual degradation would be detected earlier if performance consistency were checked periodically by quality control tests.

detailed description of how the parameters should be measured. Various accrediting bodies such as American College of Radiology (ACR) [9] and American Institute of Ultrasound in Medicine (AIUM) [10] adopted some QC procedures described in these guidelines and established a minimum set of QC tests for accreditation requirements. Although a test object is needed to perform the required QC tests, the accrediting bodies have designated no standard ultrasound phantom so far. Due to the lack of standard acceptance criteria, existing guidelines typically suggest that measurements be compared to baseline or previous measurements in order to validate the consistency of ultrasound system performance. Although this is helpful in monitoring system performance

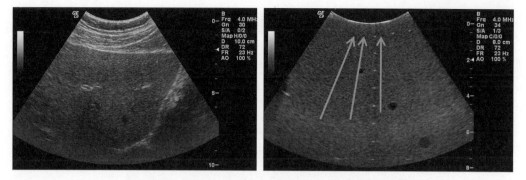

Figure 17.3 This array transducer had five broken wires since the transducer cable was rolled over by the scanner wheel (the broken wires were confirmed by an electronic transducer tester). The defect was shown on the phantom image. *Source:* Reproduced by permission of AIUM [1].

trends, questions remain concerning how to accurately measure the performance of a system and compare it to others. Although survey studies have been published to present typical ranges of the QC parameters [11, 12], criteria are usually dependent upon the model and vendor, not to mention the intra- and inter-observer variability.

17.2 System Performance

17.2.1 Phantoms for QC Testing

An ultrasound phantom is a device built with materials that have acoustic properties similar to those of human tissue so that the phantom can be used as a "simulating patient" for ultrasound imaging [13]. Important tissue-mimicking characteristics include: speed of sound propagation (which should match $1540\,\mathrm{m\ s^{-1}}$ assumed by ultrasound imagers), attenuation coefficient, backscatter coefficient, and the frequency dependence of both attenuation and backscatter within the ultrasound frequency range over which a phantom is intended to be used. Newer interests include mimicking the non-linearity parameter (B/A) for harmonic imaging, elastic properties for ultrasound elastography and thermal properties for high intensity focused ultrasound (HIFU). Typically, specification of the acoustic properties of a phantom is available to users of these phantoms. Since the acoustic properties of certain gel phantoms may drift over time, it is crucial for users to know the gel life period during which there should be no significant changes in the acoustic properties of the phantom material. Phantom storage conditions, such as the safe temperature range, should also be provided to enable proper handling of ultrasound phantoms.

There is a wide variety of tissue-mimicking materials (TMMs). Solid forms are agar, Zerdine® (a water-based polymer) and urethanes. Other materials are also used, such as epoxies to simulate bone, liquids for blood-mimicking fluid, and natural materials in custom phantoms. A variety of phantoms for testing spectral Doppler and color Doppler are available, and development is continuing. Examples are string test objects and tissue-mimicking phantoms with flow control systems of pumps and built-in flow meters.

Usually, a general-purpose or a multi-purpose ultrasound phantom is sufficient to perform the QC tests required by accrediting bodies such as ACR [9] and AIUM [10]. However, more sophisticated phantoms are required to further evaluate system performance. For example, a spherical lesion phantom is effective in evaluating both contrast and spatial resolution of an ultrasound system [14, 15]. There are also various specialized phantoms available to test tissue Doppler, 3D mode, and ultrasound-guided brachytherapy systems.

Ultrasound transducer probes come with various surface shapes, and it is essential that the probe surface remain acoustically coupled to the phantom for QC tests. Simple phantoms with curved or half-cylinder windows (Figure 17.4(a) and (b)) are useful in performing uniformity checks for curved array transducers and endocavity transducers. A phantom for ultrasound-guided brachytherapy has a curved surface for coupling with endocavity transducers (Figure 17.4(c)). A clever alternative to these phantoms is a simple homemade liquid phantom that works well with various transducers (Figure 17.4(d)) [16]. Also, a comprehensive QC phantom with cone-shaped scanning windows on two sides has been designed to fit curved linear array transducers with various radii (Figure 17.4(e)) [1].

Over time, there is a potential problem of dehydration with water-based TMMs. Some examples of desiccated phantoms are shown in Figure 17.5. Storing the phantom according to manufacturer recommendations can minimize this problem. It is also recommended that the reduction of the phantom's weight is monitored. If dehydration occurs, rejuvenation may be performed using a rejuvenation kit that can be purchased through manufacturers of phantoms.

Rubber-based phantom materials (e.g. urethane) are more stable and suitable for long-term consistency tests. However, the speed of sound propagation in urethane is only $1480\,\text{m s}^{-1}$ while the average speed of sound propagation in soft tissue is $1540\,\text{m s}^{-1}$ and that value is typically assumed in the range algorithm of an ultrasound scanner. One direct consequence of this discrepancy in sound speed affects distance measurements. Often, the targets in a rubber-based phantom are re-positioned accordingly to compensate for the mismatch in sound speed. However, this kind of

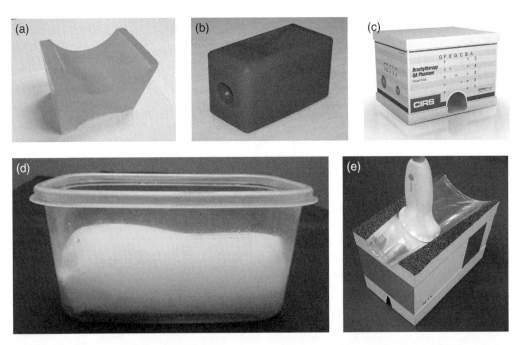

Figure 17.4 Ultrasound uniformity testing phantoms for transducers with curved surfaces. (a) ATS made for AAPM Task Group. (b) GAMMEX/RMI Model UTED. (c) CIRS ultrasound phantom for ultrasound-guided Brachytherapy QC test. (d) Home-made liquid phantom for uniformity test. *Source:* Reproduced by permission of IOP Publishing [16]. (e) UW-Madison phantom. *Source:* Reproduced by permission of AIUM [1].

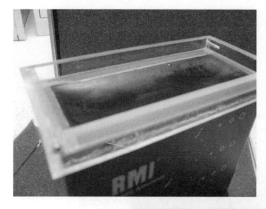
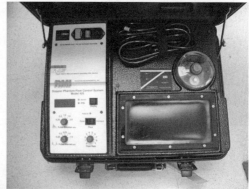
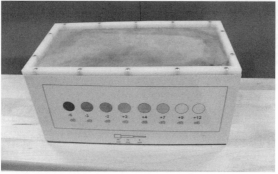

Figure 17.5 Examples of phantom desiccation are shown. The problem of dehydration over time can be minimized by following closely the manufacturer's recommendations of storage and handling.

target shifting may work differently for different transducer types when linear-, phased-, convex-, and vector-array transducers are considered [17]. Therefore, the targets in a rubber-based phantom cannot be repositioned to correct all distance measurement errors for all transducer types. Another consequence, probably more important, is that mismatch of the sound speed causes beam defocusing affecting image quality assessment [17]. This effect is well demonstrated both in a simulation study [18] and in a phantom study [19]. Users are cautioned when using QC phantoms made of rubber-based materials. While these phantoms may be very good for consistency testing, the problems caused by the mismatched sound speed must be noted.

17.2.2 Metrics for QC Testing on B-Mode

The majority of the QC tests described below are performed with a phantom that represents a "constant patient." Images and measurements taken of the phantom over periods of time can be utilized to monitor system performance changes.

1) **Image geometry:** Accurate size measurement is crucial for diagnostic ultrasound. For example, crown rump length is used to estimate gestational age. Typically, this test assesses the accuracy of distance measurements along the sound beam axis (vertical) and lateral direction (horizontal). Built-in filament targets with known distances are scanned and measured as shown in Figure 17.6. *Tips:* It is important to not press the transducer down too hard because the majority of phantom materials are elastic. Too much pressure may introduce errors in vertical distances among filament targets. *Tolerance:* The suggested defect level is ≥2 mm or

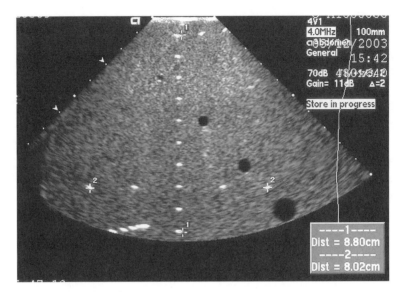

Figure 17.6 Image geometry test: distance accuracy test in horizontal and vertical directions.

a 2% error for vertical distance accuracy and ≥ 3 mm or a 3% error for horizontal distance accuracy, whichever is greater [5]. The suggested action level is ≥ 1.5 mm or a 1.5% error for vertical distance accuracy and ≥ 2 mm or a 2% error for horizontal distance accuracy, whichever is greater [5].

To verify 3D spatial measurement accuracy, AIUM standards [20] require special phantoms with volumetric egg-shaped or wire-targets (Figure 17.7) to measure perimeters, volumes, and surface areas. The caveat is that more operator skills are needed to scan volumetric egg-shaped targets. Therefore, wire target phantoms are the preferred objects to make QC testing easier and quicker.

2) **Maximum depth of penetration (system sensitivity):** This test evaluates the sensitivity of an ultrasound scanner by comparing the gradually weakening echo texture to electronic noises near the bottom of the phantom image. From this comparison, one can determine the maximum depth at which the weakest echo signal is clearly detected and displayed (Figure 17.8). This is one of the ultrasound tests without standard pass/fail criteria. Existing guidelines

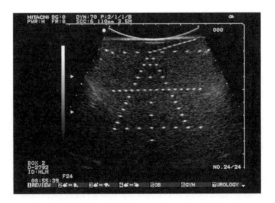

Figure 17.7 Image geometry test: 2D and 3D spatial measurements. *Source:* http://www.cirsinc.com/ products/ultrasound/zerdine-hydrogel/ultrasound-phantoms-for-2d-3d-evaluation/.

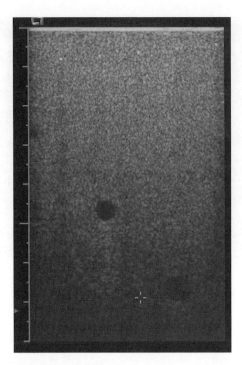

Figure 17.8 Maximum depth of penetration test.

typically suggest that the measurements must be compared to baseline or previous measurements to validate consistency of the ultrasound system performance. Since this is a consistency check, system presets need to be fixed in order to minimize variations. The reproducibility of this test is important, so efforts have been made to develop automated ultrasound QC software in this area [1, 21, 22]. One such example is described in an AIUM publication [1] (Figure 17.9). *Tips:* This test should be done with the field of view just large enough to permit a maximum depth of visualization. The system should be at maximum transmit power, maximum focal depth and proper receiver gain and time gain compensation (TGC) to allow a visible echo texture in deep regions. Obviously, this QC parameter also depends on phantom attenuation properties. Transducers with low frequencies are better tested using $0.7\,\mathrm{dB\,cm^{-1}\,MHz^{-1}}$ phantoms and other frequencies with $0.5\,\mathrm{dB\,cm^{-1}\,MHz^{-1}}$ phantoms. *Tolerance:* The suggested defect level is over 1 cm of change from the baseline and the suggested action level is over 0.6 cm of change from the baseline [5]. This approach does not consider the transducer frequency factor. It has been noted that a 1 cm of loss in the maximum depth of penetration is a much more severe problem for high operating frequency transducers than for low operating frequency transducers. A better criterion is to consider both the depth of change and the transducer operating frequency and to take action when a 5 dB change in sensitivity is measured [6].

3) **Image uniformity and artifact survey:** The image-uniformity test is a visual assessment that involves looking for various image artifacts and non-uniformities including: vertical or radially oriented streaks, horizontal bands, dropouts, reduction of brightness near the edges of the image and the brightness transitions between focal zones (Figure 17.10). In cases of an element dropout, the defect may be detectable by the "in-air" scans (Figure 17.11). Therefore, some would use an in-air approach for a quick uniformity assessment. However, we should understand that the "in-air" only approach has limited sensitivity, especially for sector and vector

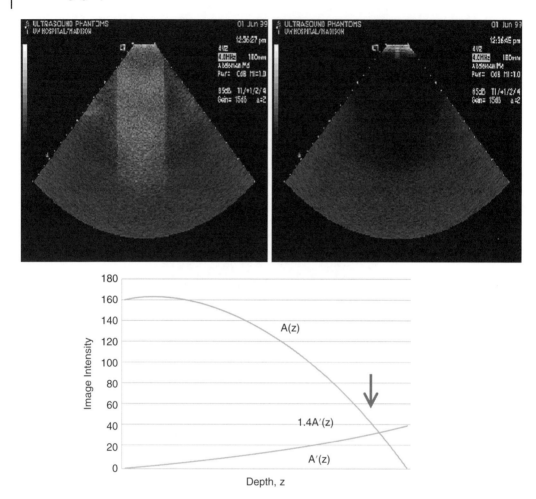

Figure 17.9 Automated QC software to measure the maximum depth of penetration. *Source:* Reproduced by permission of AIUM [1].

transducers. Therefore, a uniform phantom scan is needed for a more thorough uniformity test. Even though one can often work around minor non-uniformities in clinical applications, these defects should be seen as a potential large problem and the source that causes the non-uniformities should be investigated. Non-uniformities may be caused by defects in transducer elements, cable wires, connectors, the scanner transmitter, or TGC, among other reasons. *Tips:* Make sure the coupling gel is good. Turn off the compound imaging feature to heighten the sensitivity of non-uniformity detection. Vary the field of view (FOV) and use both single and multiple focal zones during this test. Live images are more sensitive than frozen images in detecting non-uniformities. Selecting a shallow depth setting is good for detecting transducer dropouts due to the reduced aperture. *Criteria:* The criterion for this test is subjective because the threshold may vary from operator to operator. However, any noticeable non-uniformity should be documented and monitored.

This is an area to which ultrasound QC software has been applied [23]. This method has great potential for automated QC if it can be fully integrated to ultrasound systems. One report found [12] that transducer element failure is the most frequent deficiency of modern ultrasound

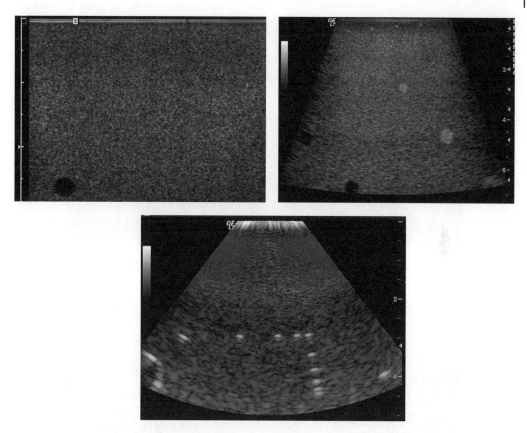

Figure 17.10 Image non-uniformity examples.

imagers. An automated QC method, would be efficient in catching element dropouts at a very early stage before they manifest themselves in clinical imaging.

4) **Ring down:** This test specifies the distance from the surface of a transducer to the first distinguishable echo signal. It outlines the shallow region where no useful echo data can be collected. Therefore, it is also known as a "dead zone" test. During this test, the portion of the QC phantom that contains a group of filament targets at close separations from the top of the phantom is utilized (Figure 17.12). As a transducer scans across the top, the distance from the transducer to the first completely imaged reflector is equal to the dead zone distance. *Tips:* Scan the phantom with a small FOV and set the focal zone to the minimum depth. *Criteria:* The dead zone should be less than 3 mm for frequencies above 7 MHz, less than 5 mm for frequencies between 3 and 5 MHz and less than 7 mm for frequencies lower than 3 MHz [5]. This appears to be a test for old technologies when near field reverberations obscure target visualization near surface. Recent technology has significantly improved clarity in this region. However, sometimes looking at these targets near the surface can reveal defects that would otherwise have been missed. In Figure 17.13, ghost images are seen in the ring down test caused by a flawed transducer probe.

5) **Anechoic lesion detectability:** This test examines the ability of an ultrasound system to detect and accurately display cystic objects of various sizes (Figure 17.14). It usually employs a phantom with cylindrical anechoic objects of various sizes located at different depths. *Tips*: Record the smallest visible anechoic object at a specific depth. Grade the visibility of the

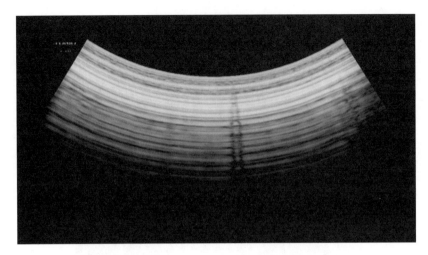

Figure 17.11 The "in-air" image acquired with the transducer surface contacting just air.

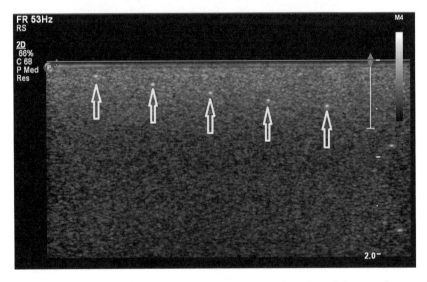

Figure 17.12 The ring down or dead zone is the distance from the front face of the transducer to the first identifiable echo. The shallow portion of an ultrasound phantom that contains a group of filament targets placed at close separations from the top of the phantom (such as 1–8 mm) is utilized for this test.

anechoic objects such as clear, fill-in, jagged edge and other noticeable characteristics. *Tolerances:* There should be no major distortion or fill-in on the anechoic object display. Changes from the baseline of the anechoic void perception should be monitored.

A huge improvement is to have spherical lesions instead of cylindrical lesions. A spherical lesion phantom consists of simulated focal lesions embedded within echogenic TMMs [14, 15]. Usually, slice thickness is worse than axial resolution or lateral resolution. If the diameter of a small sphere is much less than the "slice thickness," it may not be detectable, whereas a cylinder of the same composition and diameter but aligned perpendicularly to the scanning plane, could be easily detected. Therefore, spherical lesion phantoms add the additional aspect of testing the spatial and contrast resolution in all three dimensions. In the example shown in Figure 17.15, a

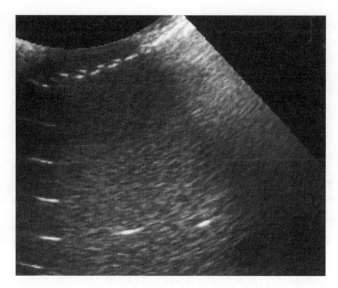

Figure 17.13 Ring down test may reveal transducer defects which otherwise would have been missed. As shown in this example, ghost images of the pins are seen caused by a flawed transducer probe.

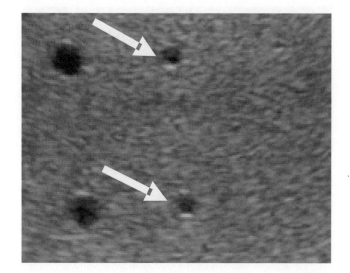

Figure 17.14 The anechoic lesion visibility test is to examine the system's ability to detect and accurately display round, negative contrast objects of various sizes. Typically, a phantom has cylindrical lesions; thus only good for 2D assessment.

conventional linear array transducer typically has a wide slice thickness near the surface; thus it cannot detect the spherical lesions at a depth of 1 cm or less. A "1.5D" array transducer with additional rows of elements can dynamically focus the beam in elevation; it thus has better detectability near the surface.

6) **Spatial resolution**: Spatial resolution measures the ability of an ultrasound system to distinguish closely spaced objects. Since spatial resolution is depth dependent, this is often measured at several depths for a transducer. Approximately, axial and lateral spatial resolution may be

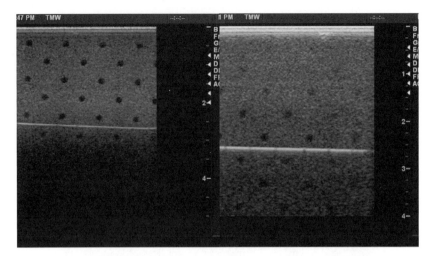

Figure 17.15 Lesion detectability test can be improved by having spherical lesions instead of cylindrical lesions. This test visually assesses the aspects of spatial and contrast resolution. In this example, a "1.5D" array transducer with additional rows of elements (left) performs better than a conventional linear array transducer (right) because it can dynamically focus the beam in elevational dimension; thus has better detectability near surface. *Source:* James A. Zagzebski.

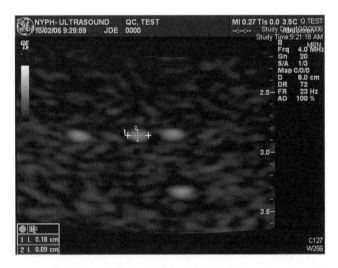

Figure 17.16 The axial and lateral resolution can be measured by imaging targets which are arranged at progressively close spacing and determining the minimal target spacing that can be "resolved" on the gray-scale image. Or we can measure the pin size in axial and lateral directions using the scanner's digital calipers.

evaluated through closely spaced filament groups in a phantom (Figure 17.16). For a rough estimation, count the number of distinguished targets in a lateral and axial direction and document the minimum target spacing. To be more quantitative, one may measure the size of the target in a lateral and axial direction. Decrease the gain to barely visualize the peak of the target. Then, increase the gain by 20 dB. The measured target size is approximate to the full width at a tenth-maximum (FWTM) of the target profile. *Tips:* System settings should be the same for periodic QC tests to monitor changes over time. Be aware that doubling artifacts may appear on

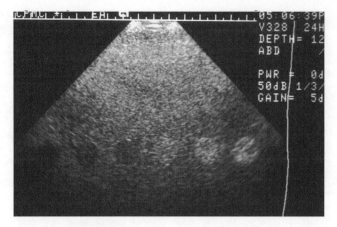

Figure 17.17 A phantom with built-in low contrast targets is used to assess contrast resolution.

axial resolution images for frequencies greater than 5 MHz. *Tolerance:* In general, axial resolution measured by filaments in tissue-mimicking phantoms should be ≤1 mm for operating frequencies greater than 4 MHz and ≤2 mm for operating frequencies less than 4 MHz [5]. It should remain stable over time. Lateral resolution should be less than

$$\lambda \times \frac{Focal\_Length(mm)}{Aperture(mm)}$$

where λ is the wavelength [5], although, in general, information about the aperture is not known to users.

7) **Contrast resolution:** Contrast object detectability is used to assess the contrast resolution of an ultrasound system. A special phantom with built-in low contrast targets is needed for this test (Figure 17.17). The test result relies heavily on display devices. In general, this test is done by comparing a new image with the baseline image. Therefore, it is more of a consistency check than an absolute measurement of system performance because there is no definitive pass/fail criterion.

8) **Soft copy and hard copy image fidelity:** This test concerns all the hard copy recording devices and the soft copy viewing monitors on an ultrasound scanner as well as the ones in reading rooms. Since these devices operate independently from one another, it is important to properly set up each device to ensure agreement between image features on the system monitor and the features on the monitors in reading rooms. The consistency of image display monitors should be periodically checked. The standards and guidelines for diagnostic display monitors in general should also apply to display monitors for ultrasound imaging [24]. Typically, tests should be done for maximum and minimum luminance, luminance uniformity, resolution, and spatial accuracy. The majority of the ultrasound imaging systems have built-in test patterns, such as the SMPTE pattern [25] and TG18 test pattern [26] that can be used for testing various prospects of soft/hard copy devices (Figure 17.18). *Tips:* For quick follow-up testing, grayscale bar patterns on clinical image displays can be used (Figure 17.19). However, a simple 15-step grayscale bar pattern may not be sensitive enough to detect subtle but problematic deficiencies in monitor agreement. *Criteria:* The shades of gray, weak, and strong echo textures should be optimized and made consistent between the monitor on an ultrasound scanner and the photographic hard copies or soft copy viewing monitors in

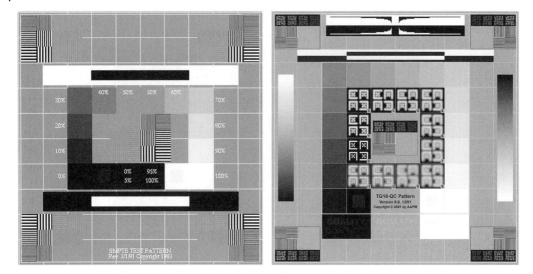

Figure 17.18 Image test patterns (SMPTE pattern and TG-18 pattern) are normally available on the machine and can be used to check the monitor display [24–26].

reading rooms. The number of grayscale steps should not vary from the baseline by more than two over time [5].

9) **Physical and mechanical inspection:** During routine QC testing, physical checks related to equipment are worth attention. This assures the mechanical integrity of an ultrasound system, and the safety of both patient and operator. This test includes: checking for any cracks or delamination in transducers, noting loose and frayed electric cables, loose handles or control arms, checking the working condition of wheels and wheel locks, making sure all accessories (such as video cassette recorder (VCR), printer, etc.) are securely fastened to the system, making sure image monitors are clean and air filters are not dusty. Certain physical damage to a transducer may be revealed simply by careful visual inspection of the transducer. For example, a hole in the transducer lens that was possibly punctured by biopsy needles can be revealed by this test (Figure 17.20(a)). Other examples of deficiencies revealed by this simple test include cracks in the transducer housing, cuts in the transducer cable possibly as a result of being rolled over by the wheel of the ultrasound scanner, missing or broken pins in a transducer connector, or other issues with the mechanical integrity of the equipment (Figure 17.20(b) and (c)).

17.2.3 Metrics of QC Testing on Doppler Ultrasound

Although there are simplified Doppler ultrasound devices, such as standalone continuous wave (cw) device or standalone pulsed wave (pw) devices, the clinical ultrasound systems of our emphasis here are duplex systems that include a combination of B-mode and Doppler mode. An example is given in Figure 17.21. A line in the B-mode image indicates the Doppler ultrasound beam and a range gate outlines the echo data segment for pulsed Doppler measurement. A cursor aligned by an operator to be parallel to the vessel wall measures the Doppler angle. The flow information is displayed on the lower portion of the image. Doppler ultrasound QC tests involve two major aims: to ensure consistent flow velocity measurements among various Doppler ultrasound systems; and to ensure consistent flow velocity measurements of a Doppler ultrasound system over time. Both are critical for clinicians to use the measured results for diagnosis.

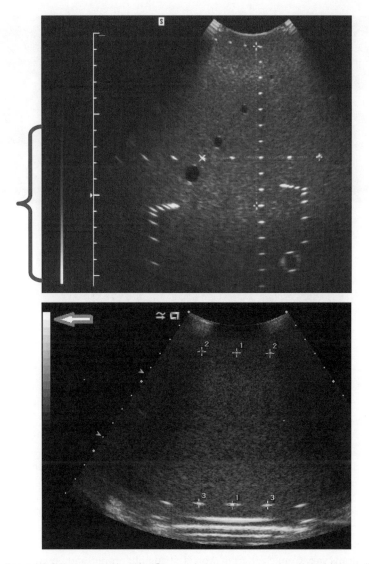

Figure 17.19 For quick follow-up testing, the Gray-scale bar pattern on the clinical image display (continuous bar or 15 discrete steps) can be used to ensure what is visible on display monitor on the ultrasound scanner is also visible on the soft/hard copy devices.

There are a large number of tests to evaluate the performance of a Doppler ultrasound system. Some are not suitable for testing Doppler systems in the clinical environment. Typically, measurable quantities for Doppler QC in the clinical environment are as follows [3, 8, 27]:

1) Doppler signal sensitivity
2) Doppler angle accuracy
3) Directional discrimination
4) Range-gate accuracy
5) Accuracy of peak-velocity readings

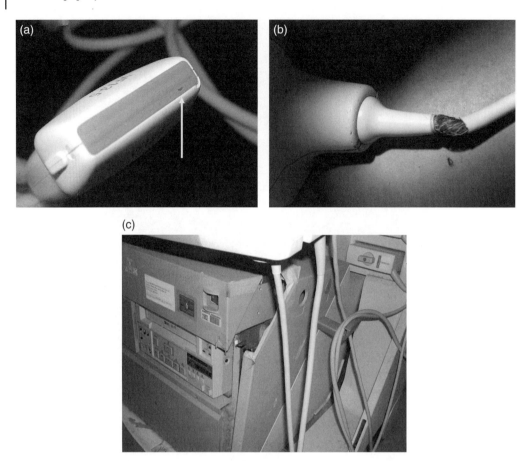

Figure 17.20 Deficiencies revealed by simple test of physical and mechanical inspection.

Although these parameters are used primarily for testing duplex Doppler instruments, applications to other types of Doppler devices (e.g. color Doppler and power Doppler) are also possible. These tests are not currently included in accreditation required QC tests.

Doppler phantoms vary from oscillating targets, string phantoms, and flowing fluids to complex tissue-mimicking phantoms with flow control systems. Take a Doppler phantom with a flow control system (Sun Nuclear/Gammex Inc., Middleton, Wisconsin) for example [27]. The background material in the phantom is tissue-mimicking with a sound speed of $1540\,\mathrm{m\,s^{-1}}$ and an attenuation coefficient slope of $0.5\,\mathrm{dB\,cm^{-1}\,MHz^{-1}}$. The flow of the phantom is formed by pumping a blood-mimicking fluid through a latex vessel. A microprocessor-based controller with a digital flow rate readout is employed to control the amount of the flow in the vessel. The phantom can produce both constant flows and pulsatile flows. The flow rate is measured and displayed in real-time; thus the velocity accuracy of a Doppler ultrasound system can be checked.

1) **Doppler signal sensitivity:** Doppler signal sensitivity is determined by measuring the maximum range of penetration of Doppler signals. This is done by scanning the flow in the diagonal vessel of the phantom with the output power at its maximum level and the receiver gain adjusted to its highest value without excessive noise on the display. The Doppler signals get progressively weaker as the depth increases, finally lessening to a point where the signal pattern

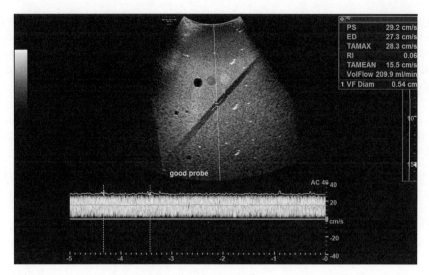

Figure 17.21 Duplex B-mode and Doppler ultrasound image obtained from a Doppler phantom with flow control system.

can barely be discerned from the background noise. This is where the maximum range of penetration is set. The pulsatile flow mode of the phantom is used to make the signal pattern easier for recognition from background noises.

2) **Doppler angle accuracy**: Doppler angle accuracy is tested by aligning the central line of the display with the built-in vertical column of the reflectors in the phantom and the angle-correction cursor line parallel to the diagonal vessel wall (Figure 17.21). The measured angle from the unit should agree with the built-in angle in the phantom [27]. Additional tests of Doppler angle accuracy can be performed by comparing the measured angle from the Doppler unit with the angle measured by using a protractor on a hard copy of the image, or using angle measurement tools on a picture archiving and communication system (PACS).

3) **Directional discrimination**: Directional discrimination adequacy is assessed by placing the Doppler sample volume cursor in the vessel where a single direction flow is assured, and inspecting whether a mirror image appears on the display. If a reverse flow is presented, errors might have occurred in the phase shifting circuitry of the Doppler unit.

4) **Range-gate accuracy**: The range gate accuracy test concerns the accuracy of the position of the Doppler sample volume cursor. In this test, the cursor is moved slowly across the vessel while simultaneously observing the Doppler signals. The strongest Doppler signal and the highest peak-velocity are expected when the cursor is at the center of the vessel. The range gate accuracy of a Doppler unit is important when small vessels are studied in clinical applications.

5) **Accuracy of peak-velocity readings**: Although a Doppler flow phantom may provide flows different from those encountered in real clinical applications, the phantom peak-velocity accuracy test measures the ability of a Doppler unit to produce accurate readings of idealized flows. Since the flow can be controlled, the test can be repeated. Unfortunately, the built-in flow meter of the phantom can only provide readings of the flow rate, not of the peak-velocity. Therefore, the following equation is used to estimate peak-velocity Vp:

$$Vp = 2F / S$$

Where F is the flow rate on the digital display of the phantom and S is the cross-sectional area of the vessel. The assumption of a laminar flow with a parabolic velocity profile is made for the flow in the vessel. This assumption may not be true for a Doppler phantom under certain conditions. Therefore, vendor specifications of the operating conditions for the parabolic velocity profile should be provided to users of the phantom.

17.2.4 Metrics of QC Testing on Ultrasound-Guided Prostate Brachytherapy Systems

Ultrasound imaging has been utilized effectively not only for diagnostic purposes but also for guiding therapeutic procedures. Transrectal ultrasound imaging has long been utilized in prostate brachytherapy for treatment planning, image guidance during the seed implantation, and verification of the seed distribution after the seed implantation is completed. QC testing of such an ultrasound system needs to include additional tests beyond the QC tests discussed earlier in this chapter. Since ultrasound-guided prostate brachytherapy has been widely accepted as a primary tool for treating prostate cancer, guidelines of ultrasound QC testing for this particular application were examined by Task Group 128 of the American Association of Physicists in Medicine. A detailed report was published addressing quality assurance requirements specific to transrectal ultrasound used for guidance of prostate brachytherapy [28]. Some of the suggested QC tests are the same as those described for B-mode ultrasound QC, namely:

1) **Grayscale visibility (soft copy and hard copy image fidelity)**
2) **Maximum depth of penetration (system sensitivity)**
3) **Axial and lateral resolution**
4) **Axial and lateral distance measurement accuracy (image geometry)**

   Additional QC tests are suggested specifically for transrectal ultrasound-guided prostate brachytherapy systems:
5) **Area measurement accuracy**: Since the accuracy of area measurement is crucial for prostate brachytherapy treatment, verification of area measurement is a pivotal part of the QC program for this type of equipment. This test requires a phantom with a target of a known cross-sectional area to verify the measured results by an ultrasound system. For an area measurement accuracy test, the target in the phantom needs to be traced on an ultrasound system and the result verified. The action limit for this test is described as follows [28]: "The calculated value should be within 5% of the nominal target area." It is suggested that this test be performed annually.
6) **Volume measurement accuracy**: The accuracy of the volume measurement directly affects the dosimetry calculation for prostate treatment. This test requires a phantom with a three-dimensional target of known size. The volume is measured following typical clinical protocols to use the stepper on the prostate treatment ultrasound system and contour the target at each step location. The action limit for this test is described as follows [28]: "The calculated value should be within 5% of the nominal target volume." It is suggested that this test be performed annually.
7) **Needle template/electronic grid alignment**: An ultrasound system for prostate seed implantation provides an electronic grid pattern superimposed on the ultrasound image. Typically, this grid pattern consists of a matrix of points with a point-to-point spacing of 5 mm. On the other hand, a needle template where holes are arranged accordingly to correspond to the electronic grid pattern on the ultrasound image is attached to the ultrasound probe and the stepper device. The template allows the seed implant needle to follow predefined trajectories.

Therefore, it is very important that the electronic grid pattern be aligned with the actual needle template. It is noted by AAPM TG128 that it will need a phantom with "an array of high contrast targets for verification of the electronic grid" [28]. Unfortunately, such a phantom is not currently available. However, a simple technique using a tank of degassed water at room temperature has been published to be effective in aligning the needle template to the ultrasound image grid pattern [30]. If inaccuracy is noted, the transducer probe support usually allows adjustment in three orientations – lateral, anterior–posterior, and rotational dimension. The action limit is 3 mm in alignment [28]. The frequency for this test is recommended to be annual for pre-planned implants and optional for intra-operative planning.

8) **Treatment planning computer**: This test is recommended during the acceptance testing of an ultrasound system and/or treatment planning computer [28]. It inspects the integrity of the treatment planning software using ultrasound images from the ultrasound system. Specifically, the prostate volume measured on the ultrasound system should match the volume measured on the treatment planning computer. Otherwise, the dosimetry plan created by the treatment planning computer cannot reflect the actual dosimetry received by the treated prostate. A phantom with a built-in volume target can be utilized for this test. The ultrasound images of the volume target can be imported into the treatment planning computer. The volume target can also be traced and contoured to measure the volume using the treatment planning software and be compared to the result measured by the ultrasound system. The volume rendered by the computer shall agree with that of the ultrasound system to within 5% [28].

The above mentioned QC tests outline the issues of primary importance to QC testing on ultrasound-guided prostate brachytherapy systems. Although the AAPM TG128 did not designate a QC phantom in this category, commercial phantoms are available and may be useful for the QC tests discussed above.

17.3 Testing Paradigm and Clinical Implementation

17.3.1 Acceptance Testing and Commissioning

Acceptance testing and commissioning should include a set of high level performance tests that can determine whether or not the system is performing adequately according to the manufacturer's specifications. The measurements should cover a sufficiently wide range of features that best indicate the system performance, even allowing meaningful comparison among ultrasound systems. In addition, these tests generate the baseline data for future QC tests.

All of the metrics described above should be tested during the acceptance testing when applicable. As an ultrasound system typically has multiple transducers, the acceptance testing can be time consuming. The importance of testing image display monitors should be emphasized. It is crucial to have the optimal image quality on the system monitor because image acquisitions are done based upon the image display on the system monitor. On the other hand, it is also crucial to have consistent image display between the system monitor and the monitors in reading rooms because critical interpretation is done on reading room monitors. Additional safety concerns are necessary during the acceptance testing, such as checking the environmental conditions including electrical environment (power line, grounding, etc.).

For medical physicists, it is important to have detailed manufacturer's specifications of system performance at the time of acceptance testing.

Table 17.1 Quality Control Levels [1–8].

	Testing Effort	Testing Frequency	Testing Personnel	QC Test Examples
Level 1	Quick checks with no special tool	Daily or weekly or monthly	By ultrasound users and overseen by medical physicists	• Physical and mechanical inspection • Display monitor visual inspection
Level 2	Quick QC tests with a simple phantom	Quarterly or semi-annually	By ultrasound users and overseen by medical physicists	• Image uniformity and artifact survey • Image geometry • Soft copy and hard copy image fidelity
Level 3	Comprehensive QC tests with multiple phantoms	Annually or bi-yearly	By medical physicists	• Maximum depth of penetration • Ring down • Anechoic lesion detectability • Spatial resolution • Contrast resolution • Comprehensive image display monitor QC • Doppler ultrasound QC

17.3.2 QC Testing

Three levels of QC testing are proposed in the IEC standard (Table 17.1) [23]. AIUM and ACR guidelines have similar suggestions [2, 4]. In ultrasound imaging, some changes may happen abruptly and need frequent monitoring to detect the problem in time. Level 1 tests are quick checks to be performed very frequently (i.e. daily, weekly, or monthly) by ultrasound system users and require no special equipment. Level 1 tests include visual inspection of the integrity of an ultrasound system and simple consistency checks of the image display monitor. Failure in level 1 tests may activate level 2 or level 3 tests.

Level 2 tests need a simple phantom and are performed less frequently (quarterly or semi-annually) by ultrasound system users. The image uniformity and artifact survey test is a level 2 test. The image geometry test is another QC test that may be performed at level 2 [23]. Failure in level 2 tests may activate level 3 tests.

Level 3 tests are more comprehensive and require more sophisticated testing tools. Level 3 tests should be performed annually or at least every two years by qualified medical physicists. Level 3 tests should include all level 1 and level 2 tests. In addition, level 3 tests include maximum depth of penetration, anechoic lesion detectability, spatial resolution and contrast resolution, ring down, and detailed display monitor testing. Acceptance testing falls in the category of level 3 tests. It should take place before the first patient is scheduled thereby establishing baseline performance values of an ultrasound system.

17.3.3 Efficacy and Sensitivity of Current Ultrasound QC

Studies have been done to examine the efficacy and sensitivity of ultrasound QC testing. The results vary. An early paper in 1984 [31] reported QC tests such as depth of penetration, axial resolution and gray scale efficacious for that time. However, a paper published in 1992 [32] reported poor correlations between their subjective operator assessment of human images and QC parameters including lateral resolution, dynamic range and slice thickness. Therefore, it was suggested that other quality assurance (QA) parameters were needed to quantify good image quality and equipment performance [32]. In a paper in 1996 [33], the importance of a rigorous testing of circumference was emphasized because it was found that the testing of traditional distance accuracy in axial and lateral directions was not sufficient. The study revealed a 15% over-measurement in circumference on one of the six machines tested. One study [11] reviewed data from an ultrasound QC program over a period of three years and adjusted the testing frequency of certain QC tests in order to catch deficiencies in a more timely manner. A more recent publication [12] summarized four-year experience with a clinical ultrasound QC program. Transducer failure was found to be the most common deficiency in modern ultrasound scanners. This raised the question of how we can effectively assess array transducer performance.

With regards to the efficacy of Doppler ultrasound QC testing, one study [34] examined the accuracy of volumetric flow rate measurements on five scanners with three experienced operators and the same Doppler phantom with a flow control system. The results showed that some scanners were worse than others in flow rate accuracy and errors of up to 20% were observed. This finding is consistent with an earlier study [35] showing an average variation coefficient of 23% for measuring the peak-velocity on 17 duplex Doppler units. Although a later study [29] showed much better consistency in flow velocity measurements among the units in one institution, the necessity of Doppler QC is warranted.

17.3.4 Ultrasound Accreditation

AIUM provides voluntary accreditation programs [10] in various specialties of ultrasound practices including abdominal, breast, gynecologic, urologic, dedicated musculoskeletal, dedicated thyroid/parathyroid, fetal echocardiography and obstetric or trimester-specific obstetric. Starting on 1/1/2015, head and neck specialties were also included. With regards to quality assurance requirements, AIUM indicates that a quality assurance program should be in place. Although the AIUM accreditation document provides only limited directives for the required quality assurance program, it states that routine calibration should be conducted at least once a year and that ultrasound practices must meet or exceed the AIUM quality assurance guidelines. Based upon the AIUM guidelines on routine quality assurance [2], daily QC level 1 tests should be done by sonographers such as a visual inspection of the physical and mechanical integrity of the system. Some tests should be performed multiple times per day such as transducer cleaning and immediate cleaning anytime there is a spill of bodily fluids or hazardous material. In addition, AIUM guidelines [2] require annual tests of transducer uniformity, maximum depth of visualization, target detection and distance measurement accuracy tests. These annual tests should be conducted by a physicist, an engineer or sonographer.

ACR [9] currently provides accreditation for breast ultrasound (including ultrasound guided breast biopsy) and general ultrasound in various specialty areas including: general, obstetrical, gynecological, vascular, and combination of the above. Effective June 1, 2014, documentation of ultrasound QC is required as part of the accreditation application package. All facilities applying for accreditation must comply with the minimum QC testing requirements. As part of the accreditation application, facilities must demonstrate compliance with the ACR QC requirements by providing: (i) A report from the most recent annual survey performed by a qualified medical physicist or "appropriately trained personnel with ultrasound imaging equipment experience" who has been approved by the lead interpreting physician [9]; (ii) Documentation of corrective action if the annual survey identifies performance problems. The required QC tests must be performed at least annually on all machines and transducers in routine clinical use. The annual QC tests include physical and mechanical inspection, image uniformity and artifact survey, geometric accuracy (optional), system sensitivity, scanner display monitor performance, primary interpretation display monitor performance, and optional contrast and spatial resolution. There is also a recommendation for sonographers to perform an optional component of routine QC tests recommended semiannually. The optional semiannual QC tests include: physical and mechanical inspection, image uniformity and artifact survey, geometric accuracy (only for mechanically scanned transducers) and visual assessment of display monitor performance. There is currently no ACR-designated ultrasound phantom. Synchronizing the format of ultrasound accreditation with other imaging modality accreditations, ACR [9] ultrasound accreditation also uses a summary form for medical physicists to submit their reports and an evaluation form for oversight of the site's routine QC as conducted by sonographers.

17.4   Medical Physics 1.5

17.4.1   Electronic Transducer Tester

As mentioned earlier, transducer failure was found to be the most common deficiency of modern ultrasound scanners. One important ultrasound QC approach worth mentioning is to test the transducer separately from the system through electronic means. This approach is different from visual assessments of system performance utilizing tissue-mimicking phantoms. A transducer testing device has been developed to focus on testing the array transducer alone in a quantitative and objective manner [36–38]. A list of measurements provided by this device includes: element sensitivity, element center operating frequency, element fractional bandwidth, pulse shape, pulse duration and element and cable capacitance. Since the transducer is separated from the ultrasound scanner for a direct element-by-element evaluation, the device is much more efficient in identifying defects in transducers than phantom tests that inspect the integral performance of the entire imaging chain of the ultrasound system. This device is efficient in detecting problems with array transducers as follows: dead and reduced sensitivity elements; acoustic lens delaminations; lens swelling; matching layer delamination; backing material delamination; fluid infiltration into or behind the acoustic stack; damaged cable wires and damage to connector electronics. Figure 17.22 shows an example of the test report for one transducer that indicates several failed individual element channels. Studies [39, 40] reported using a transducer tester on 299 transducers on an annual basis for several years. The transducer arrays were tested element-by-element by the electronic transducer tester. The pass/fail criteria were set at four contiguous weak elements, three or more scattered dead elements, or two contiguous dead elements. The initial failure rate was approximately 40%. Three years after the introduction of annual transducer testing, the failure rate was lowered to 27.1%. The study demonstrated that it is difficult for users to realize when transducer function is deteriorating. Transducer failure may happen to both newer and older transducers. Remedies to reduce the transducer failure rate include correct transducer handling and reduced workload.

17.4.2   Automated Ultrasound QC Methods

The current phantom QC tests are objective and vulnerable to intra- and inter-observer variability. More reproducible and quantitative QC test results can be achieved with the aid of computerized

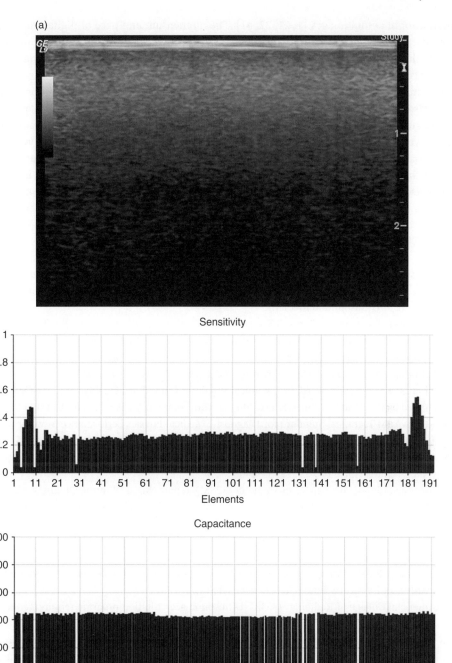

Figure 17.22 (a) The uniformity image from a transducer showed several dark streaks. (b) The report of the transducer by an electronic transducer tester confirmed several dead elements.

analysis of phantom images [1, 21, 22, 41]. The momentum and pace of digital imaging has supported the development of computerized analysis. The wide application of automated ultrasound QC methods is foreseeable if the automated method can be applied in a simple manner by ultrasound users and fully integrated into ultrasound system itself.

In summary, this chapter describes QC testing procedures currently required and/or recommended by advisory organizations and accreditation programs in diagnostic ultrasound imaging and ultrasound-guided brachytherapy. Although standard criteria of these QC tests is lacking, routine QC tests are proven to be efficacious in validating system performance consistency and monitoring system performance trends. If applied properly and diligently, ultrasound QC can detect system deficiencies before they become clinically evident. More clinical ultrasound physics support is warranted to improve overall patient care, which is discussed comprehensively in the next chapter.

References

1 Madsen, E.L., Garra, B.S., Zagzebski, J.A. et al. (2014). *AIUM Quality Assurance Manual for Gray Scale Ultrasound Scanners*. Laurel, MD: AIUM Technical Standards Committee, American Institute of Ultrasound in Medicine.

2 Boote, E.J., Forsberg, F., Garra, B.S. et al. (2008). *Routine Quality Assurance for Diagnostic Ultrasound Equipment*. Laurel, MD: AIUM Routine Quality Assurance of Clinical Ultrasound Equipment Subcommittee, American Institute of Ultrasound in Medicine.

3 Performance Criteria and Measurements for Doppler Ultrasound Devices: Technical Discussion – 2nd Edition, AIUM Technical Standards Committee, Quality Assurance Subcommittee, chaired by E. L Madsen, American Institute of Ultrasound in Medicine, Laurel, MD, 2002.

4 ACR-AAPM Technical Standard for Diagnostic Medical Physics Performance Monitoring of Real Time Ultrasound Equipment ACR Guidelines and Standards Committee, revised 2016.

5 Goodsitt, M.M., Carson, P.L., Witt, S. et al. (1998). Real-time B-mode ultrasound quality control test procedures. *Med. Phys.* 25: 1385–1406.

6 Institute of Physical Sciences in Medicine (IPSM) Report No. 71, Routine Quality Assurance of Ultrasound Imaging System, The Institute of Physical Sciences in Medicine, Ultrasound and Non-Ionising Radiation Topic Group, chaired and edited by Price R, 1995.

7 Institute of Physics and Engineering in Medicine (IPEM) (2009). Quality Assurance of Ultrasound Imaging Systems, Report no. 102, York.

8 Hoskins, P.R., Sherriff, S.B., and Evans, J.A. (eds.) (1994). *Testing of Doppler Ultrasound Equipment*. Institute of Physical Sciences in Medicine (IPSM).

9 American College of Radiology (ACR). Ultrasound accreditation program requirements https://www.acraccreditation.org/Modalities/Ultrasound (accessed 12/23/2019).

10 American Institute of Ultrasound in Medicine (AIUM). Ultrasound practice accreditation requirements. http://www.aium.org/accreditation/accreditation.aspx (accessed 28 August 2016).

11 Dudley, N.J., Griffith, K., Houldsworth, G. et al. (2001). A review of two alternative ultrasound quality assurance programmes. *Eur. J. Ultrasound* 12 (3): 233–245.

12 Hangiandreou, N.J., Stekel, S.F., Tradup, D.J. et al. (2011). Four-year experience with a clinical ultrasound quality control program. *Ultrasound Med. Biol.* 37 (8): 1350–1357.

13 Zagzebski, J.A., Edmonds, P., Stiles, T. et al. (2014). *Methods for Specifying Acoustic Properties of Tissue-Mimicking Phantoms and Objects*. AIUM Technical Standards Committee.

14 Kofler, J.M. and Madsen, E.L. (2001). Improved method for determining resolution zones in ultrasound phantoms with spherical simulated lesions. *Ultrasound Med. Biol.* 27 (12): 1667–1676.

15 Kofler, J.M. Jr., Lindstrom, M.J., Kelcz, F., and Madsen, E.L. (2005). Association of automated and human observer lesion detecting ability using phantoms. *Ultrasound Med. Biol.* 31 (3): 351–359.

16 King, D.M., Hangiandreou, N.J., Tradup, D.J., and Stekel, S.F. (2010). Evaluation of a low-cost liquid ultrasound test object for detection of transducer artefacts. *Phys. Med. Biol.* 55: N557–N570.

17 Goldstein, A. (2000). The effect of acoustic velocity on phantom measurements. *Ultrasound Med. Biol.* 26 (7): 1133–1143.

18 Chen, Q. and Zagzebski, J.A. (2004). Simulation study of effects of speed of sound and attenuation on ultrasound lateral resolution. *Ultrasound Med. Biol.* 30 (10): 1297–1306.

19 Dudley, N.J., Gibson, N.M., Fleckney, M.J., and Clark, P.D. (2002). The effect of speed of sound in ultrasound test objects on lateral resolution. *Ultrasound Med. Biol.* 28 (11–12): 1561–1564.

20 Carson, P.L., DuBose, T., Hileman, R. et al. (2004). Standard Methods for Calibration of 2-Dimensional and 3-Dimensional Spatial Measurement Capabilities of Pulse Echo Ultrasound Imaging Systems, AIUM Technical Standards Committee, American Institute of Ultrasound in Medicine, Laurel, MD.

21 Gorny, K.R., Tradup, D.J., and Hangiandreou, N.J. (2005). Implementation and validation of three automated methods for measuring ultrasound maximum depth of penetration: application to ultrasound quality control. *Med. Phys.* 32: 2615–2628.

22 Thijssen, J.M., Weijers, G., and de Korte, C.L. (2007). Objective performance testing and quality assurance of medical ultrasound equipment. *Ultrasound Med. Biol.* 33 (3): 460–471.

23 International Electrotechnical Commission (IEC) TS 62736 Ed. 1.0 Ultrasonics – Pulse-echo scanners – Simple methods for periodic testing to verify stability of an imaging system's elementary performance. 2016.

24 ACR-AAPM-SIIM technical standard for electronic practice of medical imaging. https://siim.org/page/practice_guidelines (accessed 29 November 2019).

25 Gray, J.E., Lisk, K.G., Haddick, D.H. et al. (1985). Test pattern for video displays and hard-copy cameras. *Radiology* 154: 519–527.

26 AAPM On-line Report No. 03, Assessment of display performance for medical imaging systems, by AAPM Task Group 18 chaired by E Samei, 2005. http://www.aapm.org/pubs/reports/OR_03.pdf (accessed 28 August 2016).

27 Boote, E.J. and Zagzebski, J.A. (1988). Performance tests of Doppler ultrasound equipment with a tissue and blood-mimicking phantom. *J. Ultrasound Med.* 7: 137–147.

28 Pfeiffer, D., Sutlief, S., Feng, W. et al. (2008) AAPM Task Group 128: Quality assurance tests for prostate brachytherapy ultrasound systems. *Med. Phys.* 35: 5471–5489.

29 Groth, D.S., Zink, F.E., Felmlee, J.P. et al. (1995). Blood flow velocity measurements: a comparison of 25 clinical ultrasonographic units. *J. Ultrasound Med.* 14 (4): 273–277.

30 Mutic, S., Low, D., Nussbaum, G. et al. (2000). A simple technique for alignment of perineal needle template to ultrasound image grid for permanent prostate implants. *Med. Phys.* 27 (1): 141–143.

31 Donofrio, N.M., Hanson, J.A., Hirsch, J.H., and Moore, W.E. (1984). Investigating the efficacy of current quality assurance performance tests in diagnostic ultrasound. *J. Clin. Ultrasound* 12: 251–260.

32 Metcalfe, S.C. and Evans, J.A. (1992). A study of the relationship between routine ultrasound quality assurance parameters and subjective operator image assessment. *Br. J. Radiol.* 65: 570–575.

33 Dudley, N.J. and Griffith, K. (1996). The importance of rigorous testing of circumference measuring calipers. *Ultrasound Med. Biol.* 22 (8): 1117–1119.

34 Hoyt, K., Hester, F.A., Bell, R.L. et al. (2009). Accuracy of volumetric flow rate measurements. *J. Ultrasound Med.* 28: 1511–1518.

35 Kimme-Smith, C., Hussain, R., Duerinckx, A. et al. (1990). Assurance of consistent peak-velocity measurements with a variety of duplex Doppler instruments. *Radiology* 177: 265–272.

36 Moore, G.W., Gessert, A., and Schafer, M. (2005). The need for evidence-based quality assurance in the modern ultrasound clinical laboratory. *Ultrasound* 13: 158–162.

37 Powis, R.L. and Moore, G.W. (2004). The silent revolution: catching up with the contemporary composite transducer. *J. Diagn. Med. Sonography* 20: 395–405.

38 Weigang, B., Moore, G.W., Gessert, J. et al. (2003). The methods and effects of transducer degradation on image quality and the clinical efficacy of diagnostic sonography. *J. Diagn. Med. Sonography* 19: 3–13.

39 Martensson, M., Olsson, M., Segall, B. et al. (2009). High incidence of defective ultrasound transducers in use in routine clinical practice. *Eur. J. Echocardiogr.* 10: 389–394.

40 Martensson, M., Olsson, M., and Brodin, L. (2010). Ultrasound transducer function: annual testing is not sufficient. *Eur. J. Echocardiogr.* 11: 801–805.

41 Gibson, N.M., Dudley, N.J., and Griffith, K. (2001). A computerised quality control testing system for B-mode ultrasound. *Ultrasound Med. Biol.* 27 (12): 1697–1711.

18

Clinical Ultrasonography Physics: Emerging Practice

Nicholas J. Hangiandreou[1], Paul Carson[2], and Zheng Feng Lu[3]

[1] Department of Radiology, Mayo Clinic Rochester, Rochester, MN, USA
[2] Department of Radiology, University of Michigan, Ann Arbor, MI, USA
[3] Department of Radiology, University of Chicago, Chicago, IL, USA

18.1   Philosophy and Significance

Diagnostic ultrasound has long been viewed as a "safe" modality, posing minimal practical risks when used for diagnosis. This may help explain why, as described in Chapter 17, testing requirements for ultrasound (US) practices to maintain compliance with accrediting bodies have been extremely minimal historically, and testing requirements to maintain compliance with federal or state regulations have been limited or non-existent. This, in turn, may explain the lack of medical physics support of any type provided in US practices, especially when compared with other modalities.

This current situation presents enormous opportunity for increasing the levels of medical physics involvement in US imaging practices. There are significant benefits that physics involvement can offer over a wide range of areas in the clinical US imaging practice, including performance testing for pre-purchase technology assessment; system acceptance and routine, ongoing quality control (QC) testing; protocol and scanning preset optimization for imaging and Doppler-based measurements of velocity and volume flow rate; introducing innovative imaging and measurement technologies into clinical practice; and education of sonographers and physicians. Also, the value of increased physics support will increase with time as US systems become more complex over time. However, the current state of minimal physics support in ultrasound practices also presents a significant practical challenge: *Physicists must be prepared to demonstrate to the clinical practice the value of any additional proposed services*; i.e. show how service cost is reasonable while increased practice quality or efficiency are useful for better serving the patient. This is an important consideration for physicists in every modality, but it is especially acute for ultrasound because the current paid level of physics support in many US practices may be non-existent. The remainder of this chapter will discuss opportunities for expanded physics support to increase quality and efficiency of US practices, and strategies for cost-effective implementation.

Clinical Imaging Physics: Current and Emerging Practice, First Edition. Edited by Ehsan Samei and Douglas E. Pfeiffer.

18.2 Metrics and Analytics

In this section, optimization and expansion of the traditional US image quality assessment techniques and approaches described in Chapter 17 will be discussed. Then the application of more sophisticated task-based model observer methods to ultrasound images will be considered.

18.2.1 Intrinsic Performance

The traditional performance metrics reviewed in Chapter 17 will continue to be useful in many testing scenarios. In particular, these measurements of individual performance metrics form the backbone of acceptance test and QC testing programs. In general, these metrics would benefit from (i) automated or semi-automated commercial software for obtaining performance measurements, (ii) documentation of detailed measurement protocols including image acquisition and data analysis, and (iii) data validating measurement properties; e.g. the accuracy or sensitivity, reproducibility, and stability of these metrics versus common imaging parameters (necessary when comparing performance between systems from different vendors). Both shareware (e.g. QA4US, http://music.radboudimaging.nl/index.php/MUSIC_qa4us) and commercial (e.g. UltraIQ, www.cablon.nl) software packages for image analysis are becoming available. However, definition of the entire process for obtaining performance metrics (including detailed phantom and protocol for acquisition of the ultrasound test images), and documentation of their properties are critical elements to allowing these metrics to be compared between clinical sites, and for meaningful performance standards to be determined and possibly included in future regulatory or accreditation requirements. This level of description for these methods is currently lacking. Metrics defined as described here should be developed to accommodate 2D and 3D grayscale imaging, and color and power mode Doppler imaging. Similar methods are needed for assessment of common quantitative measurements, such as spectral Doppler peak, mean velocity, and volume flow rate. Also, although some work to develop assessment methods for quantifying the severity of axial artifacts, e.g. due to transducer element or data channel component degradation, has been reported [1, 2], commercial tools and validated protocols to perform this function are also needed.

Although the same metric, e.g. maximum depth of penetration (DOP), may be included in protocols for both acceptance testing and ongoing QC, more consideration should be given in the future to the potential development of different measurement protocols to support these two different testing scenarios. At acceptance, the goal is to determine at the time of purchase if the device is operating at a sufficient level for payment to be issued. Precise methods that require greater care and time to execute, e.g. those that require data export from the scanner and subsequent computer analysis, are acceptable since these tests are performed infrequently. For periodic QC testing, where the goal is to detect clinically significant changes in performance since the last testing session, a greater premium is placed on lowering the costs of testing in terms of equipment cost and operator time, and simple visual approaches may be best. It should be noted, however, that time and cost savings might be recognized by performing very fast, very simple scans that are later autonomously analyzed and reported. Similarly, acceptance testing methods performed by a physicist or physicist assistant should have a very high sensitivity so even subtle issues are detected, while QC measurement performed by a clinical sonographer might benefit from methods with reduced sensitivity, so that issues that will clearly not require any action are not detected (since revealing minor problems could cause increased time to be invested by less-experienced personnel, with no potential clinical benefit).

There continues to be a need for meaningful performance benchmarks for both acceptance testing and QC applications, recognizing that these standards may be different from one another.

Performance standards for initial equipment acceptance are more straightforward. Vendor specifications, where available, provide clear performance thresholds, but care must be taken to assure that assessment techniques used to define the specification and for acceptance testing are comparable. Another very useful acceptance criterion that can be used when multiple identical equipment items are being purchased involves consistency of performance, requiring each device to operate within some tolerance of the median performance level for the group. This approach has practical clinical importance as the results of an exam should not depend in any significant way on which particular imaging system was used to perform the exam. Measurement methods with excellent reproducibility are required. Since the same price is being paid for each device, it seems reasonable to require that none perform at a significantly lower level than any others, even if this threshold performance level for acceptance is more demanding than one that might be considered as acceptable during later routine QC testing.

Further development of clinically meaningful performance benchmarks for ongoing QC testing is needed. Equipment issues that impact patient or operator safety are straightforward and must be addressed without delay. Managing more subtle equipment flaws is more difficult, and performance thresholds and action levels in these cases will ideally be established in partnership with the clinical practice, considering specific practice needs. One example of this would be to relate reductions in linear distance measurement accuracy to practical clinical impact in obstetric image practices, where these values are related to published databases of normal values and play a key role in patient management [3]. In general, reductions in various aspects of system performance, e.g. DOP or axial artifacts due to damaged transducer elements or channel components, can negatively impact the practice in several ways. (i) Effective QC testing can reveal the presence of axial artifacts that are not evident during clinical scanning. Although some work has begun to quantify the impact these might have on diagnostic performance, e.g. on Doppler velocity measurement accuracy and precision [4], much more data on these potential impacts is needed to allow effective risk assessment. Similarly, even modest reductions in DOP might indicate subtle increases in overall image noise, however, the practical impact on diagnostic performance has not been widely studied. (ii) Easily visible axial artifacts and DOP reductions can limit the effective useful field of view for a probe, but could leave clinically adequate image quality in the remaining image field. (iii) Visible artifacts or image degradation of any type present a risk to the reputation of the clinical practice when images are provided to patients and referring physicians outside of the imaging practice. (iv) Visible artifacts, especially if only intermittently observed, could present a distraction or annoyance to the sonographer, and result in reduced practice efficiency. In all cases, the clinical practice must play a strong role in determining when any of these potential impacts reaches an unacceptable level and require equipment repair or replacement. The cost of repair or replacement will also affect performance action levels, and so action levels may well be different depending on the service plan in force, e.g. payment for time and materials versus an annual service contract. When a service contract is present, the action level for some performance problems may even vary with time during the year. (Incidentally, it is worth noting here that even if only visible flaws are of concern to the clinical practice, it has been shown that a QC program provides significant benefit for detecting these issues, over and above simple reliance on the system operators to identify them [5, 6].)

18.2.2 Qualimetry

In general, additional performance measurement methods over and above those described above are needed in order to perform effective, comprehensive technology assessments of imaging systems being considered for purchase, or for image protocol and preset optimization. Techniques that provide an overall assessment including combined contributions of spatial resolution, contrast, and noise would be particularly useful, as would methods that are more directly correlated with actual clinical use of the imaging system. When performing pre-purchase comparisons of candidate imaging systems in our practice, in addition to measurements based on standard US phantoms, we have included imaging of normal volunteers and patients, with collection and analysis of image quality rating data from clinical sonographer and radiologist staff [7]. These comprehensive physics-led assessments have been judged as valuable contributions to the selection process. Our complete evaluation also includes assessment of connectivity-related functions, including DICOM structured report functions for measurement export, quality and format of live video out, and compatibility of all exported data with radiology department picture archiving and communication system (PACS) and institutional image archives.

Images of human subjects definitely present the most realistic and challenging imaging situation when evaluating ultrasound systems for purchase, but the images do not naturally lend themselves well to computer analysis. Collecting observer rating data from staff is feasible, but it is time-consuming and is generally more variable than computer analysis. Also, unless all candidate scanners are present at the same time, different patients will be scanned with the different scanners, so the challenges to different system candidates will not be the same. Normal volunteers also present realistic imaging challenges to the scanner, however there are not typically clinical findings present, which can be quite limiting when evaluating systems for lesion sensitivity. Images from the same volunteer can also vary from day to day, so different scanners may still be not presented with a standard, uniform challenge.

An extremely useful addition would be the inclusion of task-based assessments using model observers and corresponding clinically-relevant phantoms and targets ("tasks") [8]. Although human observers could be used as described above for pre-purchase technology assessments, use of computer-based model observers would be extremely valuable for this, and especially post-purchase for ongoing image optimization work. Model observer applications in ultrasound have been previously reported for imaging system evaluation and system design optimization (see, for example, [9–15]). Phantom targets used include echogenic cones imaged in cross section, anechoic spheres, and anechoic cylinders, while computational observers used include matched filters, the ideal observer, and target segmentation (in [14] via Canny edge detection). Figure 18.1 shows an example of a commercial phantom designed for task-based system assessment and typical regions-of-interest automatically generated during an automated SNR calculation.

(a) (b) (c)

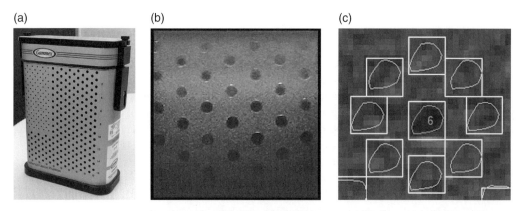

Figure 18.1 (a) Example of a commercial ultrasound phantom containing co-planar arrays of spherical targets with two different diameters. (b) Ultrasound image of the array of large spherical targets. (c) Results of an early automated analysis program geared to computing target signal-to-noise ratio.

Although they have been reported in the literature for many years, these methods have not yet been developed to the point that they can serve as standard tools for the clinical medical physicist. To make this transition, as described above for intrinsic performance methods, these model observer methods would require commercial software for obtaining performance measurements, documentation of detailed measurement protocols, and data validating measurement properties. Another improvement needed for imaging system assessment would be the development of commercial phantoms with a wider variety of targets, to better mimic a wider variety of clinical tasks. A simple example in mammography is the Mammography Quality Standardization Act (MQSA) phantom, which presents sets of targets of three specific types: specks, rods, and masses. The mammography system is evaluated based on the ability of the medical physicist to detect each of these target types in a phantom image. Reference [16] reports a set of clinically-relevant *simulated* targets for design of breast ultrasound systems, but for system evaluation, *physical* phantoms containing these targets are needed. As reported there, clinical tasks should be defined in close consultation with clinical imaging staff. Target sets may be specific to particular clinical applications. Also, protocols designed for ultrasound system evaluation should take into account the fact that clinical patient imaging may generally include survey or search phases, during which regions of the body are scanned dynamically to identify abnormalities or suspicious regions, and also characterization phases where the scan settings are optimized to best demonstrate detected abnormalities. Optimized scanner settings for demonstration of a lesion may have inadequate temporal resolution for dynamic survey, so phantom targets may need to be imaged separately to test both search and characterization capabilities.

18.2.3 Radiometry

Adherence to Food and Drug Administration (FDA)-mandated power output and intensity levels for diagnostic ultrasound imaging devices is asserted by the equipment manufacturer in documentation provided to the FDA prior to making a system commercially available. Information pertaining to power output and intensity is provided to the user as part of the system documentation, and mechanical and thermal indices are annotated in the image display to provide the user a mechanism to acquire images in a manner adhering to the "as low as reasonably achievable" (ALARA) principle. Traditionally, power output of the ultrasound system has not been independently verified in the field by clinical medical physicists. Equipment to map acoustic fields is common in research environments, but currently is not typically available to the clinical physicist. In principle, it may be possible to use measurements of image signal-to-noise ratio (SNR) and maximum DOP [16] or measurements of harmonic signal content from contrast agents or similar materials in a phantom to track changes in power output as part of the QC program, assuming that other imaging factors can be controlled for. The importance of assessing scanner and probe output as part of future acceptance testing or QC is unclear, but needs may emerge especially when therapeutic ultrasound systems are considered.

18.3 Testing Implication of New Technologies

Performance measurement methods and tools that can accommodate newer and future diagnostic devices with improved imaging and measurement capabilities are needed. The same is true for scanner functions that may have been previously available on commercial imaging systems, and whose use has thus far been limited but is expected to expand rapidly in the near future. Examples include structured report integration with PACS for general imaging applications (not limited to obstetric or vascular exams), as well as the use of ultrasound contrast media in radiology practices in the United States.

Phantom scan surface sizes and target configurations must allow easy coupling and measurement of a very wide variety of probes, from small footprint high-frequency devices designed for use in the operating room, to very long linear arrays incorporated into automatic scanning assemblies, e.g. those designed to allow automated breast scanning. Phantom scan surfaces should allow 3D probes to scan in both standard "axial" and "sagittal" orientations, and internal features to facilitate accurate probe positioning may be helpful [17]. As the scope of clinical physics support extends to other practices beyond radiology, a wide variety of bi-plane, intracavitary, and endoscopic probes will be encountered, that may challenge phantom designs in terms of efficient and effective coupling.

Fundamentally new imaging and measurement modes will clearly require new performance measurement methods to be developed, including test objects and analysis tools. Examples include elastography imaging, both strain imaging and shear wave methods, and B-mode flow imaging. New testing methodologies are also needed for assessment of new quantitative measurements, for example shear wave speed or Young's modulus, and strain ratio.

In recent years, many new imaging system developments have been geared toward imaging of "difficult to scan" patients, and this trend is expected to continue. For example, for imaging a generally larger patient population, systems with increased SNR and sensitivity are being developed using a variety of engineering approaches that, for example, can allow abdominal probes operated at their highest user-selectable frequency to image to depths greater than 20 cm. Phantoms with clinical attenuation coefficients and depths of 20 cm or less do not allow measurement of DOP for these probes. Other characteristics that tend to reduce ultrasound image quality are superficial tissue layers that cause excessive scattering and reflection and image clutter, attenuation that limits imaging depth, and variations in sound speeds away from the typically-assumed 1540 m s^{-1} that can reduce spatial resolution. System features such as harmonic imaging and spatial compounding have been introduced with the primary goal of reducing artifacts and improving image quality in difficult-to-scan patients. A newer feature with similar aim is speed of sound optimization. Current common ultrasound phantoms are relatively simple to scan and simulate simple, "glass-bodied" patients, and do not generate the same types of echo patterns seen when scanning many real-world patients. The utility of these phantoms for providing pre-purchase system assessment data relevant to actual clinical use is thus significantly limited. Their utility for optimizing clinical imaging protocols and presets is likewise limited. These comments apply equally well to traditional B-mode and color Doppler imaging, traditional measurements such as Doppler peak velocity, and newer imaging and measurement modes such as those related to elastography. Phantoms that allow better simulation of imaging of real-world patient populations are sorely needed. One possible approach to increasing the value of performance assessments made with simple, commercial phantoms would be to develop a set of layers of phantom materials that could be added to the phantom scan surface, either singly or in combination. These layers could contain scattering, reflecting, attenuating, or aberrating materials (or combinations), to provide a more challenging imaging situation. "Control" layers of standard phantom material could be provided to simply adjust the depth to specific targets. Curved phantom material layers to vary the scan surface geometry to better mimic patient surface contours and angles of approach to phantom targets might also prove useful. These capabilities could be extremely helpful to increase the real-world clinical relevance of both traditional performance metrics and newer task-based assessments, and could be used to improve tests of both imaging and measurement capabilities. This general approach has been used to extend the utility of phantoms used for radiation dosimetry [18].

Ultrasound systems are being designed more and more to automatically adjust to the anatomy and tissues present when imaging specific body parts, to produce good image quality with a minimum of operator adjustment. Terms such as "tissue specific" imaging and "plop-ability" have been coined to describe this characteristic. Automatic and semi-automatic functions for optimization of gain and time-gain compensation in patient images are common. Similarly, automatic measurement tools for detecting the peak velocity envelope and mean velocity of spectral waveforms are becoming common, but will likely work best when presented with physiologic waveforms from human arteries and veins. Anthropomorphic phantoms would allow objective assessment of these capabilities in a consistent manner over time (as opposed to the use of human volunteers or patients). Two examples of commercial anthropomorphic test phantoms for ultrasound are shown in Figure 18.2.

A greater diversity of tests is also needed to allow assessment of new capabilities of ultrasound systems that go beyond the fundamental imaging and measurement functions discussed above. One example would involve adjunct systems integrated with the US imaging platform to track transducer position. These allow calibrated freehand acquisition of 3D volumes and fusion of

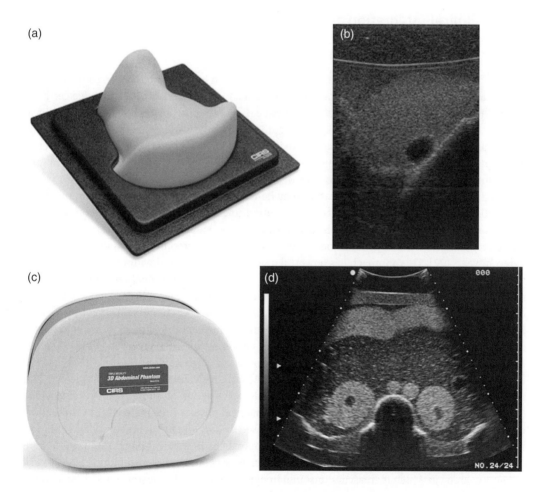

Figure 18.2 Commercial anthropomorphic ultrasound phantoms of the (a) neck and (b) abdomen, along with examples of corresponding ultrasound images.

real-time ultrasound images with prior computed tomography (CT) or magnetic resonance (MR) (or ultrasound) exams [19, 20], and are now offered by several commercial US system vendors. Another non-imaging function experiencing growing use is DICOM structured report data export [21], covering the gamut of ultrasound measurements and clinical applications. Verification of the completeness and accuracy of these transmitted measurements is important, as is the appropriate utilization of the measurement on PACS (e.g. in the case of OB measurements, relating the measurement to a published database of normal values). These functions are not typical components of a traditional medical physics testing plan for an imaging system, but all contribute to the quality of the patient information produced by the imaging system, and so should be considered by the physicist as part of any comprehensive system assessment. Another element of image quality related to PACS integration and cross site work sharing involves the live video feed out of the scanner. The utilization of this live video feed to support primary diagnosis is expected to grow as work sharing becomes more common, as it allows close consultation between the sonographer and the remote-site interpreting radiologist.

18.4 Clinical Integration and Implementation

18.4.1 Training and Communication

In academic settings, medical physicists are often called upon to provide basic ultrasound imaging physics and technology education to radiology residents to support their initial practice certification, although poor attendance is sometimes an issue. Less common are requests to provide education to staff sonographers and radiologists regarding the physics, engineering, and promising clinical application areas of new innovations in imaging technology. This type of education is critical to optimal implementation and clinical use of rapidly evolving scanner capabilities, and may be even more valuable when provided to staff of ultrasound practices outside of radiology, where imaging physics and technology education may be less highly emphasized in training programs and certification exams. Providing effective education to clinicians via traditional, common, lecture-based approaches is complicated by the intense time demands on staff and trainees who provide direct patient care. The general concept of "flipping the classroom" has become very popular in recent years [22]. This approach has powerful potential benefits for providing physics education to clinical trainees and staff [23]. Providing quality, "canned" educational content that can be reviewed on the physician's schedule then frees precious face-to-face teaching sessions for addressing specific questions, reviewing difficult concepts, and assessing comprehension. The AAPM/RSNA physics modules are a promising start, but much more optimization of these materials is needed. In our practice, we have experimented with providing videos of recorded 60 minute physics lectures to our radiology residents that can be accessed during clinical down times, but the utility of these materials was found to be limited. Alternatively, following the example of Khan Academy (http://en.wikipedia.org/wiki/Khan_Academy) a series of short, ~3–10 minute video "micro lectures," each explaining just a single key medical physics imaging concept would allow even very short breaks during the clinical day to be used to start and finish the review of an important concept. A number of promising innovative approaches to medical physics education were presented at the 2014 Annual Meeting of the American Association of Medical Physicists [24, 25].

Another arena in which increased ultrasound imaging physics and education could be beneficial is in the medical school. The use of ultrasound is becoming more and more ubiquitous in medical practices outside of radiology, but imaging technology education seems extremely limited.

Basic education to medical students on the complexity, power, and limitations of these imaging systems could potentially deliver significant patient care benefits later in their practices.

18.4.2 Optimization

Optimization of ultrasound exam, imaging, and measurement protocols and presets represents an enormous opportunity for clinical medical physicists. Optimization is required in a number of circumstances, including: (i) when initially implementing a new scanner, probe, or innovative imaging mode or processing function; (ii) when trying to standardize the calibration and reproducibility of measurements, e.g. Doppler peak velocity or volume flow rate; (iii) when trying to match the characteristics of ultrasound images and measurements between different scanner vendors or models, e.g. when exams from multiple geographically-separated practice locations are read by a single group of radiologists; and (iv) optimizing scanning protocols over time. Traditionally, clinical physicists have been intimately involved in protocol development and image optimization for many medical imaging modalities, such as screen-film radiography and mammography, digital radiography and mammography, CT, magnetic resonance imaging (MRI), nuclear medicine, and positron emission tomography (PET). This has not typically been the case in ultrasound. In our practice, optimization of scanner presets has more heavily depended on a small, core group of systems users (sonographers and radiologists) working with vendor applications support personnel. Factory presets are initially used to scan volunteers and patients, and scan parameters are adjusted and stored into the preset until the "look" of the image is aesthetically pleasing to the group, or matches that of a prior scanner. This general procedure is then iteratively applied throughout the lifetime of the imaging system, more frequently following initial introduction of the system and less frequently thereafter. It is also applied when new imaging hardware (e.g. transducers) or software processing tools are introduced though system upgrades.

This aesthetic approach has some limitations. It can actually slow the introduction of new, innovative imaging features and technologies. For example, post-processing features designed to minimize and reduce the appearance of speckle to improve low contrast detectability are often muted, as they may result in an unfamiliar, "electronic" look. Matching the image appearance of a new system to an existing one is also most conveniently done when the systems can be used side-by-side but this can be difficult for example, when integrating a system at an affiliated clinical site remote from the main practice location. Figure 18.3 illustrates the challenge presented by different image appearances from different scanner models. This situation represents a significant opportunity for medical physicists to contribute to this process by using quantitative figures of merit based on either traditional (Section 18.2.1) or task-based (Section 18.2.2) performance measures. Task-based performance metrics should be especially valuable in this application. Application of these metrics will not replace the existing process, but should complement and enhance it, for example by demonstrating improved detection performance when new features are utilized, thus encouraging their use. Initial work in this area has been recently reported [26].

Opportunities for physicists to use objective approaches to contribute to scan protocol and preset optimization efforts also exist for measurements based on Doppler spectra, e.g. peak systolic velocity. It has long been recognized that velocity measurements made with commercial ultrasound imaging systems may suffer from intrinsic errors, that can vary with respect to scan variables, transducers, and system models (see for example [27, 28]). There is great potential for clinical physicists to apply objective performance measurement techniques to optimize peak velocity accuracy and reproducibility, and standardize measurement calibration across a range of imaging

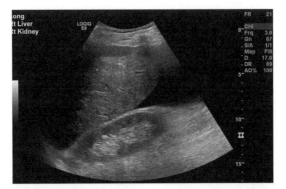

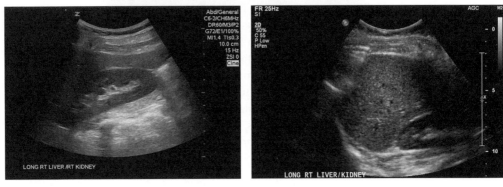

Figure 18.3 Sample liver abdominal ultrasound images obtained using different ultrasound scanner models in different clinical sites that are all part of the same distributed radiology practice. Matching the different overall contrast levels, echotextures, and other factors across different scanners used in the same clinical practice should facilitate effective cross-site exam interpretation.

systems that may exist across an integrated health care system, thus improving patient care that depends on these Doppler velocity measurements [29]. The quality of this work depends on versatile phantoms that can accurately mimic a variety of clinical applications, ranging from measurements with higher Doppler angles of large superficial carotid arteries to measurements of smaller, deeper renal arteries using lower Doppler angles. Another aspect of improved modeling of real-world patients for more clinically-relevant performance measurement (as discussed earlier in Section 18.3) involves mimicking both healthy and diseased states. The Doppler optimization work described here would definitely benefit from flow phantoms containing conduits without and with obstructions mimicking disease. Finally, assessment of automated peak velocity envelope detection tools as well as the study of peak velocity estimation by human sonographers in a clinically meaningful way requires physiologic Doppler phantom waveforms similar to those seen in the carotid and other human vessels. Current commercial flow phantoms or string phantoms that may be very well suited for acceptance testing or QC may be limited for these tasks [30]. Similar opportunities for practice improvement by the clinical physicist also exist for measurements of volume flow rate [31, 32] and potentially measurements of absolute shear wave velocity or elastic modulus, and strain ratio.

Clinical medical physicists have commonly facilitated the management of optimized imaging and measurement protocols in other modality areas. This includes distribution of the protocols and other scanner configuration information across all scanners in the practice, maintenance of back-up copies of this information, and implementation of processes for distribution to remote imaging systems, change-control, and storage of change history. These would be valuable clinical physics functions for ultrasound practices as well.

18.4.3 Automated Analysis and Data Management

Automated methods of image analysis for ultrasound performance assessment have been previously reported [33–38]. However, in our experience, fully automated techniques are not robust and are prone to failure due to a variety of factors, including: a wide variety of probe and image formats; a lack of specific information localizing ultrasound pixel data in the overall image; wide diversity in data present in public fields of the DICOM image headers by different system vendors; a general dearth of information in the DICOM header public fields; 8-bit image pixels that are prone to pixel value saturation; and logistical difficulties in routing data from the scanner under evaluation to the computer performing the image analysis. However, significant opportunity exists for future implementation of tools for ongoing QC assessments on the scanner itself, which can potentially avoid many of these pitfalls. It has been proposed that useful assessments of probe element and channel functionality might be done by analyzing the interference pattern observed in an image obtained "in air," i.e. without any coupling media or phantom present [6, 39, 40]. This suggests one opportunity for fully automated quality testing that could be performed by the US scanner (although there are undoubtedly also many other possibilities). This specific test would be especially helpful in light of reports that these types of problems are most prevalent in current US systems [5]. Optimal implementation would involve collaboration between clinical physicists and system engineers. Engineers could implement scan modes optimized to reveal possible system flaws, e.g. exciting sector (or vector) arrays like sequential linear arrays to overcome their intrinsic tendency to hide these artifacts when operated in their normal scan modes [39]. Clinical physics involvement is needed to assure that performance thresholds and action levels are meaningful with respect to clinical practice needs. Ideally, these thresholds would be available to the practice to configure. Measurement results, not simply pass/fail assessments, could be provided via DICOM structured report or a DICOM image "report page" such as those provided by clinical calculation packages. In general, user-configurable, on-board, automated QC tools would be of tremendous value to the clinical ultrasound practice.

There has been significant recent interest in comprehensive extraction of metadata from DICOM object headers, and analysis of this information to track dose, exam efficiency, and other imaging and practice characteristics (see, for example, [41, 42]). Automated DICOM header data mining and analytics should be especially valuable in ultrasound practices that will still be mainly dependent on manual image optimization and acquisitions into the foreseeable future. Potential applications in the ultrasound practice would include tracking of: efficiencies of specific exams; scanner and room utilization; utilization of specific probes for specific clinical applications; utilization of added-cost imaging functions, such as extended field-of-view imaging and elastography; use of standard exam protocols; and general use of good scan practices. As noted earlier, there is typically a highly variable and sparse assortment of data available in the public fields of DICOM image headers, so maximizing the availability of practice analytics in the short term will require collaboration between clinical physicists and ultrasound image system manufacturers. Vendor tools can reveal an extremely rich data set, potentially consisting of all of the scanner control settings used to acquire each image, that may be made available in private fields of the DICOM header. This information can potentially open the door to practice improvement efforts to optimize image and measurement protocols, image quality, and sonographer efficiency.

18.4.4 Meaningful QC

As described in the introduction to this chapter, emphasizing the value introduced by physics services in ultrasound imaging practices is critical. This begins with design of the QC program. The fact that clinical diagnostic ultrasound systems have been used for decades without a high incidence of major safety incidents in the absence of widespread quality testing programs does not rule out the value of some level of routine QC evaluation to assure proper operation of these complex imaging systems over time. This accurate, historical observation of overall safe use ignores the risks and consequences to the patient of a poor exam and possible misdiagnosis due to incorrect equipment function [43]. A wide variety of variables are available for optimizing value in the US QC program, including the following:

- *Tests included in the program.* A wide variety of ultrasound imaging performance tests have been reported, but not all of these are valuable components of a QC program where the goal is to detect changes in performance over time (as opposed to providing absolute performance benchmarks).
- *Testing methods.* Some specific tests (e.g. image uniformity) may be included in protocols for pre-purchase technology assessment, acceptance testing, and ongoing QC. However, the test methods may be different, adapted to goals of each testing application. For QC testing, methods that are simple and efficient to apply are generally preferred.
- *Frequency of QC tests.* Test frequency must consider a variety of factors including the clinical significance of the particular defects a specific test is designed to detect and the rate of progression of the defect. Different tests may be performed with different frequencies, e.g. some performed quarterly while others may only be performed annually.
- *Personnel performing the hands-on tests.* A wide variety of personnel may be considered, ranging from equipment service personnel, clinical sonographers, physicist assistants, and clinical physicists. Ideally, cost-effectiveness will be increased if more frequent testing can be performed by personnel already present in the practice, e.g. sonographers or service personnel performing preventive maintenance.

The goal of the QC program is not to detect all equipment flaws that may be present at any given time, but rather to identify the majority of actionable defects found in proportion to the total cost of the program (including equipment, personnel, travel, etc.). Defects that directly impact the safety of patients or equipment operators must be addressed at the time they are detected. However, beyond these straightforward cases, the determinations of what defects are "actionable" and when repair or replacement may be needed must be carefully aligned with the needs and perspectives of each individual clinical practice. Specific areas of risk to be considered by the practice when determining action limits were discussed earlier in Section 18.2.1.

It is critical that the clinical medical physicist be closely involved in initial design and implementation of the QC program, provide ongoing supervision, and also lead continuous quality improvement efforts for the QC program over time. Periodic reviews of program performance are essential and can reveal significant opportunities for optimization [5]. Also, as technology changes, it is important to reevaluate the tests included in the program, as well as specific test methods and frequencies. For example, new fast scanning acquisition strategies utilizing broad plane waves of ultrasound may be less sensitive to flaws in individual transducer elements than are traditional acquisition methods, thus reducing the importance of frequent, sensitive tests to detect this defect. Also, new system modes such as strain imaging will definitely require new tests as part of a technology assessment, but they may not require additional QC tests. If key system components that may be prone to failure are already evaluated in the QC program, e.g. by the image uniformity test, there may be no need to repeat a test in multiple imaging modes.

18.4.5 Support for Non-radiology Ultrasound Practices

Ultrasound is unique among planar diagnostic imaging modalities in radiology, in that there is considerably more equipment in use outside of radiology departments than inside. On our clinical campus for example, the ratio of systems outside of radiology to inside is ~4:1. The current level of clinical physics support in these practices is minimal at best. However, a few opportunities to collaborate on specific ultrasound-related issues outside of the radiology department has suggested that even modest levels of clinical physics involvement could add considerable value to these practices and the patients they serve.

There are at least two significant potential barriers to the medical physicist considering service delivery in non-radiology practices. The first is lack of familiarity with these clinical practices. Practice workflow, dataflow, and system integration can be very different and even more complex than that seen in the radiology department. The US imaging equipment designed specifically for use in these practice settings may be unfamiliar, e.g. involving intravascular or endoscopic probes, and may offer only limited DICOM capabilities. In addition, the level of physics and technology education received in formal training programs may be very limited, which can make communication difficult. Adding to this, even the terminology used to describe imaging systems, components, and artifacts may be very different that that used in radiology. All of these considerations absolutely mandate close collaboration between the physicist and the physician and technologist practice staff, as well as with equipment service personnel and equipment vendors.

The second potential barrier deals with available physics staffing resources in proportion to the sheer volume of non-radiology US systems that might benefit from some level of physics support. Here, limiting physicist hands-on involvement to areas where unique value is offered is crucial. As described earlier, design, implementation, supervision, and quality improvement of testing programs demand the greatest direct physicist involvement. In our experience, hands-on testing by the physicist is most important for technology assessment and system optimization, and less important for acceptance testing and QC. Implementing a program of annual QC testing (starting at system acceptance when possible), especially if physicist assistants or equipment service or technologist personnel can perform the hands-on testing, might be a manageable, yet valuable, starting point.

18.5 Conclusions

Ultrasound imaging is in wide use both inside and outside of radiology departments and, due in part to rapid technology development and innovation of commercial systems, clinical use of this technology is expected to grow. Physics support of radiology ultrasound practices is currently limited compared with other modality areas. However, significant opportunities exist to expand physics involvement and provide valuable practice and patient benefit. Teamwork and collaboration with clinical practice staff, equipment service personnel, and equipment manufacturers will be essential to maximize this benefit. Equally important will be an emphasis on maximizing the value of physics services, and continuous improvement of medical physics methods and testing programs.

References

1 Larson, S. (2013). AAPM Working Group on Quantitative B-mode Ultrasound Quality Control: Software for assessment of transducer artifacts. AAPM Annual Meeting, 2013. http://amos3.aapm.org/abstracts/pdf/77-22645-311436-91647.pdf.

2 Stekel, S., Hangiandreou, N., Tradup, D. (2013). American Institute of Ultrasound in Medicine 2013 Final Program, Page 129 Analysis of Uniformity Artifacts Detected During Clinical Ultrasound Quality Control.

3 Madsen, E.L., Song, C., Frank, G.R. (2013). Phantom and User-friendly Software for Rapid Periodic Quality Assurance of Gray-scale Ultrasound Scanners. AAPM Annual Meeting, 2013. http://amos3.aapm.org/abstracts/pdf/77-22645-311436-101912.pdf.

4 Vachutka, J., Dolezal, L., Kollmann, C., and Klein, J. (2014). The effect of dead elements on the accuracy of Doppler ultrasound measurements. *Ultrason. Imaging* 36: 18.

5 Hangiandreou, N.J., Stekel, S.F., Tradup, D.J. et al. (2011). Four-year experience with a clinical ultrasound quality control program. *Ultrasound Med. Biol.* 37 (8): 1350–1357.

6 Dudley, N.J., Griffith, K., Houldsworth, G. et al. (2001). A review of two alternative ultrasound quality assurance programmes. *Eur. J. Ultrasound* 12: 233–245.

7 Hangiandreou, N.J., Stekel, S.F., and Tradup, D.J. (2011). Features to consider when selecting new ultrasound imaging systems. *J. Am. Coll. Radiol.* 8 (7): 521–523.

8 He, X. and Park, S. (2013). Model observers in medical imaging research. *Theranostics* 3 (10): 774–786.

9 Smith, S.W., Wagner, R.F., MEMBER, IEEE et al. (1983). Low contrast detectability and contrast/detail analysis in medical ultrasound. *IEEE Trans. Sonics Ultrason.* 30 (3).

10 Lopez, H., Loew, M.H., and Goodenough, D.J. (1992). Objective analysis of ultrasound images by use of a computational observer. *IEEE Trans. Med. Imaging* 11 (4).

11 Insana, M.F. and Hall, T.J. (1994). Visual detection efficiency in ultrasonic imaging: a framework for objective assessment of image quality. *J. Acoust. Soc. Am.* 95 (4).

12 Kofler, J.M. Jr. and Madsen, E.L. (2001). Improved method for determining resolution zones in ultrasound phantoms with spherical simulated lesions. *Ultrasound Med. Biol.* 27 (12): 1667–1676.

13 Zemp, R.J., Parry, M.D., Abbey, C.K., and Insana, M.F. (2005). Detection performance theory for ultrasound imaging systems. *IEEE Trans. Med. Imaging* 24 (3): 300–310.

14 MacGillivray, T.J., Ellis, W., and Pye, S.D. (2010). The resolution integral: visual and computational approaches to characterizing ultrasound images. *Phys. Med. Biol.* 55: 5067–5088.

15 Nguyen, N.Q., Abbey, C.K., and Insana, M.F. (2013). Objective assessment of sonographic quality I: task information. *IEEE Trans. Med. Imaging* 32 (4).

16 IEC Standards Document 61391-2 Ed. 1.0 b: 2010. Ultrasonics – Pulse-echo scanners – Part 2: Measurement of maximum depth of penetration and local dynamic range. www.iec.ch.

17 Tradup, D.J., Hangiandreou, N.J., American Institute of Ultrasound in Medicine (2009). Final Program, Page 98. Performance Testing Methods for a Commercial Automated 3-Dimensional Breast Ultrasound Scanner.

18 Fisher, R.F. and Hintenlang, D.E. (2014). Super-size me: adipose tissue-equivalent additions for anthropomorphic phantoms. *J. Appl. Clin. Med. Phys.* 15 (6).

19 Hakime, A., Deschamps, F., De Carvalho, E.G.M. et al. (2011). Clinical evaluation of spatial accuracy of a fusion imaging technique combining previously acquired computed tomography and real-time ultrasound for imaging of liver metastases. *Cardiovasc. Intervent. Radiol.* 34: 338–344.

20 Pinto, P.A., Chung, P.H., Rastinehad, A.R. et al. (2011). Magnetic resonance imaging/ultrasound fusion guided prostate biopsy improves cancer detection following transrectal ultrasound biopsy and correlates with multiparametric magnetic resonance imaging. *J. Urol.* 186: 1281–1285.

21 Ridley, E.L. SIIM: DICOM structured reports speed ultrasound reporting. http://www.auntminnie.com/index.aspx?sec=ser&sub=def&pag=dis&ItemID=107448.

22 http://en.wikipedia.org/wiki/Flipped_classroom.

23 Prober, C.G. and Khan, S. (2013). Medical education reimagined: a call to action. *Acad. Med.* 88 (10): 1407–1410.

24 http://www.aapm.org/meetings/2014am/PRAbs.asp?mid=90&aid=23062.

25 http://www.aapm.org/meetings/2014AM/PRSessions.asp?mid=90&sid=5761.

26 Dudley, N.J. and Gibson, N.M. (2014). A case study in scanner optimization. *Ultrasound* 22: 21–25.

27 Winkler, A.J. and Wu, J. (1995). Correction of intrinsic spectral broadening errors in Doppler peak velocity measurements made with phased sector and linear array transducers. *Ultrasound Med. Biol.* 21 (8): 1029–1035.

28 Hoskins, P.R. (1996). Accuracy of maximum velocity estimates made using Doppler ultrasound systems. *Br. J. Radiol.* 69: 172–177.

29 Zhang, Y., Stekel, S., Tradup, D., and Hangiandreou, N. (2014). Analysis of variations in clinical Doppler ultrasound peak velocity measurements. *Med. Phys.* 41 (6): 447.

30 Zhang, Y., Lynch, T., Stekel, S. et al. (2014). RSNA Annual Meeting 2014 Program, page 368. Flow and String Phantoms for Clinical Medical Physics Evaluation of Doppler Ultrasound System Performance.

31 Hoyt, K., Hester, F.A., Bell, R.L. et al. (2009). Accuracy of volumetric flow rate measurements: an in vitro study using modern ultrasound scanners. *J. Ultrasound Med.* 28: 1511–1518.

32 Tradup, D., Zhang, Y., Strissel, N. et al. (2014). American Institute of Ultrasound in Medicine, 2014, Final Program, Page 42. Analysis of the Accuracy of Clinical Doppler Ultrasound Volume Flow Rate Measurements.

33 Dudley, N.J. and Gibson, N.M. (2014). Early experience with automated B-mode quality assurance tests. *Ultrasound* 22: 15–20.

34 Satrapa, J., Schultz, H.J., and Doblhoff, G. (2006). Automated quality control of ultrasonic B-mode scanners by applying an TMM 3D cyst phantom. *Ultraschall. Med.* 27: 262–272.

35 Thijssen, J.M., Weijers, G., and de Korte, C.L. (2007). Objective performance testing and quality assurance of medical ultrasound equipment. *Ultrasound Med. Biol.* 33: 460–471.

36 Rowland, D.E., Newey, V.R., Turner, D.P., and Nassiri, D.K. (2009). The automated assessment of ultrasound scanner lateral and slice thickness resolution: use of the step response. *Ultrasound Med. Biol.* 35: 1525–1534.

37 Gorny, K.R., Tradup, D.J., and Hangiandreou, N.J. (2005). Implementation and validation of three automated methods for measuring ultrasound maximum depth of penetration: application to ultrasound quality control. *Med. Phys.* 32: 2615–2628.

38 Stekel, S.F., Johnson, L.A., Tradup, D.J. et al. (2007). SIIM Annual Meeting 2007 Program, Page 78. Development, Implementation, and Initial Use of a Comprehensive System for Automated Quality Control of Diagnostic Ultrasound Scanners.

39 Tradup, D., Stekel, S., Zhang, Y., and Hangiandreou, N. (2014). American Institute of Ultrasound in Medicine, 2014 Final Program, Page 74. Feasibility of Ultrasound Uniformity Artifact Detection Using Only In-air Images.

40 Quinn, T. and Verma, P.K. (2014). The analysis of in-air reverberation patterns from medical ultrasound transducers. *Ultrasound* 22: 26–36.

41 Wang, S., Pavlicek, W., Roberts, C.C. et al. (2011). An automated DICOM database capable of arbitrary data mining (including radiation dose indicators) for quality monitoring. *J. Digit. Imaging* 24 (2): 223–233.

42 Langer, S.G. (2012). A flexible database architecture for mining DICOM objects: the DICOM data warehouse. *J. Digit. Imaging* 25 (2): 206–212.

43 Martensson, M., Olsson, M., Segall, B. et al. (2009). High incidence of defective ultrasound transducers in use in routine clinical practice. *Eur. J. Echocardiogr.* 10: 389–394.

Part VII

Magnetic Resonance Imaging

19

Clinical MRI Physics: Perspective

Douglas E. Pfeiffer

Boulder Community Health, Boulder, CO, USA

19.1   Historical Perspective

Stemming from some basic physics principles, the development of magnetic resonance imaging (MRI) presents perhaps the most contentious story in medical imaging. The underlying principles of MRI are found in the work of II Rabi, who in 1937 discovered the quantum phenomenon of nuclear magnetic resonance (NMR) on the atomic level [1]. This work earned him a Nobel Prize in Physics in 1944. In 1946, Felix Block [2] and Edward Purcell [3] independently discovered NMR in bulk samples of solids and liquids. When materials were placed in a strong magnetic field, they absorbed energy that was then re-emitted as they returned to their relaxed state. Block and Purcell measured the precessional signals in water and paraffin, earning them the shared Nobel Prize in Physics in 1952.

For the next several decades, much effort went into characterizing the NMR spectroscopic signals of many types of samples. Particularly, investigators determined the relaxation times of many biological tissues. In 1971, Raymond Damadian determined the T1 and T2 relaxation times of excised normal and cancerous rat tissue. He found that the cancerous tissue had longer relaxation times than normal tissue [4].

Developing the property of NMR into an imaging modality took place during the 1970s. In 1973, which incidentally is the same year that Hounsfield introduced computed tomography, Paul Lauterbur determined that gradients could be applied to the magnetic field of an NMR device, thereby giving spatial information as well as the NMR signal [5]. He termed his technique "zeugmatography," which comes from the Greek word meaning "that which joins together." His first image was of two 1 mm capillaries filled with water inside a 4.2 mm tube filled with a combination of H_2O and D_2O. He used simple back-projection for image reconstruction. Peter Mansfield and his group published a similar technique in 1974 [6], refining it further in 1977 [7]. Their efforts earned them the Nobel Prize in Physics in 2003.

While attending a lecture by Lauterbur, Richard Ernst realized that gradients could be applied both in the frequency and phase dimensions and image reconstruction accomplished using Fourier techniques [8]. These insights are still the basis of MRI in modern scanners. He was awarded the Nobel Prize in Chemistry in 1991.

Clinical Imaging Physics: Current and Emerging Practice, First Edition. Edited by Ehsan Samei and Douglas E. Pfeiffer.
© 2020 John Wiley & Sons, Inc. Published 2020 by John Wiley & Sons, Inc.

One remarkable aspect of Lauterbur's 1974 paper is that he did not cite the work done by Damadian, even though he had made direct reference to Damadian in notes made the day after his discovery. This oversight led to significant bitterness and a continuing fight over appropriate credit for the development of MRI. Damadian's early efforts in building a scanner attempted to map the volume point by point, generating a data map rather than an image. Slightly modifying his approach, he used his "Field Focusing Nuclear Magnetic Resonance (FONAR)" [9] method to present the first MRI of a human being, that of an associate's thorax [10]. This first image took almost five hours to collect the 106 data points forming the image. Perhaps too rashly, but true to his style, he stated in a July 20, 1977 press release that "a new technique for the nonsurgical detection of cancer anywhere in the human body has now been perfected." He was later forced to retract that statement.

He abandoned the approach in the early 1980s in favor of that taken by Lauterbur and Mansfield. He did, however, get a patent for the apparatus in 1974. He successfully sued General Electric for patent infringement 1997 in a legal fight that ended up in the Supreme Court of the United States. Damadian's effort lead him to believe that he deserved the Nobel Prize instead of Lauterbur and Mansfield, or at least along with them. He has not given up his appeal for Nobel recognition.

In spite of these controversies, MRI quickly became essential to diagnostic imaging and developed rapidly. Mansfield's 1977 work included echo-planar imaging (EPI), which is at the heart of modern rapid scanning techniques. In 1987, Charles Dumoulin developed MR angiography [11], allowing for vascular visualization without the use of contrast agents. In 1992, functional MRI was developed. This technique uses blood-oxygen-level dependent contrast [12], allowing the visualization of hemodynamic response related to energy use by neural cells (Figure 19.1). The pulse sequence uses the magnetization difference between oxygenated and de-oxygenated blood to develop the image data. Diffusion-weighted imaging (DWI, or diffusion tensor imaging, DTI) allows the mapping of molecules in biological tissues; of greatest clinical interest is the diffusion of water. Since the flow of water is modified or obstructed by membranes, macromolecules, and

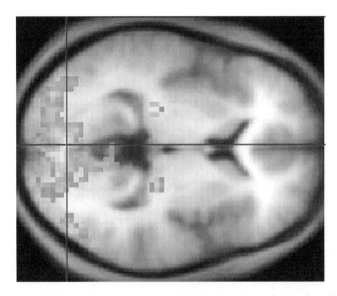

Figure 19.1 An fMRI image with yellow areas showing increased activity. *Source:* OpenStax College [CC BY 3.0 (http://creativecommons.org/licenses/by/3.0)], via Wikimedia Commons.

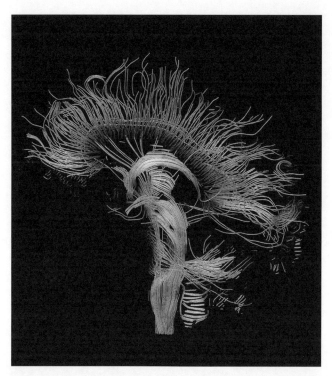

Figure 19.2 Visualization of a DTI measurement of a human brain. Depicted are reconstructed fiber tracts that run through the mid-sagittal plane. Especially prominent are the U-shaped fibers that connect the two hemispheres. *Source:* Thomas Schultz (Own work) [GFDL (http://www.gnu.org/copyleft/fdl.html), CC-BY-SA-3.0 (http://creativecommons.org/licenses/by-sa/3.0.

the like, this can provide even microscopic detail about tissue properties. Some of the most startling images are produced through DTI, as shown in Figure 19.2. This application was developed in the mid-1980s by several groups [13–15].

Clearly, much of the early development in MRI was through advances in applications and pulse sequences, allowing physicians to view the body non-invasively in ways inconceivable just a few years before. This is not to say that the equipment itself remained static. Indeed, the scanners themselves have advanced dramatically over the last few decades. The first units used relatively simple coils, such as birdcage or quadrature, for signal reception (Figure 19.3). These were prone to drift, geometric distortion, and artifacts. As computing power advanced, the complexity coils also advanced. The simple coils have been largely replaced by 8- or 16-channel coils. Multi-element arrays are becoming the common standard for newly installed units (Figure 19.4).

19.2 Current and Upcoming Technologies

While it is technically possible to construct an MRI system with permanent or resistive magnets, at least at low field strengths (<0.5 T), the weight and cost of operation make these practically infeasible. In practice, only superconducting magnets are used. These are cooled to near absolute zero with liquid helium (4.2 K). Clinical field strengths range from 0.2 T in inexpensive open systems, to 3 T. The Food and Drug Administration (FDA) has approved field strengths up to 8 T for clinical

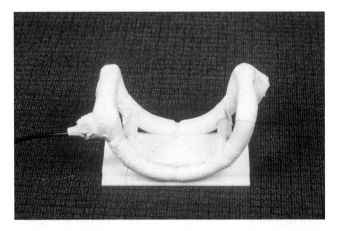

Figure 19.3 A simple extremity surface coil, shop-made at the facility, used in the 1980s. *Source:* Ronald Price.

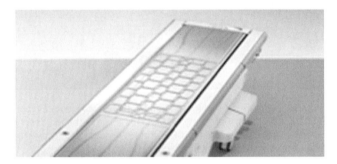

Figure 19.4 A multi-element array coil embedded in the scan table. Each element is individually selectable. *Source:* General Electric Medical Systems.

use in patients one month and older, and up to 4 T for clinical use in neonates up to one month [16], and research and developmental systems currently exceed 10 T, and higher (14 T) for small animal studies.

MRI systems can be divided into several categories: bore, open, and specialty. Bore magnets are the type most commonly seen, illustrated in Figure 19.5. These have static magnetic fields generally in the 1.0–3.0 T range. They provide excellent field uniformity and long scan ranges. They have traditionally suffered from the relatively narrow bore size, which was prohibitive to claustrophobic patients and those with large body habitus. Realizing this, manufacturers have recently been significantly increasing the bore size, up to 50 cm diameter, to alleviate those issues. Bores are also shorter now than they were a decade ago, which further addresses the claustrophobic issues.

The physics of magnetic fields dictates that a significant magnetic field extends a distance from the magnet. MR safety guidelines dictate that the five gauss line should be maintained inside the scan room when possible. To achieve this, these magnets are magnetically shielded to reduce the extent of the five gauss line. However, this active shielding has the impact of increasing the spatial gradient heading into the bore. Spatial gradients are one of the limiting factors for some MR-conditional devices.

Open magnets, as shown in Figure 19.6, are designed to provide access to patients who are claustrophobic or who maintain a larger body habitus than will be accommodated by traditional

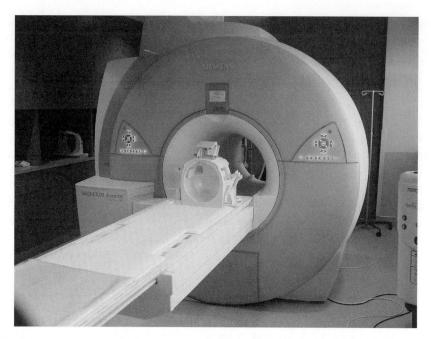

Figure 19.5   A typical superconducting 1.5 T bore magnet system used in clinical practice.

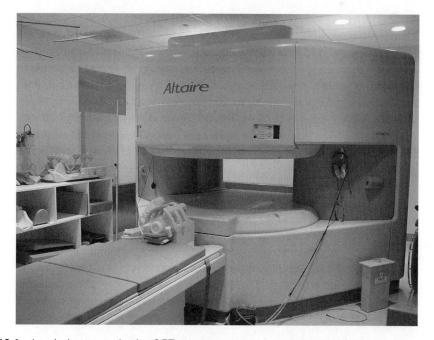

Figure 19.6   A typical superconducting 0.7 T open magnet system used in clinical practice.

bore magnets. These systems tend to be lower field strengths, up to 1 T, than found in bore magnets. For this reason, scans tend to be longer and of lower signal to noise ratio (SNR) than higher field systems. They are also limited in some of the specialty sequences that can be performed with them. However, they do serve a purpose in allowing those who might not otherwise be able to tolerate MR imaging to receive the benefits, if at some cost.

Specialty magnets are designed to serve a very specific niche. Small, extremity systems (Figure 19.7) serve the needs of orthopedic practices, for example, where whole body capability is not required. These systems can be installed in a much smaller space at a much lower cost than conventional systems. Intraoperative MRI systems, such as seen in Figure 19.8, are typically dedicated to neurological applications. Such systems can help to improve neurosurgical outcomes by ensuring complete resection of lesions and early recognition of complications.

Scanners are also being developed that are hybrids of MRI and other modalities. In particular, positron emission tomography-magnetic resonance (PET-MR) systems are showing promise in areas such as cardiac and neurological imaging. As with other hybrid combinations, it is difficult to optimize the system for both modalities [17]. PET systems use photomultiplier tubes (PMTs) in their detection systems, but PMTs are notoriously susceptible to magnetic fields. Further, PET imaging requires attenuation correction for image reconstruction, and a method for that correction is not readily available in a PET-MRI scanner. The final hurdle is the best geometry for a PET-MRI hybrid system. They could be two sequential units, similar to current positron emission tomography-computed tomography (PET-CT) systems. It could be possible to construct a PET detector array

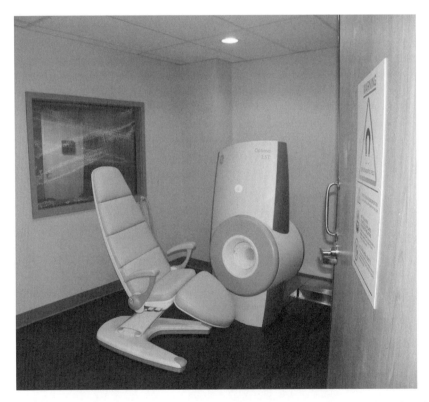

Figure 19.7 A specialty MRI imaging system. This 1.5 T small superconducting magnet is designed specifically for extremity imaging. It is installed in an orthopedic office in a ski resort town.
Source: Stephen Veals.

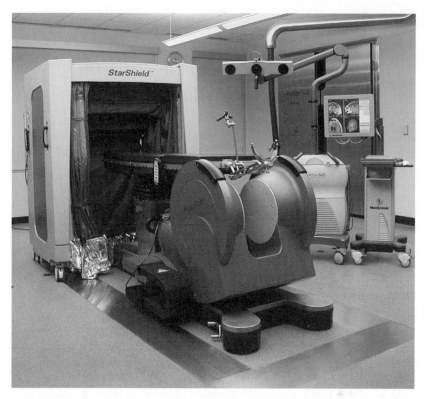

Figure 19.8 A specialty MRI system. This is a small magnet designed specifically for imaging during brain surgery.

that could be inserted into the bore of the MR magnet. The third possibility is to integrate the two systems into a single gantry. The first clinical PET-MRI systems are currently being installed.

As stated above, coils used in MR imaging have advanced significantly. Current coils largely incorporate four or eight channels. These are for both solid, shaped coils (Figure 19.9) or flexible coils (Figure 19.10). Many scanners are now incorporating arrays of coil elements that are

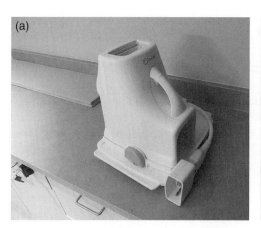
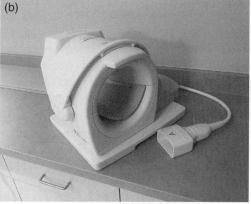

Figure 19.9 Solid, shaped coils designed for use on a specific body part. (a) Foot-ankle coil. (b) Knee coil.

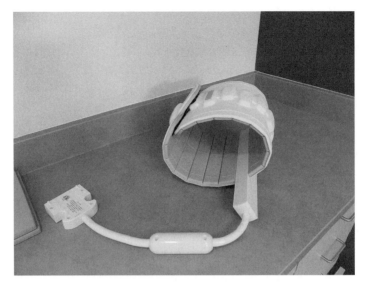

Figure 19.10   A flexible coil that may be used to conform to multiple anatomical areas.

selectively activated (Figure 19.4). Digital RF systems have allowed for much more rapid switching and short rise and fall times. Coils are also incorporating parallel RF receive and transmit, allowing for complicated pulse sequences. The number of independently addressable RF channels has been increasing steadily, and electrical and computational limits seem to be the only limiting factors. It is therefore expected that technological advances will allow for significantly denser arrays.

The applications for which MRI is used continue to drive technologies and pulse sequences. Cardiac imaging has become standard, as has MR angiography. Functional imaging is not widely implemented clinically, but its use is increasing. Spectroscopy holds promise for cancer detection and characterization. Again, it has not seen wide clinical implementation, but it remains a useful tool. Specialized efforts such as The Human Connectome Project (http://www.humanconnectomeproject.org,) could yield a wealth of clinical information and will push MR imaging to its limits. This project hopes to "construct a map of the complete structural and functional neural connections *in vivo* within and across individuals."

19.3   The Movement from 1.0 to 3.0

Medical physics support for MRI systems has primarily been focused on the meeting the requirements of the ACR MR Accreditation Program, as defined in the ACR MR QC Manual.[1] This manual defines tests to be performed and provides directions for performing those tests. Evaluations are a mixture of qualitative and quantitative, focusing on standard imaging sequences. As the manual was published in 2004, it was not written with many of the advanced capabilities and technologies in mind. It is imperative for clinical physicists to modify test protocols to evaluate scanners in a clinically relevant manner. Multi-element array coils must be tested to reveal weaknesses in any of the elements. Gradients should be pushed to reveal flaws that might be

---

1 ACR MR QC Manual.

impacting clinical scans. Transitioning from the 1.0 paradigm to the 3.0 paradigm will require looking at the scanner in different ways, determining what expected failure modes are and how to test components adequately to reveal flaws.

Pulse sequence implementation presents difficulties for many clinical medical physicists. Manufacturers release sequences at a remarkable pace, and very often the physicist is not aware that they have been installed. Sometimes the facility receives adequate training on the sequence, but not always. It is important for the physicist to verify that the sequence performs as expected on the clinical scanner. To do this, however, the physicist must understand what the sequence is intended to do, what it looks like, and how it can fail. Many physicists are not comfortable parsing out pulse sequences, having been trained mainly to look only at the images being produced in phantom and evaluating those images. In the Medical Physics 3.0 paradigm, physicists must be available to assist facilities in the evaluation and implementation of new sequences.

Medical physicists have traditionally supported facilities through the evaluation of anatomical images. While this will remain important, it is clear that applications will move MR imaging beyond the planar anatomical realm into functional and specialty imaging. At this time there are no standards for performance evaluation of such images, and the transition to the 3.0 model will require development of appropriate protocols and standards.

Safety is a large concern in MR imaging. Some aspects, such as projectile threats, are well known and generally well addressed. Manufacturers of biophysical implants are producing more devices that are deemed "MRI compatible." There is significant confusion around the use of that term and the requirements placed on these devices; efforts are being made to provide some standardization of terminology [18]. In any case, very often the final determination of whether a particular series of sequences can be used on a particular patient will depend upon information provided by the medical physicist. This is a level of support for a facility that has not traditionally been a part of medical physics services, particularly in the consultant support model. Being able to answer the question of whether a scanner and the scan sequences meet the conditional requirements may involve measurements, such as spatial gradient determination, not typically made and knowledge of the scanner, such as slew rates, that can be difficult to gain. This type of support is the more patient and facility focus that is at the heart of the Medical Physics 3.0 model.

As part of its Criteria for Significant Risk document, FDA has provided SAR levels over which use is considered to be a significant risk [16] (Table 19.1).

Since MRI has not encountered a regulatory environment such as seen in x-ray imaging, facilities will most likely look to the medical physicist for help in ensuring compliance with the guidelines in this document.

In summary, one can envision a transition from being focused mainly on equipment performance based on evaluation of anatomical images, to include broader support based on functional images, advanced image quality metrics, and patient-centric advice. This will require significant re-training for most medical physicists (Table 19.2).

Table 19.1 SAR levels posing a significant risk per FDA guidelines.

Site	Dose	Time (min) equal to or greater than	SAR (W/kg)
Whole body	Averaged over	15	>4
Head	Averaged over	10	>3.2

Table 19.2 Comparison of medical physics 1.0 and 3.0 paradigms.

Magnetic resonance imaging	1.0	3.0
Focus of MP's attention	Equipment	Patient
Image quality evaluation	Visual, subjective	Mathematical, quantitative
MP "tools of the trade" for image quality evaluation	Line pairs, simulated fibers, specks, and masses	Modulation transfer function (MTF), noise power spectrum (NPS), detective quantum efficiency (DQE), SNR uniformity, noise component analysis
Ongoing QC	Individual subjective evaluation of image quality, manufacturer-specified tests	Automated, remote of advanced image quality metrics
Patient dosimetry	SAR, audible noise	SAR, audible noise
Radiation risk estimation	Burns	Burns
Commonly used imaging technologies	Anatomical images, smaller element arrays	Functional images, large element arrays

References

1 Rabi, I., Zacharias, J., Millman, S., and Kusch, P. (1938). A new method of measuring nuclear magnetic moments. *Phys. Rev.* 53: 318.

2 Bloch, F., Hanson, W., and Packard, M. (1946). Nuclear infraction. *Phys. Rev.* 69: 127.

3 Purcell, E., Torrey, H., and Pound, R. (1946). Resonance absorption by nuclear magnetic moments in a solid. *Phys. Rev.* 69: 37–38.

4 Damadian, R. (1971). Tumor detection by nuclear magnetic resonance. *Science* 171 (3976): 1151–1153.

5 Lauterbur, P.C. (1974). Magnetic resonance zeugmatography. *Pure Appl. Chem.* 40: 149–157.

6 Garroway, A.N., Grannell, P.K., and Mansfield, P. (1974). Image formation in NMR by a selective irradiative process. *J. Phys. C Solid State Phys.* 7: L457–L462.

7 Mansfield, P. (1977). Multi-planar image formation using NMR spin echoes. *J. Phys. C Solid State Phys.* 10: L55–L58.

8 Ernst, R.R. (1975). NMR fourier zeugmatography. *J. Magn. Reson.* 18: 69–83.

9 Damadian, R., Minkoff, L., Goldsmith, M. et al. (1976). Field focusing nuclear magnetic resonance (FONAR): visualization of a tumor in a live animal. *Science* 194: 1430–1432.

10 Damadian, R., Goldsmith, M., and Minkoff, L. (1977). FONAR images of the live human body. *Physiol. Chem. Phys.* 9: 97–100.

11 Dumoulin, C.L., Souza, S.P., and Hart, H.R. (1987). Rapid scan magnetic resonance angiography. *Magn. Reson. Med.* 5: 238–245.

12 Huettel, S.A., Song, A.W., and McCarthy, G. (2009). *Functional Magnetic Resonance Imaging*, 2e, 26. Massachusetts: Sinauer ISBN 978-0-87893-286-3.

13 Le Bihan, D. and Breton, E. (1985). Imagerie de diffusion in-vivo par résonance. *C. R. Acad. Sci. (Paris)* 301 (15): 1109–1112.

14 Merboldt, K., Hanicke, W., and Frahm, J. (1985). Self-diffusion NMR imaging using stimulated echoes. *J. Magn. Reson. (1969)* 64 (3): 479–486.

15 Taylor, D.G. and Bushell, M.C. (1985). The spatial mapping of translational diffusion coefficients by the NMR imaging technique. *Phys. Med. Biol.* 30 (4): 345–349.

16 United States Food and Drug Administration (2014). Guidance for Industry and FDA Staff: Criteria for Significant Risk Investigations of Magnetic Resonance Diagnostic Devices. http://www.fda.gov/downloads/MedicalDevices/DeviceRegulationandGuidance/GuidanceDocuments/ucm072688.pdf. 6/20/2014 (accessed 24 February 20152015).

17 Daftary, A. (2010). PET-MRI: challenges and new directions. *Indian J. Nucl. Med.* 25 (1): 3–5.

18 Kanal, E., Froelich, J., Barkovich, A.J. et al. (2015). Standardized MR terminology and reporting of implants and devices as recommended by the American college of radiology subcommittee on MR safety. *Radiology* 274 (3): 866–870.

20

Clinical MRI Physics: State of Practice

Ronald Price

Department of Radiology, Vanderbilt University, Nashville, TN, USA

20.1   Introduction

The medical physicist is an essential member of the clinical team. As such, it is necessary to assure that good communication channels are established with the other team members – specifically, with the magnetic resonance (MR) technologists to design and monitor the routine quality assurance and safety programs, with the responsible physicians to optimize pulse sequences and protocols, and with the administrative staff to assure compliance with accreditation and regulatory requirements. This chapter will specifically explore the current role of the medical physicist in acceptance testing, magnetic resonance imaging (MRI) quality assurance, clinical image quality support, and MRI accreditation compliance. As part of these discussions, frequent reference is made to requirements, tests, procedures and performance standards that are specified in the American College of Radiology (ACR) MRI Quality Control Manual [1] and in the ACR-AAPM Technical Standard for Diagnostic Medical Physics Performance Monitoring of MRI Equipment [2].

20.2   System Performance

20.2.1   Intrinsic Performance

The major subsystems of an MR scanner are the main magnet (B_0 – field), the RF transmitter/receiver (B_1 – field) and the three imaging gradients. The medical physicist will generally be responsible for defining and performing tests that confirm that these subsystems are performing appropriately. In addition to the MR imaging instrumentation, the physicist is also responsible for assessing the integrity of the image display systems.

20.2.2   Qualimetry

The MR system assessments performed by the medical physicist generally include phantom testing of: magnetic field homogeneity, slice position accuracy, slice thickness (ST) accuracy, high-contrast spatial resolution, low contrast performance, RF coil performance (typically signal to noise ratio (SNR)), geometric accuracy, image signal uniformity, and an assessment of image artifacts. The image display (monitor) assessments include verification of appropriate monitor brightness, uniformity, and resolution. The medical physicist typically is expected to perform all of these assessments at least annually as well as following significant system upgrades or repair.

20.2.2.1 Magnetic Field Homogeneity

Magnetic field homogeneity is defined as the uniformity (with no patient in the magnet) of the main magnetic field strength (B_0) over a specified volume of diameter (D). Typically, ΔB_0 is specified as the spread of resonant frequencies in parts per million (ppm) over a spherical volume (DSV). Homogeneity (ΔB_0) is specified as the spread of resonant frequencies in parts per million (ppm) over a spherical volume (DSV). For example, 1 ppm for a 3.0 T magnet (resonance frequency = 123 MHz) is equal to 123 Hz. If the 1 ppm ΔB_0 were measured over a 40 cm DSV, the homogeneity for the system would be specified as <1 ppm over a 40 cm DSV. The homogeneity for the same system when specified over a larger DSV, e.g. 50 cm DSV, would generally be greater than specified for the smaller 40 cm DSV. Over the 50 cm DSV, the measured ΔB_0 may be 2 ppm (246 Hz) or greater. It is recommended that these measurements be performed with the largest available spherical phantom (Figure 20.1).

There are several significant problems that may be the result of poor field homogeneity. These may include:

1) Poor fat suppression (Figure 20.2a)
2) Spatial distortion and image shading (Figure 20.2b)
3) Reduced image intensity
4) Curved slice profiles
5) Artifacts especially with large field of view (FOV) gradient echo (Figure 20.2c)

Depending upon the specific MR system and system vendor, there are at least three testing methods that may be used by the medical physicist to assess magnetic field homogeneity. These are: spectral full width at half maximum (FWHM) method (Figure 20.3), bandwidth-difference method [3], and phase-difference method (Figure 20.4). A full description of the spectral FWHM and the phase-difference methods can be found in the ACR MRI Quality Control Manual [1].

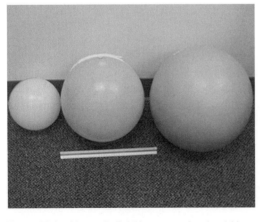 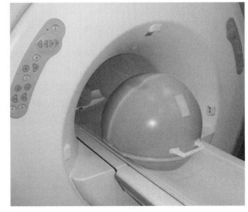

Figure 20.1 Magnetic field homogeneity should be assessed using the largest available spherical phantom.

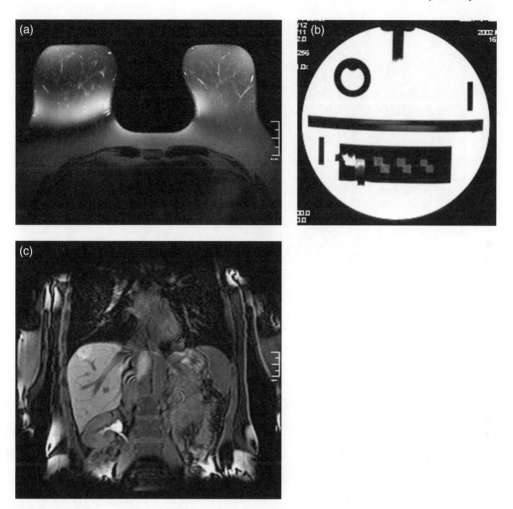

Figure 20.2 Image artifacts resulting from magnetic field inhomogeneity. (a) breast MR image illustrating non-uniform fat suppression, (b) phantom image illustrating geometric distortions and (c) large FOV gradient echo image illustrating out-of-volume signal interference producing "zebra" artifact.

The description of the bandwidth-difference method is provided in the 2006 Medical Physics article by Chen et al. [3]. The spectral FWHM method is faster than the other methods, requires no special pulse sequence and can be obtained during "prescan" coil tuning. However, the method is only an estimate of global field homogeneity and thus provides little information on the location of the discrete inhomogeneities.

The main advantage of the bandwidth-difference method is that it can generally be performed on any MRI system and the method can use either spin-echo or gradient-echo sequences. The equation for calculating the field homogeneity (ΔB_0) parts-per-million is below. A disadvantage is that the bandwidth-difference method is limited to providing homogeneity assessment only along the image frequency-encoding axis. Because of this limitation multiple image sets will be required to evaluate the spatial distribution of the field inhomogeneities. The basic measurement requires acquisition of two identical images differing only in the receiver bandwidth (BW_1 and BW_2) with the lower bandwidth being set at the lower limit for the chosen pulse sequence and the upper

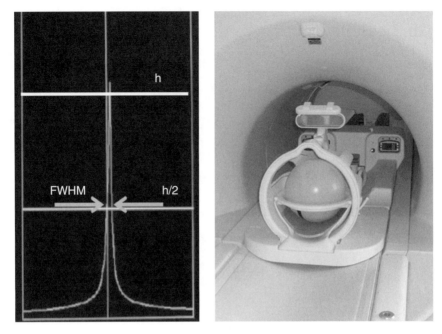

Figure 20.3 The spectral full-width at half maximum (FWHM) method for estimating magnetic field inhomogeneity.

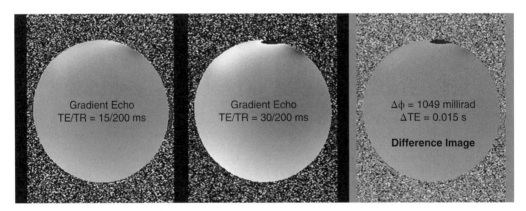

Figure 20.4 Phase-difference method for assessing magnetic field homogeneity.

bandwidth at the highest available value. The quantities d_1 and d_2 are the distances measured between corresponding points in the two images and FOV is the image field-of-view.

$$\Delta B_0\left(\text{ppm}\right) = \frac{\left(\text{BW}_1 \, x \, \text{BW}_2\right) x\left(d_1 - d_2\right)}{42.576\text{MHz/T} \, x \, B_0\left(\text{T}\right) x \, \text{FOV}_x \, x\left(\text{BW}_2 - \text{BW}_1\right)}$$

The phase-difference method can be performed with either 2D or 3D image sets and does provide detail on the location of inhomogeneities. However, it requires access to the phase images, which may not be available on all systems.

With the phase-difference method, gradient echo sequences are acquired with two different echo times (15 and 30 ms) but otherwise identical parameters. The change in phase angle per unit time ($\Delta\phi/\Delta t$) of the two images, as determined by subtracting the two images, is directly related to the magnetic field homogeneity and inversely to the gyromagnetic ratio (γ).

$$\Delta B_0 = \left(\Delta\phi / \Delta t\right)/\gamma = \left(\Delta\phi / \gamma\right)/\left(TE_2 - TE_1\right)$$

Note that in the second image (TE = 30 ms) the longer time allowed for de-phasing to take place has resulted in a phase-wrap of π−radians at the top of the phantom due to the regions higher level of field inhomogeneity. For this region, the $\Delta\phi$ in the difference image must have π−radians added to correct for the additional phase shift.

20.2.2.2 Slice Position and ST Accuracy

Slice position accuracy measurement is illustrated in Figure 20.5 with an image of the ACR large phantom. A more complete description of ST and slice position measurements can be found in the National Electrical Manufacturers Association (NEMA) ST document [4] and in the ACR QC Manual [1]. The ACR phantom contains two sets of crossed non-signal-producing ramps (arrow) located on the extreme ends of the cylindrical phantom.

The slice position ramps are non-signal producing acrylic ramps in the signal producing filler material and appear dark in the images. When the slice is positioned where the ramps cross the dark bars will appear of equal length. Any difference in length can be directly related to the error in the laser light positioning.

The factor of 1/5 (0.2) illustrated in Figure 20.6 is specific for the ACR phantom and is necessary because the slice-thickness ramps have a slope of 10:1 relative to the axial plane of the image. Other phantoms may utilize ramps with different slopes and thus will require a different factor.

20.2.2.3 High-Contrast Spatial Resolution

The same axial slice that is used for slice position and ST measurements also contains the insert used to assess high-contrast spatial resolution (Figure 20.7). The insert consists of three sets of

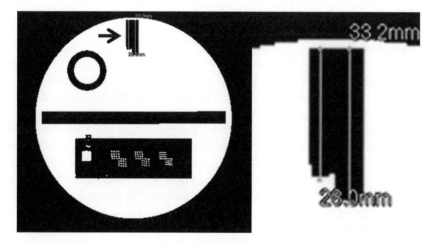

Figure 20.5 Axial MR image of the ACR phantom taken through the portion of the phantom containing the crossed slice-position ramps.

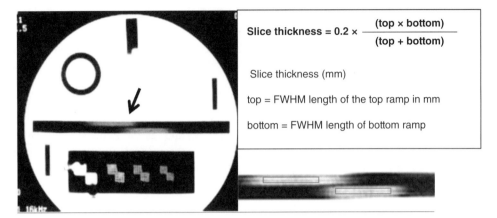

Figure 20.6 The same axial slice used for slice position accuracy also contains the crossed signal-producing ramps (arrow) used for slice thickness (ST) accuracy (also referred to as the slice profile).

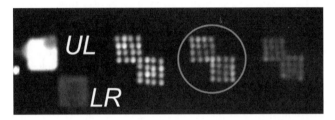

Figure 20.7 High-contrast resolution insert in the ACR phantom. Equally-spaced hole arrays are filled with signal-producing fluid. Hole spacing: left (1.1 mm), middle (1.0 mm) and right (0.9 mm.)

equally-spaced holes drilled into acrylic filled with signal-producing fluid. The spacing of the three sets are: 1.1, 1.0, and 0.9 mm. The specific set that should be resolved will depend upon the in-plane pixel size that is determined by the FOV(mm) divided by the matrix size. The reference ACR sequences have a FOV = 250 mm in both the phase and frequency axes with a square acquisition matrix of 256 × 256. With this combination, pixel size is approximately 0.98 mm × 0.98 mm and thus should be able to resolve the 1.0 mm hole pattern (red circle in Figure 20.14).

20.2.2.4 Signal-to-Noise

One of the most important tasks of the annual testing is the assessment of the performance of all clinical coils. This assessment is specifically to determine the SNR and to determine if there are any coil artifacts such as significant phase ghosting. The phantom of choice is a uniform signal-producing volume. The ACR phantom also contains a uniform section (Figure 20.8) that is free of any internal structures and can thus be used for these measurements. There are two accepted methods for calculating SNR. The first and easiest method is described in the ACR Quality Control Manual [1] and utilizes only one image. The signal is estimated as the mean signal from a large ROI centered in the phantom (Figure 20.8). The image noise is estimated as the standard deviation (SD) of an air region-of-interest (ROI). The air region should be chosen as large as possible to achieve reliable statistical results and should be chosen in a region with no signal and specifically a region with no phase ghosting (Figure 20.8a). The limitation of this method lies with its use when evaluating array coils in which image intensity correction is used to improve signal uniformity: GE(SCIC), Siemens (PURE) and Philips (CLEAR). When these image processing algorithms

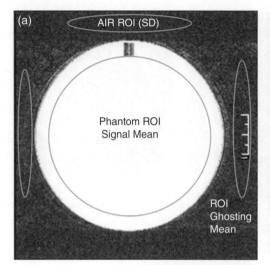
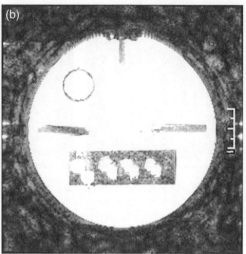
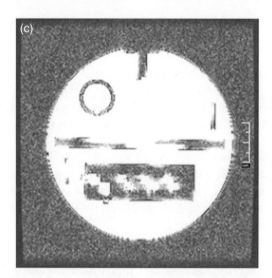

Figure 20.8 (a) A uniform signal-producing phantom free of all internal structures may be used to assess coil SNR and the presence of phase ghosting. (b) Image acquired with an 8-channel array receive-only coil that has been processed using image uniformity correction resulting in and "air" signal that is not a true representation of image noise. (c) The same image processed without image uniformity correction.

are use the air-background signal is no longer noise (Figure 20.8b) but rather a calculated value based on the combination of the data from the multiple array elements. When an image intensity correction algorithm is used, the NEMA image-difference method [5] is preferred.

$$SNR_1 = Mean\ Signal\ /\ SD$$

The NEMA image-difference method [5] estimates the image noise from an image that is the result of subtracting two images that were acquired with identical acquisition techniques with only a short time interval between (Figure 20.9). The image noise is estimated from the difference image as the SD of a large ROI in the phantom. The signal is estimated as the mean signal from one

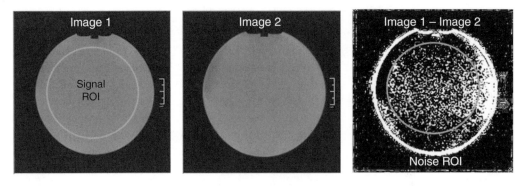

Figure 20.9 The NEMA method utilizes the image-difference method to estimate image noise. Image noise is estimated from the standard deviation of the subtraction image ROI avoiding edge effects.

of the two original unsubtracted images. In order to correct for error propagation resulting from the subtraction the above SNR equation must be multiplied by a factor of $\sqrt{2}$.

$$\mathrm{SNR}_2 = \sqrt{2} \times \left(\mathrm{Mean\ Signal} / \mathrm{SD}\right)$$

20.2.2.5 ACR Low Contrast Detectability Score

As a quick and convenient qualitative estimate of SNR [1, 6–9], the ACR has recommended using the low-contrast detectability (LCD) score for routine quality assurance measurements (Figure 20.10). The ACR phantoms contain low-contrast inserts that are imaged and scored visually. The large phantom contains four inserts (disks with 1.4, 2.5, 3.6, and 5.1% image contrast) and the small phantom contains two inserts (3.6 and 5.1%). Each insert is arranged with 10 "spokes" with each spoke containing three disks. The disk diameters in each spoke decrease progressively from 7 mm in diameter to 1.5 mm. The LCD score is defined as the number of completely visualized spokes out of the possible maximum score of 40 for the large phantom and a maximum score of 20 for the small phantom.

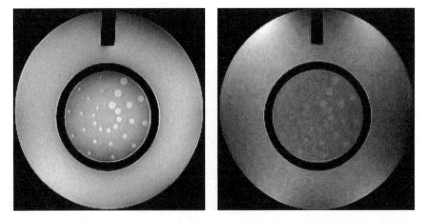

Figure 20.10 Images of one of the low-contrast inserts contained in the ACR large phantom obtained on two different MR systems. (left) LCD score for this slice is approximately =10, (right) LCD score approximately = 6.

20.2.2.6 Image Geometric Accuracy

A regular assessment of the geometric accuracy of the system is important to assure that the imaging gradients are properly calibrated and that there are no significant spatial distortions due to excessive magnetic field inhomogeneity [10]. Any phantom of known dimension can be used for the test and the assessments should always be evaluated in each of the three imaging planes. Figure 20.11 illustrates dimensional accuracy measurements made with the ACR phantom. The sagittal image (Figure 20.11a) is used to assess accuracy along the z-axis and the axial image is used to assess the x- and y-axes. In the ACR large phantom the length of the phantom in the z-axis is known to be equal to 148 mm. The dimension of the phantom in the (x, y)-axes is 190 mm. The figure also illustrates dimensions measured in the oblique directions. The ACR accreditation accuracy criterion is ± 2 mm. Depending upon the specific clinical application, it may be necessary for the medical physicist to establish a more restrictive accuracy requirement.

20.2.2.7 Image Signal Uniformity

Image intensity uniformity should be checked for coils that are designed to provide a uniform signal over a defined volume such as the head and knee coils. A NEMA [11] specified parameter used for quantifying image non-uniformity is pixel-based and is referred to as the peak deviation non-uniformity (N).

$$N = 100 \, X \left(S_{max-} S_{min} \right) / \left(S_{max+} S_{min} \right),$$

where S_{max} is the maximum signal intensity pixel value and S_{mim} is the minimum pixel signal intensity within the specified image volume. For perfect uniformity, the value of $N = 0\%$.

The ACR parameter, called the percent image uniformity (PIU), is similarly defined but in an effort to reduce the influence of image noise has chosen to define S_{max} and S_{min} as the mean signal over small ROIs positioned over regions of high and low signal intensity.

$$PIU + 100 \, X \left[1 - \left(S_{max-} S_{mim} \right) / \left(S_{max+} S_{mim} \right) \right]$$

For perfect uniformity, the ACR value of $PIU = 100\%$.

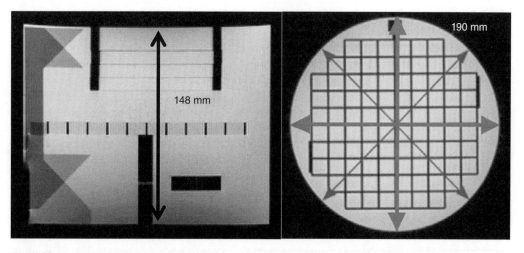

Figure 20.11 (left) Sagittal image of ACR large phantom illustrating assessment of the assessment of image dimensional accuracy in the longitudinal (z-axis). (right) Axial image illustrating measurements in the (x, y)-axis as well as oblique orientations.

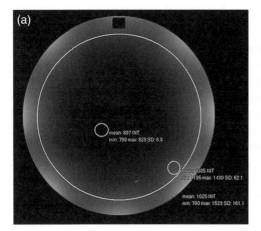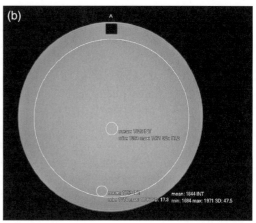

Figure 20.12 (a) Image acquired with an eight-channel receive only coil without image uniformity correction yielding PIU = 77%. (b) Image acquired with same coil with image uniformity correction (CLEAR) applied yielding PIU = 96%.

With the advent of volume coils composed of an array of small receive-only coils, the inherent uniformity is generally poor due to the depth dependent sensitivity profile of the small coils. When the signal is simply summed from the coil array, the image will typically be characterized by a low-intensity center as shown in Figure 20.12a. To achieve better image uniformity, images may be processed using propriety image uniformity correction algorithms (Figure 20.12b). As illustrated in Figure 20.8, the application of an image uniformity correction algorithm may significantly affect the non-signal producing background intensity and thus affect the SNR estimates.

The measurement of SNR and image uniformity for non-volume surface coils is discussed in detail in the ACR manual and in the NEMA-MS-6 [12] document entitled "Determination of signal-to-noise and image uniformity for single-channel, non-volume coils in diagnostic magnetic resonance imaging (MRI)."

20.2.2.8 Artifact Evaluation/Phase-Ghosting Assessment

It is well known that MR images are sensitive to phase-ghosting artifacts. These artifacts may be the result of errors in the application of the imaging phase encoding gradients or errors in the RF transmit/receive systems. These artifacts are manifest as multiple images in the non-signal producing background displaced from the signal-producing structures along the phase-encoding axis (orthogonal to the frequency-encoding axis) (Figure 20.13). In some cases, these images may appear as a fused column of low-intensity background signal. The ACR [1] has chosen to quantify the degree of phase ghosting by calculating the percent signal ghosting (PSG).

$$PSG = 100 \, X \left| \left(S_{ghost} - S_{bkg} \right) / 2 \times Mean \right|,$$

where, S_{ghost} is the mean signal in ghost ROI (Figure 20.13) located in the phase-encoding axis and S_{bkg} is the mean background signal in the frequency-encoding axis that has been specifically positioned to avoid any other artifacts that may be present in the image. PSG values are typically a small fraction of 1%. PSG should be considered unacceptable if it approaches 1%. The ACR failure PSG value is 1.5%.

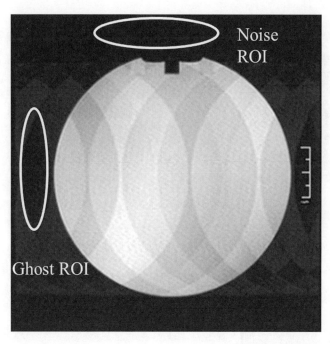

Figure 20.13 MR image illustrating phase-ghosting. In this image the phase-encoding axis is horizontal and the frequency-encoding axis is vertical. The very significant ghosting shown in this figure is still well below 1%.

20.2.2.9 Image Display Monitor Performance

The requirement for annual performance testing of display monitors has a part of the ACR accreditation process since its inception. Effective July 1, 2015, the Joint Commission has also added this requirement. Specifically, Item A23 of The Joint Commission's *Revised Requirements for Diagnostic Imaging Services* states that "... Magnetic Resonance Imaging (MRI) services: The annual performance evaluation conducted by the diagnostic medical physicist of MRI scientist ... includes testing of image acquisition display monitors for maximum and minimum luminance, luminance uniformity, resolution, and spatial accuracy." These tests will generally require a calibrated luminance meter (Figure 20.14a) and the ability to display a standard SMPTE or equivalent pattern (Figure 20.14c). These measurement procedures are described in more detail in the AAPM Task Group 18 Report [13] entitled "Assessment of Display Performance for Medical Imaging Systems" and in the ACR MRI Quality Control Manual [1]. Of the following list of four tests, the first two tests are performed using the luminance meter. Maximum (L_{max}) and minimum (L_{min}) luminance is measured while adjusting the window-level/window-width (WL/WW) control to display the maximum brightness and then repeat the WL/WW adjustment to display the image at full black, respectively. Luminance uniformity is determined from measurements made at five different locations (center and all four corners) on the display monitor (Figure 20.14b). The last two tests are typically performed while displaying the standard SMPTE pattern on the monitor. While viewing the SMPTE pattern at standard monitor setting, determine if the 5 and 95% contrast patches (arrows) are visible. The ACR suggests the display performance criteria listed below.

1) Max and min luminance (L_{max} and L_{min})
2) Luminance uniformity
3) Resolution using SMTE pattern
4) Spatial accuracy (SMTE)

(a)   (c)

(b)

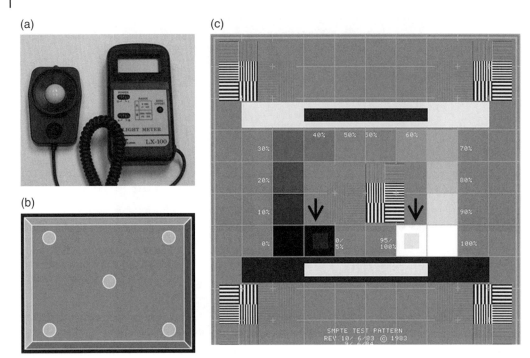

Figure 20.14 (a) Photography of a calibrated light meter (Lutron Electronics Light Meter Model LX-100, Taipei, Taiwan), (b) Illustration of the screen locations where luminance measurements are to be made for uniformity assessment, (c) SMPTE (Society of Motion Picture and Television Engineers) test pattern with arrows indicting the 5 and 95% patches.

ACR specifies the following performance requirements for MR displays. More on this topic can be found in Chapter 23.

Max luminance (WL/WW = min): $>90\,\text{Cd m}^{-2}$
Min luminance: $<1.2\,\text{Cd m}^{-2}$
Uniformity: %difference = $200^* (L_{max} - L_{min})/(L_{max} + L_{min})$
Intensity at corners must be within 30% of intensity at the center of the screen.
Resolution: display 100% contrast bar pattern of frequency = ½ monitor line frequency
Spatial accuracy: lines straight within $\pm 5\,\text{mm}$

20.3 Testing Paradigm and Clinical Implementation

20.3.1 Acceptance Testing

Though not always practical or possible, the medical physicist should be involved in the installation process and become acquainted with the local service engineer, the tools that they use and the vendor's technical specifications for the specific system. Acceptance testing, if at all possible, should ideally be performed prior to any patient studies. Of course, the primary goal of acceptance testing is to confirm that the system which is installed does in fact include all of the components and features that were agreed upon and if the system meets specified performance criteria. Since most MR services are now required to be accredited, it is also important for the medical physicist to confirm that the system meets image quality standards set by the relevant accreditation agency.

In addition, image performance results obtained during acceptance testing will establish baseline performance parameters that will be used for ongoing routine quality assurance measurements.

A detailed description of MRI acceptance testing in addition to procedures that can be used for routine quality assurance testing is provided in the 2010 AAPM Report No. 100 [14]. This report identifies tests that should be performed prior to installation as well as tests that are to performed following installation. Report No. 100 specifically recommends that these tests be performed on new systems before the first patient scan, following any major hardware or software upgrade and on existing systems that have not been previously accredited.

Pre-installation checks should include vibration and RF shield integrity testing. Each of these tests will most likely be performed by system vendor personnel; however, the medical physicist should be present to assist and to confirm that the test results are in compliance with the contract specifications. Over the years, vibration testing has become more important due to the smaller and lighter systems that are now being marketed. These smaller systems are more susceptible to vibration and the resultant phase-ghosting that may be produced.

RF shield testing is also commonly performed by the vendor personnel. Typically, RF scan room testing is performed both prior to the MR magnet installation and then repeated afterwards. The result of the RF testing is generally expressed in terms of dB signal attenuation. Typical pre-installation design specification is an attenuation of 100 dB at a frequency of 100 MHz. Typical post-installation specification is 85 db.

As part of acceptance testing, the medical physicist should check the patient monitoring and communication systems as well as an evaluation of the overall safety program. The evaluation should include magnetic fringe field mapping. Fringe-field mapping can generally be performed using a hand-held three-axis magnetometer such as shown in Figure 20.15. Also, regarding the static magnetic field, an important aspect of the site's MR safety program is access control to the various MRI service areas. It is recommended that this control be achieved by implementing the four-zone concept as defined in the ACR Guidance Document for Safe MR Practices: 2013 [15]. The four-zone concept provides for progressive restrictions in access to the MRI scanner (Figure 20.16):

Zone I: general public
Zone II: unscreened MRI patients
Zone III: screened MRI patients and personnel
Zone IV: screened MRI patients under constant direct supervision of trained MR personnel

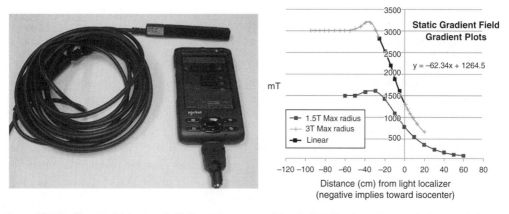

Figure 20.15 Hand-held three-axis Hall magnetometer (MetroLab Technology, Geneva, Switzerland) for magnetic field mapping.

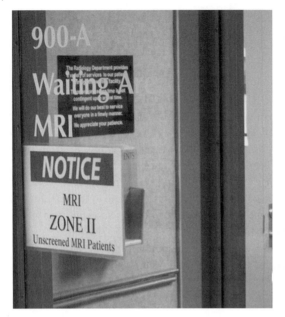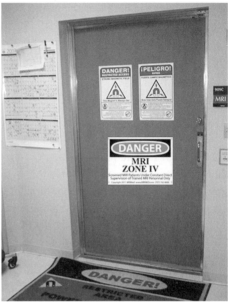

Figure 20.16 MRI Safety Zone signage (I-IV) is required by accreditation agencies including the Joint Commission. Zone I is for general public, Zone II is for unscreened MRI patients, Zone III is limited to screened patients and MR personnel and Zone IV is the MR magnet room.

Finally, the acceptance testing should include a full evaluation of available pulse sequences and image quality assessment. Image quality assessments should include checks of: magnetic field homogeneity, image geometric accuracy, ST and slice position accuracy, PIU, SNR or alternatively LCD, PSG. All of these image quality assessments are also a specified part of the accreditation process and will be discussed in greater detail in the section on accreditation requirements.

Unfortunately, there is no general consensus on specific acceptance criteria for most of the acceptance tests. The medical physicist will have to use information from the vendor of the specific MR system along with any specifications that are contained in the purchase contract to determine the appropriate acceptance criteria.

20.3.2 Quality Control

At most clinical sites it is the responsibility of the medical physicist to implement and monitor the routine image quality assurance program. It is generally the responsibility of the site's quality control technologist to perform and record the required quality control (QC) measurements.

The first steps required of the medical physicist in implementing the quality image quality assurance program is to choose which phantom will be used, determine which pulse sequences will be monitored and the frequency at which measurements will be made. The most commonly used phantoms are the ACR phantoms (Figure 20.17a and b). A vendor provided phantom or other commercially available phantom (Figure 20.17c) may also be used provided this phantom also meets the requirements of the site's accreditation agreement.

If the site is an accredited site, the medical physicist must assure that the proposed QC measurements and documentation (Figure 20.18) meet the requirements of the specific accrediting agency.

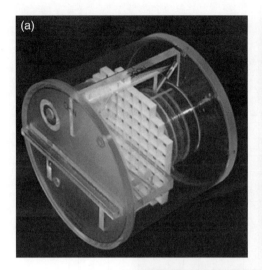
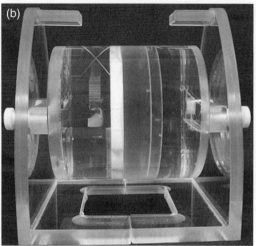
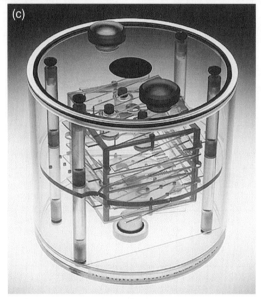

Figure 20.17 Possible phantoms for routine daily/weekly MRI image quality assessment. (a) The ACR large QC phantom (190 mm inner diameter), (b) ACR small phantom (100 mm) and (c) Magphan SMR 170 phantom (The Phantom Laboratory, Salem, NY).

The next step for the medical physicist is to work with the technologist to implement the imaging QC protocol, to establish baseline image quality parameters and appropriate action limits.

It is necessary for the medical physicist to determine parameter action limits for each MRI system. It should be noted that whatever action limits are chosen, they must be at least as restrictive as required by the accreditation agency.

To get started with establishing the initial action limits:

1) The service engineer should run all vendor tests to assure system is performing to vendor specifications
2) Establish baseline during acceptance testing (AAPM Report 100)

DATA FORM FOR WEEKLY MRI EQUIPMENT QUALITY CONTROL

MR Facility Name _____

MR Scanner Identifier _____

1 Date of Test Year	2 Table OK?	3 Console OK?	4 CF (Hz)	5 TX Gain/Atten-uation (dB)	Phantom Distances(mm) Sag Loc Length	Axial Slice #5 ← Diameters →		Slice 1 HR Holes#		Slice # ___ Number of LCD Spokes	Artifacts ?	Test By
					6 H/F (148)	7 A/P (190)	8 R/L (190)	9 UL	10 LR	11	12	13
Action Limits →												

NOTES

MRI Quality Control Manual

Reviewed by: _____   Qualified Medical Physicist/MRI Scientist   Date of Review _____

Figure 20.18 The ACR weekly QC log.

3) Collect QC data for 10–20 successive (ideally daily) determinations of the following:

- Central frequency
- Transmitter gain / attenuation
- Geometric accuracy
- High contrast resolution
- Low contrast resolution or SNR
- Other parameters as determined by the medical physicist

4) Record these "Baseline" values in the system QC log

   The action limits are then determined from these baseline measurements. A typical approach is to determine the action limits based upon the variability of the parameter, generally by using the mean and SD of each parameter. It is common to choose ± 1–$2\,$SD from the mean as the action limit. The exact values must be determined by the medical physicist considering the stability for the system. The ACR has established several action limits for their accreditation program that are based specifically on the ACR phantoms and the ACR reference sequences [6–9]. The medical physicist should review the current status of the ACR action limits at the ACR website (https://www.acraccreditation.org).

- Central frequency expressed in ppm
  (action limit $< \pm 2$–$3\,$ppm successive measurements, e.g. $3\,$ppm @ $1.5\,$T $\sim 200\,$Hz)
- Transmitter gain or attenuation (typically in dB)
- Geometric accuracy
  (ACR action limit: $\pm 2\,$mm using ACR phantom and ACR reference parameters.)
- High-contrast resolution
  (ACR action limit: at least $1\,$mm using ACR sequence and phantom)
- LCD
  (ACR action limit: low contrast object count or SNR ± 1–$2\,$SD)
- Artifacts

  (any artifacts noted in the QC log and image saved for further evaluation)
  A reference for parameters that should be routinely monitored, the ACR accreditation program requires at least weekly measurements of the following:

1) Center frequency and RF gain/attenuator (obtained as part of the phantom pre-scan)
2) Table positioning accuracy (verification of table position and laser alignment accuracy)
3) Setup and scanning (verification of system functionality)
4) Geometric accuracy (measured in both sagittal and axial planes)
5) High-contrast resolution
6) Low-contrast resolution
7) Artifact analysis
8) Visual check list (performed monthly)

20.3.3 Clinical Support

One of the more important roles of the medical physicist is to provide timely technical assistance and advice to the clinical staff. It is generally the medical physicist who has the best fund of knowledge regarding: what controls contrast, resolution and SNR in pulse sequences (Figure 20.19), the origin and resolution of artifacts (Figure 20.20), MR safety and accreditation requirements.

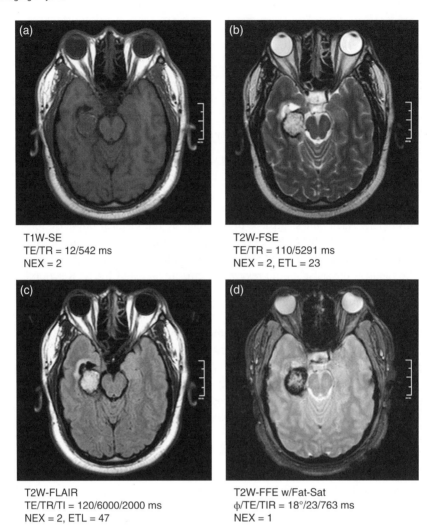

T1W-SE
TE/TR = 12/542 ms
NEX = 2

T2W-FSE
TE/TR = 110/5291 ms
NEX = 2, ETL = 23

T2W-FLAIR
TE/TR/TI = 120/6000/2000 ms
NEX = 2, ETL = 47

T2W-FFE w/Fat-Sat
φ/TE/TIR = 18°/23/763 ms
NEX = 1

Figure 20.19 (a) Spin-echo T1-weighting parameters will depend upon the field strength. Rapid gradient-echo T1-weighted images will often be achieved using inversion-recovery pre-pulses., (b) T2-weighted fast-spin-echo (FSE) sequences will depend upon the echo-train length (ETL) which also may affect spatial resolution, (c) Long inversion time (TI) fluid attenuated inversion recovery (FLAIR) sequences will often times require trial and error to select the correct TI value to provide good CSF suppression, and (d) Good quality fat-suppressed FFE sequences will require good magnetic field homogeneity typically evaluated by the physicist.

As illustrated in Figure 20.19, a typical MRI head protocol will generally require multiple sequences to generate a range of different tissue contrasts (T1-weighted, T2-weighted, CSF suppression [FLAIR] and fat-suppression). These sequences have multiple interacting acquisition parameters (TE, TR, TI, flip-angle φ, echo-train-length) that must be optimized to achieve the desired tissue contrast. In addition to assisting with the optimization of routine clinical protocols, it may be necessary for medical physicist to review all clinical images being submitted as part of the accreditation application, to confirm that appropriate acquisition parameters have been used. Since each clinical module has its own specific technical requirements (Figure 20.21) for resolution, ST and acquisition times, it is often necessary for the medical physicist to review the DICOM

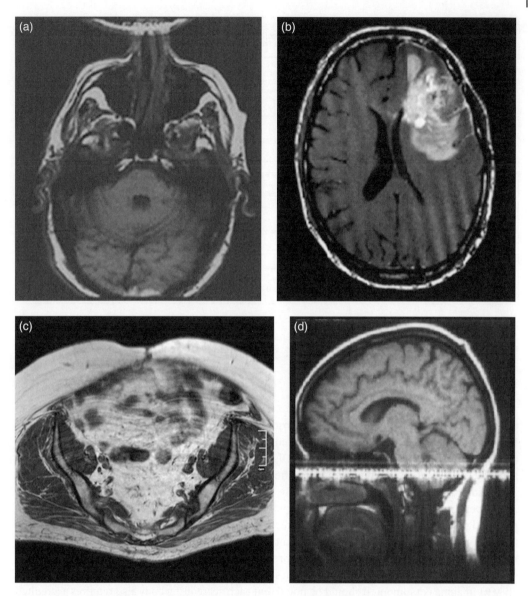

Figure 20.20 The medical physicist should assist in identifying image artifacts and in providing advice for artifact resolution. (a) Wrap artifact can be eliminated by increasing the FOV. (b) Artifacts resulting from data spikes and be result of static electricity arcs, coil arcing, or loose connections. (c) Respiratory motion artifacts can be reduced with spatial saturation bands or breath-hold sequences. (d) RF artifacts can result for open scan room doors and from breaks in the RF shield.

header information to confirm that the submitted sequences meet the specified minimum requirements. This is of particular significance for submission of the 3D image-sets required as part of the ACR Breast MRI accreditation process. Of particular concern, is the requirement that the acquired non-interpolated ST be ≤3 mm. In some cases, this determination may be difficult for the clinical staff. At the time of the DICOM review, the physicist should also check all images for unacceptable artifacts. The contributions of the medical physicist can often be extremely beneficial in minimizing accreditation problems.

Brain for TIA – maximum examination time ≤ 35 minutes			
Required Sequences	Category A: Pulse Sequence and Image Contrast	Category C: Anatomic coverage and imaging planes failure *to meet these specifications will result in failure*	Category D: Spatial Resolution
Sagittal, axial or Coronal dark fluid	Must have good discrimination between the brain and cerebral spinal fluid (CSF)	• Axial must cover the entire brain • Sagittal must cover the entire brain from left to right and the top of the brain to the C2 level • Coronal must cover the entire brain from the anterior cranial vault to the posterior cranial vault • The midline cut must be through the aqueduct	Slice thickness ≤ 5.0 mm Gap ≤ 2.5 mm if coronal Gap ≤ 2.0 mm if axial or sagittal In plane pixel (read) ≤ 1.0 mm In plane pixel (phase) ≤ 1.2 mm Pixel area ≤ 1.2 mm^2
Axial diffusion weighted imaging (DWI)	Must have a B value greater than 800	Axial must cover the entire brain	Slice thickness ≤ 5.0 mm Gap ≤ 2.0 mm In plane pixel (read) ≤ 2.0 mm In plane pixel (phase) ≤ 2.0 mm Pixel area ≤ 2.0 mm^2
Axial or coronal T2 FLAIR	Must have good contrast between the gray matter and white matter The CSF must be hypo or isointense with the white matter	• Axial must cover the entire brain • Coronal must cover the entire brain from the anterior cranial vault to the posterior cranial vault	Slice thickness ≤ 5.0 mm Gap ≤ 2.0 mm In plane pixel (read) ≤ 1.0 mm In plane pixel (phase) ≤ 1.2 mm Pixel area ≤ 1.2 mm^2
Axial bright fluid	The CSF must be hyperintense relative to the brain Must have good contrast between the gray matter and white matter	• Axial must cover the entire brain	Slice thickness ≤ 5.0 mm Gap ≤ 2.0 mm In plane pixel (read) ≤ 1.0 mm In plane pixel (phase) ≤ 1.2 mm Pixel area ≤ 1.2 mm^2
Axial or coronal T2* weighted gradient echo	The CSF must be hyperintense relative to the brain	• Axial must cover the entire brain • Coronal must cover the entire brain from the anterior cranial vault to the posterior cranial vault	Slice thickness ≤ 5.0 mm Gap ≤ 2.5 mm In plane pixel (read) ≤ 1.0 mm In plane pixel (phase) ≤ 1.2 mm Pixel area ≤ 1.2 mm^2

Figure 20.21 This is an example of the required sequences and imaging parameters MRI brain scans acquired for evaluation of TIA. This table was taken from the ACR "MRI Accreditation Program Clinical Image Quality Guide" available at the ACR website: www.acr.org.

20.3.4 Accreditation

As of July 1, 2015, the Centers for Medicare and Medicaid Services (CMS) has required that all medical facilities providing advanced diagnostic imaging (ADI) services that are billed through Part B of the Medicare Physician's Fee Schedule, must be accredited by one of the four CMS approved accreditation organizations. The ADI modalities are MRI, CT and nuclear medicine/PET and the accreditation organizations are the ACR, the Join Commission, the Intersocietal Accreditation Commission (IAC) and RadSite. These MRI accrediting bodies have many similar image performance standards, significant among these is the requirement for the services of a qualified medical physicist. The required medical physics credentials can be found on the agency's respective websites. (www.acr.org, www.jointcommission.org, www.intersocietal.org and www.radsite.com.) Also, a common feature of the programs of the four agencies is the requirement that a medical physicist or MRI scientist conduct a system performance evaluation at least annually on all MRI imaging equipment. It should be noted that each accrediting body also requires accredited sites to have implemented an active MRI safety program and, in most cases, the medical physicist must include a safety program review as part of their annual performance evaluation.

20.3.4.1 Annual Medical Physicist Equipment Performance Testing

The specific image quality tests and assessments required for the medical physicist's performance testing is quite similar across the various accrediting bodies. A general description of typical test procedures and phantoms was presented in Section 20.2.2 (Qualimetry). These assessments included the following: magnetic field homogeneity, slice position accuracy, ST accuracy, high-contrast spatial resolution, RF coil performance (typically SNR), geometric accuracy, image uniformity, artifact assessment and soft copy display integrity (monitors: brightness, uniformity and resolution). The accrediting agencies generally require that a medical physicist perform all of these assessments at least annually for each accredited system.

However, there are some differences between the various agencies. The specifics are available at the respective websites listed above. For example, the IAC requires submission of a complete acceptance testing report that includes testing of all of the above system parameters; however, the required annual measurements is a subset of the acceptance testing requirements and is referred to as "Annual Preventive Maintenance." The preventive maintenance measurements may be performed by any qualified individual including the vendor's service engineer. The preventive maintenance testing specifically identifies testing of SNR, field homogeneity, RF coil calibration for all coils, spatial resolution and artifact assessment. The RadSite and Joint Commission accreditation requirements are very similar to the ACR and specifically identify the qualified medical physicist as the appropriate individual to make the annual performance measurements. A conveniently available source that provides a detailed description of each of the tests listed above can be found in the ACR's "Magnetic Resonance Imaging (MRI) Quality Control Manual" [1]. The current ACR manual was published in 2015 and can be obtained from the website: https://www.acraccreditation.org and at the respective websites for the three other agencies.

20.3.4.2 ACR MR Medical Physics 1.5

The clinical utilization of MRI continues to increase along with the development of numerous new pulse sequences, techniques and instrumentation. As a result of these new developments, the medical physicist will be required to define and implement new quality control procedures. Among these new developments are parallel imaging and image acceleration algorithms (SENSE, GRAPPA, ASSET ...) made possible by multi-channel receivers and multi-element coil arrays. Other developments include the increased clinical use of EPI sequences and the use of parallel RF transmission (Transmit SENSE). EPI is now in common use for diffusion imaging and somewhat less frequently for surgical-planning fMRI studies. EPI sequences are highly dependent on the performance of the imaging gradients and are highly susceptible to N/2 ghosting. The medical physicist will generally be expected to provide routine evaluation of EPI artifacts and SNR performance. A discussion of EPI performance testing and N/2 ghosting can be found in AAPM Report 100 [14]. Similarly, new clinical pulse sequences that utilize image acceleration should also be evaluated and the performance characterized for both SNR and artifacts. Multi-channel RF transmission systems provide improved B1-field uniformity and image signal uniformity [16] and are common component of new high-field installations. The determination of the most appropriate performance tests for multi-channel RF-transmit and multi-channel receive systems continue to evolve but as always, will rely on contributions from medical physicists.

In summary, the medical physicist is an important member of the MRI service team. Their contributions to routine quality assurance and equipment performance testing can be essential for assuring that the MRI equipment is performing at a level that allows the site to provide the best possible diagnostic information and patient care. Regular safety assessments by the medical physicist may also significantly reduce the risk of patient injury and system damage.

As of January 1, 2012, the contribution of a qualified medical physicist is required for compliance with CMS for all sites that offer ADI services that are billed under Part B of the Medical Physician Fee Schedule. As of July 1, 2015, similar medical physics contributions will also be a requirement for Joint Commission Accreditation.

The evolution of new MRI hardware designs and pulse sequences in turn, leads to new clinical applications. It will be the responsibility of the medical physicist to monitor this evolution and in response, to continuously modify and update performance tests to assure optimal equipment performance.

References

1 Weinreb, J.C., Bell, R.A., Clarke, G.D. et al. (2004). American College of Radiology Magnetic Resonance Imaging (MRI) Quality Control Manual, ISBN 1-55903-146-8, 1891 Preston White Drive, Reston, VA 20191-4397. www.acr.org.

2 American College of Radiology (2019). ACR–AAPM technical standard for diagnostic medical physics performance monitoring of magnetic resonance (MR) imaging equipment. https://www.acr.org/-/media/ACR/Files/Practice-Parameters/mr-equip.pdf?la=en.

3 Chen, H.H., Boykin, R.D., Clarke, G.D. et al. (2006). Routine testing of magnetic field homogeneity on clinical MRI systems. *Med. Phys.* 33 (11).

4 National Electrical Manufacturers Association (2010). NEMA-MS-5. Determination of slice thickness in diagnostic magnetic resonance images: MS 5-2010. Rosslyn, VA: NEMA.

5 National Electrical Manufacurers Association (2008). NEMA-MS-1. Determination of SNR in diagnostic magnetic resonance images: MS 1-2008. Rosslyn, VA: NEMA.

6 American College of Radiology (1997). Site Scanning Instructions for Use of the MR Phantom for the ACR MRI Accreditation Program. Reston, VA: ACR.

7 American College of Radiology (1998). Phantom Test Guidance for the ACR MRI Accreditation Program. Reston, VA: ACR.

8 American College of Radiology (2008). Site Scanning Instructions for Use of the Small MRI Phantom for the ACR MRI Accreditation Program. Reston, VA: ACR.

9 American College of Radiology (2008). Phantom Test Guidance for Use of the Small MRI Phantom for the MRI Accreditation Program. Reston, VA: ACR.

10 National Electrical Manufactuers Association (2008). NEMA-MS-2. Determination of two-dimensional geometric distortion in diagnostic MR images: MS 2-2008. Rosslyn, VA: NEMA.

11 National Electrical Manufacturers Association (2008). NEMA-MS-3. Determination of image uniformity diagnostic magnetic resonance images: MS 3-2008. Rosslyn, VA: NEMA.

12 National Electrical Manufacturers Association (2008). NEMA-MS-6. Determination of signal-to-noise ratio and image unifomity for single-channel, non-volume coils in diagnostic magnetic resonance imaging (MRI): MS 6-2008. Rosslyn, VA: NEMA.

13 Samei, E., Badano, A., Chakraborty, D. et al. (2002), Assessment of Display Performance for Medical Imaging Systems. Report of the American Association of Physicists in Medicine (AAPM) Task Group 18, version 9.0 October 2002.

14 American Association of Physicists in Medicine (2010). AAPM REPORT No. 100: Acceptance testing and quality assurance procedures for magnetic resonance imaging facilities. College Park, MD: One Physics Ellipse.

15 Kanal, E., Barkovich, A.J., Bell, C. et al. (2013). ACR guidance document on MR safe practice: 2013. *J. Magn. Reson. Imaging* 37 (3): 501–530.

16 Katscher, U., Bornert, P., Leussler, C., and van den Bring, J.S. (2003). Transmit SENSE. *Magn. Reson. Med.* 49 (1): 144–150.

21

Clinical MRI Physics: Emerging Practice

David Pickens

Department of Radiology, Vanderbilt University, Nashville, TN, USA

21.1 Philosophy and Significance

Magnetic resonance imaging (MRI) has evolved very quickly to become a highly versatile and necessary imaging method that is found in many hospitals and medical centers worldwide. The ability of MRI to provide excellent soft tissue contrast from a variety of techniques present physicians with superb diagnostic information with no ionizing radiation. Additionally, new techniques have evolved to create imaging methods that are impossible to duplicate with other standard imaging systems. Furthermore, MRI is an integral part of many imaging research programs where new techniques are being developed that will find their way into clinical use. With such important and advancing capabilities and changes in protocols that follow the evolution of the technology, the medical physicist who is usually responsible for clinical image quality verification and documentation is tasked with keeping up with the latest developments in hardware, software, and methodologies. Simultaneously, the medical physicist is responsible for maintaining current knowledge of evolving regulations and requirements imposed by various organizations that review and accredit imaging practices.

The medical physicist has the training and experience to follow the developments of MR hardware, software, and pulse sequences in order to enhance the evaluation of these systems and provide increased clinical service to patients and radiologists. From a practical standpoint, this means that the old techniques that have served well over the years will need to be modified or replaced with improved methods, most likely highly automated, that will serve to increase efficiency as well as verify and document system performance. In addition, there are new regulations that will likely affect how the medical physicist interacts with other colleagues in providing the best overall use and safety of the MR systems while improving clinical benefits for patients.

As highly regarded members of the clinical team in the era of MRI 3.0, medical physicists will have to learn and understand new technologies in order to best serve as a resource to their clinical colleagues in the use of these new developments for optimized imaging. Each medical physicist supporting advanced MRI systems will need to understand the latest pulse sequences from the various manufacturers because they will be the resource for solving problems with patient imaging that arise. Advice on efficiency and throughput along with documentation of image quality, patient and staff safety, and regulatory compliance will be what the medical physicist will provide to each imaging site.

Clinical Imaging Physics: Current and Emerging Practice, First Edition. Edited by Ehsan Samei and Douglas E. Pfeiffer.
© 2020 John Wiley & Sons, Inc. Published 2020 by John Wiley & Sons, Inc.

Lastly, the medical physicist will be faced with new uses for MRI that include interventional and therapeutic applications, among others. Examples of technology applications developing into clinical products are the use of high energy ultrasound for treatment and ablation of tumors and the incorporation of linear accelerators into cancer therapy treatment delivery systems where monitoring of soft tissue beam positioning is performed in real time using an integrated MR imager. Other applications include image-guided surgical techniques for neurological and prostate surgery, which will be part of the routine practice in imaging centers in the future.

All these emerging opportunities for the use of MR imaging will place increased burdens on the medical physicist. Continuing education will be even more important than it is currently, since the field is evolving rapidly, and appropriate use of these systems will change as new applications become the standard of care. Additionally, medical physicists who operate in a consulting role to single-installation facilities will have to recognize the need to establish programs for addressing all the issues that arise with the use of these advanced systems when they are not on site. For all these situations, the use of advanced communication technologies and automated evaluation programs can serve the users and the medical physicists well in the future.

Current requirements for medical physics support of magnetic resonance facilities typically use the consultation model where the physicist provides testing and recommendations on a periodic basis. This model has the physicist testing the systems using a relatively simple phantom that evaluates general performance metrics such as low contrast detectability, spatial resolution, homogeneity, and spatial distortion, among others. These are important characteristics to evaluate, but are not going to be enough to provide the best service to sites in the future. There are two reasons for this. The first is that the medical physicist needs to be part of a team effort in close collaboration with the technologists, radiologists, and therapy providers, where guidance and advice can be given on operations with systems that are becoming vastly more complex and are performing much more complicated procedures than in the past. The incorporation of adjunct imaging or therapy system components within the MR environment for simultaneous image acquisitions or treatment greatly complicates the MR system environment in which the medical physicist will work. The second reason is that the requirements for achieving appropriate image quality or treatment performance from new system configurations will require that testing procedures for an increasingly regulated environment must be much more efficient. Documentation of the results from these evaluations must be made available quickly as part of the interaction of physicists with their medical colleagues. Thus, simple phantom measurements will not suffice and manual reporting several days or weeks after testing cannot provide the type of ongoing quality and timeliness that will be necessary.

In the requirements for the credentialing of individuals who test and evaluate the performance of clinical MR imaging systems, the need for training, background education, and certification is currently specified as part of system accreditation. A person who can perform testing on MR imaging systems and advise clinical facilities about the use of MRI systems meets the qualifications of a board-certified qualified medical physicist (QMP) or is classified as an MR-scientist by such groups as the American College of Radiology (ACR. Reston, VA) or The Joint Commission (TJC. Oakbrook Terrace, IL). In this document, reference will be made to QMPs as defined by the American Association of Physicists in Medicine (AAPM. Alexandria, VA), but an MR scientist can also be expected to provide some of the same services to an MR site. However, an MR scientist will not be able to provide other services such as those related to testing computed tomography (CT) systems or other radiation-based imaging or therapy systems, which may be part of the same clinical instrument or facility. Thus, the QMP will be the only qualified individual who can evaluate the technical aspects of combined imaging systems for accreditation purposes in the current regulatory environment.

21.2   Metrics and Analytics

A significant part of a QMP's duties with respect to MR systems is to provide performance evaluations of these systems, ensuring that the images made on patients will be of the highest quality and will be consistent over time. Historically, these evaluations have followed guidelines of the ACR MRI Accreditation Program, which involves the use of a particular phantom and follows specific steps found in the ACR MRI Quality Control Manual, published in 2015 [1]. In some cases, protocols and phantoms provided by the manufacturer to evaluate their systems are used either instead of or as an adjunct to the ACR-required MRI testing phantom. In cases where accreditation is required, either through ACR, through the Intersocietal Accreditation Commission (IAC. Ellicott City, MD), through TJC, or RadSite (Annapolis, MD), specific protocols and phantoms may be specified by a program that are used in the evaluation process or may be at the discretion of the site's medical physicist.

21.2.1   Intrinsic Performance

Many different capabilities of MR systems and imaging methods will require specific new techniques to ensure proper function and attendant safety of patients. While existing phantoms and testing methods can provide an overall evaluation of basic functionality, expanded use of acquisition methods that are quantitative rather than qualitative require much more detailed testing and close collaboration with users. Routine quantitative imaging will be performed in the knee joints, body, and in the head, using techniques for studying the brain and brain function, such as functional MRI– fMRI, diffusion techniques including advanced diffusion tensor imaging (DTI) and its associated fiber tracking methods (tractography), advanced cardiac imaging, ultrafast imaging techniques, and the evolution of MR spectroscopy into a form that is routinely available in most clinical environments. Approaches to testing both acquisition hardware and software as integrated systems will be necessary to ensure function of the entire process rather than testing each element as a separate component. Integrated approaches will expand the need for the medical physicist to be able to understand not only the functions of the parts, but also the characteristics of the images that are produced. An example of the future needs for such integrated approaches is the development of suitable hardware phantoms to simulate white matter tracts. Such phantoms must simulate a complete acquisition resulting in images that can be used to calibrate appropriate analysis tools, since the results will be known. These types of phantoms test the entire evaluation chain to verify that accurate and consistent quantitative evaluation of diffusion tensor images of the brain and the fiber tracts occurs in clinical images.

New hardware capabilities are expanding the functionality of these systems. While most current MR imagers operate at 1.5 or 3.0 T, worldwide there are more than 40 systems currently operating at ultrahigh fields, those over 3.0 T. These systems are found in research installations using mostly 7.0 T systems, although there are other, higher field systems in several labs including at this writing, a 10.5 T human whole-body imaging magnet in operation and an 11.7 T human imaging magnet under construction. As has been the case over the 35-year use of clinical MRI, the evolution toward higher field strengths will continue. Recently, 7.0 T systems have been approved and installed for use clinically in the United States. These systems employ advanced receiver systems implementing multi-channel parallel methods for adequate uniformity and image quality. Added to this capability is the routine use of B1 shimming, where the B1 RF field is manipulated to achieve better uniformity within the imaged section of the body using multiple RF transmit channels. Determining the accuracy and performance of these systems is likely to be a difficult but required part of the system evaluation.

As the field strengths increase and the transmit/receive systems become more complex, the use of MR systems will be extended beyond the usual imaging found in radiology departments. Development and testing of MR systems coupled with therapeutic devices such as linear accelerators (MR-LINAC) is ongoing and has led to the first commercial systems being installed in clinical environments. In these applications, the goal is to use the MR imaging capability to locate the selected area and monitor the treatment of that area while the therapeutic system delivers energy to a target. The integration of these types of capabilities requires that the medical physicist be responsible not only for image quality, but also for the proper and precise monitoring and delivery of therapy to the patient. To be effective in this role, the medical physicist must be part of the treatment team and closely monitor procedures done on these and other integrated systems. Temperature monitoring capability and treatment volume representation accuracy are required for these systems as part of the routine quality evaluation procedures, since the therapeutic subsystems could do considerable harm to the patient if not properly evaluated.

Other technologies requiring interaction of the medical physicist includes the development of hybrid imaging systems. These machines use two different imaging modalities tightly coupled within a single gantry so that the strengths of each system can be used to address aspects of a clinical imaging problem. An example of this sort of integration is the recent development of PET-MR systems where a positron emission tomography (PET) scanner is integrated into the bore of an imaging magnet so that both units can operate simultaneously with perfect physical registration of the images for later fusion. Verification of this registration requires the use of phantoms designed to produce signals for both modalities with capabilities to demonstrate resolution and contrast characteristics from both sections measured without moving the phantom. With such rich sources of data about brain function available, the dual capabilities of imaging both function and structure with these systems allow investigations of clinical and research problems that were often impractical due to the lack of temporal coherence. Thus, the medical physicist must be expert in PET imaging and proper testing of both systems for maximizing the quantitative information available while ensuring safety of patients and staff.

21.2.2 Quantitative Metrics of Image Quality

Determining image quality quantitatively is difficult unless the image is of an object of known characteristics and configuration. In clinical images, one usually has the option of characterizing the image with several techniques by reviewing aspects of the background noise, signal, and overall contrast. Spatial resolution is more difficult to measure without structures of known size and characteristics. Information content is usually not practical to measure without advanced image processing, which is not typically available for images in a clinical environment. Some measures have been described that can provide quantitative evaluation of image quality. In one approach, it was proposed that the minimum time needed to achieve a useable contrast-to-noise ratio (CNR) could be found such that an image could be evaluated quantitatively immediately after acquisition [2]. This proposed method uses the fact that the signal-to-noise ratio (SNR) in an image is proportional to the $\sqrt{t}$ where t is time. CNR is then proportional to the magnitude of the signal difference between two tissues divided by the noise:

$$\text{CNR12} \propto \frac{|S1 - S2|}{\text{Noise}} \propto \sqrt{t} \text{ where } S1 \text{ and } S2 \text{ are different tissues}$$

Such a measurement evaluates the efficiency of a pulse sequence in accumulating CNR and leads to the determination of minimum acceptable time for the detection of specific pathology:

$$T_{\min} = \left(CNR_{\text{thresh}} \frac{\Delta \sqrt{t}}{\Delta CNR} \right)^2 \quad \text{where } \frac{\Delta \sqrt{t}}{\Delta CNR} \text{ is a constant}$$

This type of formulation could lead to improved clinical image quality through automatic analysis at the point of acquisition before the patient is removed from the machine, giving the technologist the opportunity to repeat the study, if needed. For this type of system to function well, the medical physicist must be part of the clinical group that determines the threshold CNR for different pulse sequences used for specific imaging studies. The availability of real-time image quality assessment would lead to more refined and efficient pulse sequences for different disease processes and ensure better image quality more consistently.

Other techniques have been proposed as well, including the use of human observer models. In these approaches, image quality is evaluated by a mathematical structure that models the behavior of the human visual system in some way. These models have been implemented in computer software to evaluate specific characteristics of the image quality such as the presence of artifacts from parallel MRI reconstruction. In one study, an artifact-perceptual difference model was used to evaluate four different types of artifacts that included noise, blurring, aliasing, and over-smoothing in images from compressed sensing reconstruction and generalized auto-calibrating partially parallel acquisition (GRAPPA) parallel reconstruction [3]. These types of systems have the potential to provide automation for the assessment of image quality characteristics for both clinical images and, as importantly, to assess image quality for automated quality assurance procedures that extend beyond the direct methods currently available, comparing favorably to human observers [4]. One could visualize a system using model observers designed to evaluate some characteristics of clinical images as they are prepared for presentation to the radiologist that would evaluate and log changes in image quality compared to previous similar images or to a standard as has been done in automatic evaluation of x-ray mammography images for computer-aided detection (CADe). Emerging techniques employing neural network software may be ideal systems to achieve the goals of automatic image quality assessment.

21.3 Testing Implication of New Technologies

21.3.1 High and Ultrahigh Field Systems

A significant number of installed standard magnet strengths are represented by 1.5 T superconducting imagers, although there are several systems with lower fields or higher fields and various configurations. With all these systems, but especially those with higher fields extending above 3 T, it becomes very important to understand the extent of fringe magnetic fields. These can be evaluated initially by looking at the manufacturer's specifications and installation materials. However, the static magnetic fields may need to be measured in order to determine where in the magnet room certain field levels can be found or to verify manufacturer's specifications. Static gradient fields as one approaches the bore of a superconducting magnet are of concern as well and should be included in the verification of the specifications for each system. Measurements of these fields will require specialized instrumentation for accurate characterization. A typical instrument for these measurements, a three-axis gauss meter calibrated to 14 T, is shown in Figure 21.1, which permits careful mapping of iso-gauss lines in and around the magnet room. Applications for smart phones are available for measuring magnetic fields as well, but not with the precision of a calibrated dedicated instrument. The clinical medical physicist will need to become familiar with

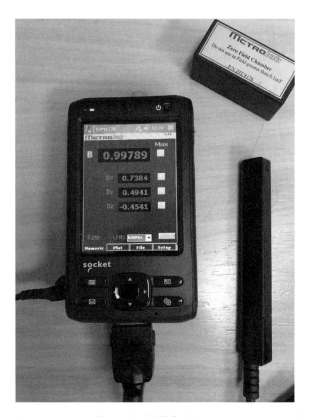

Figure 21.1 A three-axis gauss meter calibrated to 14 T. Such instruments are capable of high accuracy measurements of static magnetic fields and are portable.

these types of devices to verify the safety of the magnetic environment outside of the magnet's bore and to understand where gauss lines are located within the scan room for each installation.

Other issues with high and ultrahigh field systems are associated with concerns about RF energy absorption by the patient. The specific absorption rate (SAR) increases approximately quadratically with field strength, so at high and ultrahigh fields, pulse sequences must be very carefully designed to not cause unacceptable heating. For clinical systems with Food and Drug Administration (FDA) approval not operating under research protocols, the vendor provides an estimation of the SAR for a given pulse sequence. Unfortunately, the estimation methods are proprietary and tend to overestimate the SAR, resulting in limits to the use of certain types of pulse sequences. Additionally, scanner estimates of SAR are not useful for RF exposure testing for implanted devices, peripheral areas of the body, or for use in interventional procedures.

As these high-performance imagers become more common, it will be incumbent on the medical physicist to be knowledgeable of other ways to evaluate the RF output of scanners during clinical imaging. This will likely take the form of independent monitoring of RF output separate from the stated SAR provided by the imager as well as the use of very sophisticated RF simulation software to provide useful estimates of the SAR for different configurations of RF systems. Some RF dosimeters have been proposed at university sites that can be used to measure average SAR independent of the MR systems. One such device developed at Johns Hopkins University is designed to simulate a body-equivalent coil load so that the whole-body torso SAR can be measured completely independent of the SAR values reported by the scanner [5]. This dosimeter would require independent calibration and its use would be analogous to measuring CT scanner output for x-ray dose estimation purposes. To date, such test systems are in experimental development, but will likely become part of the instrumentation used by the medical physicist in the future along with advanced electromagnetic field simulation software to accurately characterize the SAR for different situations and coil configurations.

Also important will be the increased use of multi-channel or parallel array RF transmission systems. These systems have been under study for several years and the importance of parallel RF at ultrahigh fields has been discussed at length in the literature. RF inhomogeneity issues at wavelengths approaching the size of the human body can create standing waves, which likely contribute to dielectric artifacts represented by signal loss or gain in the images made with single source RF systems, thereby reducing image quality. Coil performance becomes a function of the object being imaged as well as its specific characteristics so that different imaging sessions, even with the same subject, will show different results. While these effects are visible in high field (3.0 T) images, they can be substantial at ultrahigh field strengths above 3.0 T. At these fields, more complex RF transmission techniques become crucial to reduce B1 inhomogeneity [6]. These issues can be mitigated by beam steering approaches (RF shimming) or using full temporally independent coil arrays with multiple channels for transmission, somewhat analogous to parallel receive systems commonly available [7]. In one recent study of RF shimming, extensive modeling of RF homogeneity and power deposition were validated in a complex head-sized phantom at 7 T to demonstrate that accurate prediction of RF coupling and power deposition as well as the B1 field can be demonstrated experimentally, lending credence to the concept that modeling and phantom work can be used in evaluation of these advanced capabilities [8].

With true parallel RF transmission, there are a few significant potential problems that require attention. For full performance and safety, these systems require sequential calibration with local control of power deposition over the entire sample, since the NMR response to the transmitted RF energy is usually not a linear one [9]. Additionally, there are significant concerns with safety validation and control to reduce the likelihood of exceeding the SAR values. Poor attention to these issues can have severe consequences for the patient with likely increases in local SAR within the body [9, 10]. In comparison to SAR from a quadrature transmit coil, a worst-case scenario using an 8-channel head array in simulation demonstrated about a factor of 10 increase in SAR. Therefore, independent monitoring and simulations need to be available for the medical physicist to provide useful information to the medical team about RF shim performance, requiring that the medical physicist become very aware of such techniques and potential safety issues for these systems.

21.3.2 Quantitative Imaging

Quantitative imaging is complex and can be difficult with current systems. With the increased capabilities of new hardware, especially equipment to speed up the acquisition process and the use of higher fields, the medical physicist must fully understand the needs of particular quantitative imaging situations. Of concern are four aspects that can be applied to any quantitative imaging system, but are especially challenging with quantitative MR imaging methods [11]: (i) imaging accuracy, (ii) imaging reproducibility, (iii) imaging bias, and (iv) patient accuracy. Imaging accuracy addresses the issues of changes that can occur with MR systems over time. An accurate system will image the same phantom with minimum variance of the results each time. In many studies it will be necessary for the patient or subject to be imaged on different systems, so a concern with quantitative imaging is how to ensure that the data gathered on one system can be compared to the same study done on a different system. This is especially important when quantitative MRI is performed at multiple sites on the same manufacturer's systems. Furthermore, one must be assured that the results in a phantom study on one vendor's system will produce the same or very similar results on a different vendor's system. Finally, the medical physicist must know how much variation will occur when the same patient is scanned on the same machine multiple times. Accurate quantitation of results from MR systems is challenging and requires carefully thought out methods for producing consistently useful results in both phantoms as well as in patient studies over time and place.

Quantitative MRI is important currently and will be much more important in the future. Among the reasons for developing quantitative techniques are the need for better disease staging, especially in diseases such as various cancers including brain, liver, prostate, and breast. Techniques have been described for quantitative evaluation of many tissues including skeletal changes in bone and cartilage. Imaging techniques and evolving methods in MR spectroscopy provide information that allow for tracking the performance of drug therapies as well as understanding the efficacy of new drugs. Increasingly, quantitative MR images are providing information directly used for therapy treatment planning in radiation oncology settings, leading to quantitative tracking of the treatment process [12].

Other uses of quantitative imaging are found in radiation oncology settings with the integration of MR imaging and linear accelerators (LINACs) that allow for treatment verification during the therapy process. Manufacturers have demonstrated non-integrated systems where a common treatment bed is shared between a conventional MR imager and a heavily magnetically-shielded LINAC in a treatment room. However, an integrated MR-LINAC system as described by Raaymakers et al. and others [13] moves the treatment and verification process into a different league, both in the design of the system and its potential uses with the incorporation of the LINAC into the magnet structure. These systems require the medical physicist to have both intimate knowledge of LINAC calibration and safety, as well as MR quality assurance and safety.

For quantitative imaging, significantly higher performance is needed along with careful assessment of that performance. QMPs will be tasked with the duties of verifying both the acquisition and post-collection processing performance so that quantitative information provided by these systems is both accurate and precise. Additionally, careful testing will verify repeatability and effective quality assurance programs will ensure overall long-term performance. Quantitative MRI requires specialized phantoms, often designed for specific capabilities necessary for a particular imaging situation and new image analysis techniques. These phantoms provide the standardization and calibration information needed for quantitative imaging. For successful quantification to be done, there is an increasing need for physics support to ensure the required quality and performance, especially over time once the MR manufacturer's training representatives have left.

21.3.3 Parallel Imaging in MR

One of the most exciting developments over the last few years has been in parallel receive imaging capabilities. When using multi-coil receive systems, the transmitted RF signal is produced by the quadrature body coil, while multiple small coils are used to acquire signals in parallel that are used to reconstruct images. There are various techniques wherein the data are combined from all the receive coils either in frequency space or image space to produce the final images. The great advantage is that by intentionally undersampling k-space by reducing the number of phase-encoding steps, it is possible to reduce the scan time significantly at the expense of more complex reconstruction of the undersampled data from each coil. These approaches are used currently in clinical imaging on high performance imagers, but are expensive to implement compared to the older quadrature coil systems because of the need for separate receive channels for each small coil and additional reconstruction software. Current systems can be equipped with as many 128 or more channels.

While the speed increases allowed by parallel technology are important and have essentially displaced the conventional quadrature transmit-receive coil except for the body resonator, testing of these systems is equally important and can be very time consuming if each of the small coils is tested individually. Each small coil has its own noise characteristics, so the noise propagation is spatially heterogeneous and is correlated between multiple small coils. Noise covariance matrices can be used to describe these noise characteristics. SNR depend on the acceleration factor, R, as well as the geometry factor, $g \geq 1$, for both the sensitivity encoding (SENSE) image-based technique and the GRAPPA k-space technique [14, 15]. However, the equation below can be used to describe an SNR for images made with either method.

$$\text{SNR}_R = \frac{\text{SNR}_0}{\left(g\sqrt{R} \right)}$$

This equation yields a variable SNR, which complicates the testing requirements, since the current ACR methods are applicable to systems with Rician noise distributions [16]. Since parallel systems do not exhibit Rician noise distributions, the conventional approaches do not provide an accurate SNR measurement. This leads to difficulties comparing image quality between different protocols and different systems. Furthermore, manufactures often use correction measures to improve image quality at the expense of altered noise characteristics, complicating accurate measurement even more.

The medical physicist will need to develop familiarity with better methods for evaluation of noise in parallel receive systems. Fortunately, a method has been developed by the National Electrical Manufactures' Association (NEMA. Arlington, VA) that can be used with coil arrays used for parallel receive [17]. This method permits calculation of the noise in an image that is corrected for non-Gaussian distributions found with parallel receive systems. In this approach, a region-of-interest (ROI) is taken from most of each image of a pair acquired five minutes apart. These ROIs are centered and encompass about 90–95% of each image through the center of a spherical phantom (Figure 21.2). The noise figure comes from the subtraction of the two images and the calculation of the corrected noise value as follows:

$$SD = \left[\frac{\sum_{i=1}^{n} \sum_{j}^{m_i} \left(R(i,j) - \bar{R} \right)^2}{\sum_{i=1}^{n} \left(m_i \right) - 1} \right]^{\frac{1}{2}}$$

where SD is the corrected noise, $R(i,j)$ is the value of an individual pixel, $\bar{R}$ is the average value of the ROI, and n, m are pixel row and column, respectively. This approach is known as NEMA Method 1 and is readily applicable to current and future systems using parallel receivers for each coil. Signal is found by adding the two images collected five minutes apart and dividing the result by two to form an average image. An ROI of 75% gives the value for signal in the image. From these data an SNR can be derived that is more applicable to parallel receive configurations.

Another measurement that is complicated by parallel receive capabilities is the measurement of uniformity. Parallel systems demonstrate spatially dependent sensitivities due to the variable characteristics of the different RF coils. Added to these are the previously mentioned correction measures for improving both SNR and intensity uniformity used by some manufacturers. NEMA again has developed techniques that can be applied to these systems as a whole, rather than attempting to test each element separately. The approach as discussed and modified by Goerner et al. is referred to as NEMA Method 2, the gray scale uniformity map [18]. This technique works with different parallel imaging paradigms and is most consistent for describing decreased uniformity with increasing R, the acceleration factor. A spherical phantom (17.8 cm diameter is typical) is used with an echo-planar imaging (EPI) acquisition from which uniformity measurements are made.

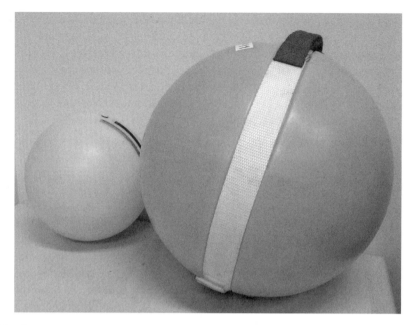

Figure 21.2 Spherical phantoms used in MRI quality assurance measurements. These are available with different diameters to fit different sizes of coils.

In the modified NEMA Method 2 Gy scale uniformity map technique, pixels are binned into five assigned gray level representations, labeled A-E based on comparison to the mean, S, in a 75% ROI. Each pixel value, I, is assigned to different bins as follows:

$$A \rightarrow I \leq S \times 0.8$$

$$B \rightarrow S \times 0.8 < I \leq S \times 0.9$$

$$C \rightarrow S \times 0.9 < I \leq S \times 1.1$$

$$D \rightarrow S \times 1.1 < I \leq S \times 1.2$$

$$E \rightarrow S \times 1.2 \leq I$$

Pixels are then grouped into G_0 (bin C), G_1 (bins B + D), and G_2 (bins A + E). These groups contain the number of pixels within 10% of the mean, between 10 and 20% of the mean, and > or <20% of the mean, respectively. The percent image uniformity, UN_2, is computed from the number of pixels in each group:

$$UN_2 = 100\left(1 - \left(0.5 \times G_1 + G_2\right)\right)$$

In this method uniformity varies with different parallel imaging configurations at different R values. However, this technique can accommodate these different methods and different acceleration values. It should be useful for more extensive parallel receive systems where testing each coil as currently recommended by accreditation programs will become impractical as the number of elements increases.

21.3.4 Ultrafast Imaging

Ultrafast imaging is usually considered to be either an implementation of single- or multi-shot EPI or of spiral imaging where two- and three-dimensional acquisitions as fast as 22 msec per image can be obtained [19]. Historically, Cartesian EPI produced fast images that were likely to experience lower spatial resolution, increased geometric distortion, additional blurring, poor image contrast, Nyquist ghosting, and signal voids. Spiral imaging for fast acquisitions can be affected by gradient timing and eddy currents, yielding reduced image quality in the form of blurring, signal voids, and magnification ghosts [19]. With these types of ultrafast approaches, testing of the gradient systems becomes highly important to ensure that these advanced imaging capabilities are functioning properly. Gradient stability and linearity are especially important, as are slew rates.

Evaluation of systems performing ultrafast acquisitions requires highly specialized methods and phantoms. Given that there are increasing numbers of fast imaging techniques available, medical physicists will have to be prepared to address new methods to ensure that imagers can operate within specifications for these types of pulse sequences. Ghosting is a significant problem in EPI imaging due to uneven phase shifts between even and odd echoes during an acquisition, leading to N/2 (or Nyquist) ghosts in the image. Phase errors are either zeroth order between even and odd echoes caused by B0 eddy currents, asymmetrical analog filter responses or other factors, or are first order, due to time shifts between centers of odd and even echoes from group gradient timing delays in addition to eddy currents. Zeroth-order ghosting produces a uniform ghost image while first-order ghosting has a null in the center of the ghost from a sinusoidal intensity modulation [20]. Ghosting can be evaluated using spherical homogeneous phantoms from which a ghosting ratio is computed with a current recommendation not to exceed 3% for single shot EPI.

Geometric distortion can be evaluated for ultrafast sequences as well, again using a spherical homogeneous phantom. Comparing the actual dimensions of the phantom, measured with a conventional spin-echo pulse sequence, allows for the testing in high performance mode where shear, compression or dilation, or image shifts can be evaluated. Comparisons are made of changes in the frequency encoding direction as a result of poor gradient performance. Thus, in Figure 21.3 from AAPM Report 100, l_x is the width of the phantom in the spin-echo image and this measurement is used as a comparison for images made with the ultrafast pulse sequence [21]. Distortions can be measured with respect to the distance changed from this measurement and scaled to yield a percent distortion, which typically should be less than 3%.

Overall stability is another concern, especially for repeated applications of ultrafast pulse sequences such as found in fMRI acquisitions. For stability measurements, signal intensity, ghosting intensity, and ghosting ratios over a significant time period should be evaluated. Since typical fMRI studies at 1.5 T might yield signal changes of about 1–4%, then the coefficient of variation for stability should be less than 0.25%. For ultrahigh field systems these types of measurements are likely to be very important, since the uses of the systems often will be to acquire data as fast as possible.

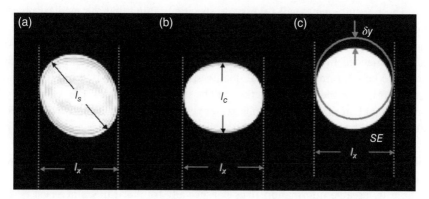

Figure 21.3 Different types of distortion that can be seen in EPI images: (a) sheer distortion, (b) compression or dilation distortion, (c) image shift. *Source:* Ref. [2]. Used with permission from AAPM.

21.3.5 MR Spectroscopy

MR spectroscopy is a challenging area of ongoing research that has had some acceptance in clinical imaging, especially for use in the brain. Single voxel spectroscopy and spectroscopic imaging techniques are being developed where the processed data provides quantitative information about metabolites in a volume of tissue. More work has been done on proton spectroscopic methods than on other nuclei, due to the more widely available equipment necessary to do spectroscopy at proton frequencies and the relatively higher signals. Higher field systems of 3.0 T and above allow investigation of hard-to-detect metabolites such as glutamine (Gln), glutamate (Glu), and gamma-aminobutyric acid in the brain. There is considerable evidence that MR spectroscopy contributes to the understanding of many clinical brain diseases including various neoplasms, demyelinating diseases, and infections [21]. Ongoing research and development is leading to other applications in the clinic in diverse areas of the body including musculoskeletal, prostate, breast, and liver. However, full reimbursement by third party payers will be required for spectroscopy to move into mainstream use.

The clinical medical physicist supporting MR spectroscopy facilities will be in a position of needing to evaluate the MR imaging system equipped for spectroscopy and spectroscopic imaging very carefully. Detailed attention to RF coil functions, dynamic shimming functions, water suppression, spurious echo suppression, and other aspects of the acquisition process are very important in achieving spectral quality suitable for routine diagnostic use. In single voxel spectroscopy, each spectrum should be inspected as part of the quality measures for each study, a difficult and time-consuming task if done manually. However, automated spectral evaluation software has been developed, but must itself be evaluated prior to clinical use. Furthermore, sets of model spectra must be produced for evaluating the system at a given field strength, for a given pulse sequence, and for other acquisition parameters [21]. Sets of reference images in age-matched subjects are likely to be needed as well. All these requirements place a burden on the facility and the medical physicist to ensure that the infrastructure is operating properly before clinical spectroscopy is performed.

Using spectroscopy in the clinical environment requires planning and, as these techniques become more distributed, requires careful oversight to avoid issues of systems and software variations that can disrupt accurate quantitation of metabolite concentration. Stable metabolic-product-containing phantoms such as the "Braino" phantom (GE Healthcare, Chicago, IL) are required and should be used in a consistent fashion so that subtle changes in machine performance do not adversely affect the study outcome. Quantitative quality measurements are necessary to identify metrics whose minima must be achieved before a study is deemed clinically acceptable. These requirements will necessitate specific training that the medical physicist may need to acquire and will necessitate an ongoing commitment to quality assurance by the facility.

There are many tests that can be performed for quality assurance of MR spectroscopy. At a minimum, as recommended in AAPM Report 100, volume-of-interest location accuracy should be demonstrated to be ±1.0 mm and spectral quality should be evaluated with a tissue-mimicking phantom appropriate for the metabolites that will be studied [9]. Water suppression, eddy current correction, fitting of Lorentzian peaks, global water peak (FWHM <7 Hz), and SNR of spectra from the phantom should be characterized. Additionally, long term stability is a concern, so extended testing by evaluating the same phantom with the same protocols consistently over time is necessary. While it is likely that many evaluations can be done automatically in the future, it will be up to the experienced medical physicist to ensure correct application of the needed techniques to produce clinically useable information. This is especially true for MRS, since best performance often requires manual shimming that only an expert operator can provide. Furthermore, software changes to the automatic analysis systems that will be widely available for spectrum analysis will need to be evaluated every time an update is performed to ensure that quantitative results are not changed.

21.3.6 Hybrid Imaging Systems and MR-Guided Interventions

Among the capabilities that are becoming available are systems that combine what traditionally had been two separate imaging instruments into a single device. Such hybrid systems follow the path set forth by the incorporation of CT scanners into PET systems. The combination of the two imagers together provides superior information to what would be available in separate devices. Integration of this type has led to medical physicists who do primarily nuclear medicine physics learning the physics of CT and the behavior of the combined, hybrid PET-CT systems. The PET-CT hybrid systems have been so successful that PET systems alone are usually not sold without the CT component.

In the research community over the last few years, the technology of PET has advanced such that a PET system can be integrated within the bore of an MR imager. This arrangement allows for simultaneous imaging with both systems, offering the superior temporal and spatial resolution only available in such in an instrument capable of coaxial simultaneous imaging. Such devices are available from some manufacturers currently, having received FDA approval for clinical use. As more uses that have direct clinical applications are developed, the prices will come down and more systems will be found in major medical centers [22]. These installations place a new burden on the medical physicist because of the need to understand the operation of both systems interacting together. Quality assurance becomes a combined project where both MR methods and PET radiopharmaceutical quantitation must be evaluated. Thus, the medical physicist must learn and understand both technologies as well as their interaction in these systems.

Hybrid systems will require expanded quality assurance methods and the development of phantoms that can be used for both. In the pre-clinical area, hybrid single photon emission CT SPECT-MRI systems have been built, and like the PET-MRI systems, require new skill sets from the physicist to properly evaluate them. Among the needs with hybrid systems to complement the phantoms and evaluation methods used for these systems separately, are new phantoms that provide signal information to both parts of the imager so that the proper registration of the images is assured while appropriate testing of image quality can be done on each subsystem. An example of a combination resolution phantom, suitable for both MR and SPECT imaging has been demonstrated by Hamamura et al. [23]. As with other combined imaging systems, the medical physicist will be the expert reference point for the users who may be less familiar with the operating principles of one system compared to the other.

21.3.7 MRI Therapeutic Systems

New technologies have moved the use of MRI into the realm of clinical intervention and therapeutic uses of systems that combine the imaging capabilities of MR with integrated therapy delivery systems. These integrated systems are used simultaneously where the images provide guidance and monitoring for biopsies or provide position and temperature monitoring while the therapeutic system is used to ablate a tumor or other mass. Examples of this can be found in the literature [24] and in commercial development of techniques and equipment for treating many organs of the body. All these approaches couple new equipment with MRI, sometimes in an operating suite, which provide new challenges for the medical physicist in terms of testing and quality assurance support for these combined systems. Additionally, there are new issues of safety that can arise if the environment is not as tightly controlled as is usually the case in a radiology department MR imaging suite. Moving forward as these new methods are developed and manufacturers provide the enhanced capabilities of biopsy and therapy using MRI to guide the process, these systems will provide new standards of care in larger medical centers and hospitals.

A specific example of an integrated therapeutic system that requires considerable support and expertise from a medical physics perspective is the use of high intensity focused ultrasound for thermal treatment of diseased tissue. Known as MR-guided high-intensity focused ultrasound (MRgHIFU), this technology places a high output ultrasound therapy system into the patient bed of an MR imager so that the MR system can provide real-time localization and temperature monitoring of tissues undergoing treatment by a high energy focused ultrasound beam. Several tissues have been treated successfully in clinical trials including uterine leiomyomas, bone metastases, and brain tumors. Other applications are in research and development including applications in prostate, liver, and breast. In these systems, the delivery of tissue heating by the ultrasound system must be very precise and the temperature of the tissue undergoing treatment must be very carefully monitored by the MR system to adequately heat the target tissue without damage to normal tissues. In order to test these systems, several aspects of MR performance must be reviewed as well as the capabilities of the ultrasound system. Thermal recording capability, treatment transducer positioning, and image quality all are important. Specialized phantoms have been proposed that mimic tissue and allow testing of the system as an integrated unit as shown in Figure 21.4 [25]. The specialized treatment table containing the ultrasound unit is configured so that it can be placed in the bore of a conventional MR imager as shown in Figure 21.5 [26]. As more of these configurations enter clinical trials and receive approval by the FDA for clinical use, the medical physicist will need to be closely involved in the initial testing and development of the quality assurance program needed to ensure the proper ongoing functioning and safety of such systems.

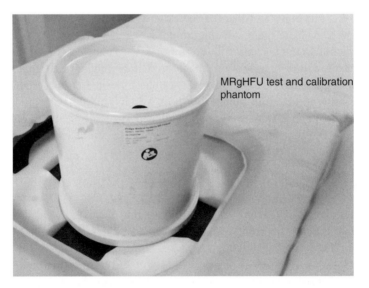

MRgHFU test and calibration phantom

Figure 21.4 Tissue-mimicking phantom designed for use in quality assurance testing and calibration of MRgHIFU systems where positioning of the therapeutic ultrasound beam is important as well as accurate temperature measurements by the MR system.

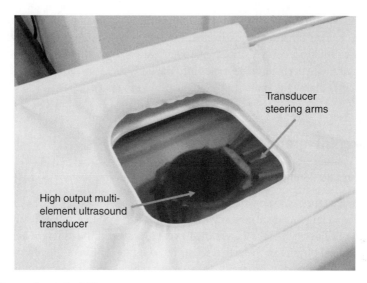

Figure 21.5 Photo of an MRgHIFU system bed insert for a conventional MR scanner. The high intensity ultrasound unit is designed to be aimed under MR imaging control with real-time temperature monitoring of the tissue being treated.

21.3.8 Pulse Sequences and Acquisition Methods

With the new developments for imaging and therapy at increasing field strengths, there comes a need for significant pulse sequence development to collect suitable data for all types of new imaging requirements. New techniques using parallel transmit and receive hardware along with the desire for more dynamic and real-time imaging applications will require new pulse sequences that take advantage of the capabilities of the hardware. Non-Cartesian acquisition schemes and improved spatial accuracy will become more important as systems are used for treatment planning and intervention. New quantitative methods will be in use, especially in the evaluation of cancer using both conventional imaging methods and magnetic resonance spectroscopy. Many new techniques that are currently in the research arena will likely be in routine clinical use including specific bio-marker imaging.

Among the more exciting research developments, which could appear in clinical practice in the next few years, is the use of hyperpolarization techniques for increasing sensitivity in MR imaging of metabolically important species. Such sensitivity increases approach theoretical maximums of five orders of magnitude, which would make practical imaging of ^{13}C or ^{15}N-labeled substrates that currently are not practical [27]. Likewise, such approaches allow hyperpolarized gas lung imaging with ^{3}He and ^{129}Xe as well as ^{129}Xe brain and biosensor imaging [28]. Especially for lung imaging, the use of ^{3}He and ^{129}Xe permit imaging that is specifically sensitive to ventilation and gas exchange processes, which are notoriously difficult to capture with conventional ^{1}H MRI.

Technical requirements for these methods include the use of a polarizer apparatus and wideband MRI system. Polarization requires non-equilibrium optical pumping such as spin-exchange optical pumping (SEOP) to polarize the nuclei of the noble gas in use. This brings into the clinical environment a new piece of highly specialized equipment, with which the clinical physicist must be familiar. Hyperpolarized ^{129}Xe is most likely to be the dominant gas for clinical use due to the expense of 3He, although quantitation methods for determining ventilation defect volume are currently an issue [28]. As these techniques are refined and approved for use in clinical environments for quantitation of lung function and diffusion imaging of the brain, specialized methods will be needed for proper quality assurance. Especially important is evaluation of the amount of polarization prior to use, since hyperpolarization can be lost in transport. Additionally, the introduction of the hyperpolarized species into the body requires verification of the lack of any sort of contaminants that would potentially be harmful to the patient.

21.4 Clinical Integration and Implementation

21.4.1 Training and Communication

The medical physicist for each site will fall into one of two categories: either they are an employee of the facility, often a large medical center with multiple MRI systems, or a consultant who visits a smaller site with one or two systems a few times a year. Because of the different nature of the clinical practice of medical physics in these two scenarios, the interaction of the physicist with the site will, of necessity, be somewhat different. In a large medical center with multiple systems, the medical physicist can access systems for testing relatively easily with the clinical load being transferred to one of the other machines. For the smaller facility with a single system, this becomes much more of a scheduling issue. As systems become more complex and the medical physicist's testing is required to be more extensive, the down-time for all the systems will be more and more of a concern with both types of facilities, but especially in the case of the single system sites. The consulting medical physicist may very well find that testing is done at varied times starting early in the morning or late at night when the disruptions are minimized. This poses some issues for the consulting physicist who may not be at the site when technologists and physicians are present and, therefore, may have more of a challenge participating in maintaining image quality while providing operational direction and evaluating patient safety. It is likely in the future that the consulting medical physicist will be using remote access technologies for quality assurance phantom analysis and reporting. Likewise, tele-conferencing will be used to offer the same types of consultations that large medical centers can receive from their in-house medical physics staff. Such electronic meetings will most likely be the only practical way that sites can receive the added medical physics services that will be required with the evolution of MR imaging and the spread to smaller facilities and the only way that the clinical medical physicist can communicate consistently with both technical staff and radiologists.

With high and ultrahigh field MRI systems becoming more widely distributed, the issues related to regulatory body interactions with each site in each country become an important area requiring the expertise that a clinical medical physicist can provide. There are several bodies that provide reference materials related to exposure to fields at 3 T and above. The International Electrotechnical Commission (IEC, Geneva, Switzerland) provides standards for many electrical and electronic systems including standards for MRI. These standards include standards for static field exposure, which vary by nation and "dose limits" describing acceptable exposure times on a daily basis. The International Commission on Non-ionizing Radiation Protection (ICNIRP, Oberschleissheim, Germany) lists guidelines for flux densities as well as describing limits on time-varying electrical and magnetic fields from 1 Hz to 100 kHz. Other bodies such as the European Union provide information on exposure to electromagnetic fields as well [29]. Finally, the US FDA (Silver Spring, MD) specifies no significant risk from MRI systems below 8 T (adults, children, and infants older than one month) or 4 T for infants one month old or less in a non-binding guidance document [30]. While the FDA currently provides recommendations and regulations for MR systems in the

United States, the influence of the international standards bodies will likely increase over the coming years as new technologies incorporating increased field strengths, RF output, gradient intensities, and slew rates are incorporated into MR imaging and understandings of safety evolve.

Day-to-day patient and staff safety are concerns for which a clinical medical physicist must be continuously cognizant. There are documents provided by the ACR and others that describe issues of MR safety in the current clinical environments [31, 32]. As more and more high and ultrahigh field systems are installed, issues of safety become more important. Sources of concern for patients and staff are related to gradient pulse noise from current and new pulse sequences, biological effects from switched and static electric and magnetic fields, long-term exposure to these fields, as well as issues related to implanted devices, which are proliferating. Additionally, increased stress for the technical staff due to more complex environments are among the issues that the medical physicist will be called upon to help sites address. The medical physicist is the responsible party who provides understanding and information on the new clinical environments that will come with the use of advanced MR imaging systems. Thus, the medical physicist must be prepared to work directly with technologists and radiologists as needed to ensure their understanding of the changing technology. Furthermore, the clinical medical physicist will be part of the team that establishes the institutional requirements for MR testing and safety that meet accreditation standards and institutional requirements.

21.4.2 Optimization

A significant function of the medical physicist is to assist facilities in obtaining images that meet the needs of the radiologist in an efficient manner while ensuring the safety of patients and staff. Among the tasks that will undoubtedly fall into the realm of the medical physicist are occupational measurements for the working environments of MR imaging facilities housing imaging systems of various configurations. These measurements include static field strengths and static gradient strengths, time-varying fields, sound levels, and can include measurements related to interactions with the static fields including peak static field measurements, time-weighted average static fields, field-time products, and instantaneous and peak dB/dt. Such measurements usually are made with specialized equipment with which the medical physicist will need to become familiar. These devices can include magnetometers with search coils or three-axis coils for making vector measurements of time-varying fields and integrators for magnetic flux density measurements. In addition, staff members may be equipped with personal magnetic field dosimeters consisting of Hall effect sensors or induction coils to monitor their exposure, which will require detailed record keeping and monitoring as well as offering advice on exposures. These additions to measurement and monitoring of the magnetic environments could become a requirement in the future, especially around ultrahigh field imaging systems, analogous to x-ray dosimetry monitoring with which the clinical physicist is experienced.

Many of the techniques that will be used regularly by clinical medical physicists are likely not methods for which training or experience has been available. Because of this, clinical medical physicists will find that there is a considerable educational component to remaining up to date with improving monitoring equipment and techniques. Specifically, medical physicists may need to be able to use RF modeling software and monitoring equipment. They may be asked to run simulations of pulse sequences for SAR compliance, something that currently is provided only by the system manufacturers. Additionally, the medical physicist may be called upon to make measurements of environmental noise characteristics upon addition of each new clinical system or updated pulse sequence. Exciting work by manufacturers has led to the introduction of low sound output pulse sequences, but these may not always be appropriate at higher field strengths where rapid gradient switching will still generate unacceptable sound pressures in the bore of the magnet and in the magnet room.

In addition to new software and hardware tools, the medical physicist will need to be familiar with optimized phantoms for specialized applications. These phantoms will be especially important in hybrid imaging systems to verify that both imaging components produce registered images suitable for quantitative analysis. Dynamic, quantitative imaging will require phantoms demonstrating flow, diffusion, or perfusion in simulated tissues. Such phantoms will impose financial burdens on imaging sites or on consulting physicists who are expected to have the appropriate phantoms during testing appointments.

With all the issues related to new capabilities, equipment, regulations, and needs of each clinical site, the burden on medical physicists will increase substantially as they are integrated into the clinical environment. Each medical physicist will need to be part of the team consisting of radiologists, technologists, and possibly clinical managers who will create, review, and implement imaging protocols involving new capabilities for imaging and for image-guided treatment that will be part of routine MR imaging. The technical background of the medical physicist will provide invaluable capabilities added to the required team approach to running an MR center. Among the tasks to be considered are the implementation of efficient workflow and use of the equipment, proper implementation of pulse sequences for the desired imaging result in consultation with radiologists, effective quality control procedures to ensure consistency and performance for each patient of a particular protocol, and efficient manipulation, post-processing, and storage of the image information for review. In the latter case, since in all likelihood, many protocols will be expected to produce quantitative results to be presented to the radiologist in numeric form or as parametric images, often with a temporal component, the burden to ensure the functioning of the post-processing chain to produce the desired output will also be the purview of the medical physicist.

This close involvement in all aspects of the imaging process will place a special burden on medical physicists who are consultants, not based at a site, to use electronic communications to interact with the site regularly. In this way, they can understand on-going issues of work flow as well as become aware of concerns requiring interaction, either through remote review of images, pulse sequences, or protocols, or through a return visit to the site. In future imaging environments, however, one would expect that much useful consultation can be provided by electronic means between required visits, allowing the consulting physicist to provide their skillset to multiple sites.

21.4.3 Automated Analysis and Data Management

A major challenge for the clinical medical physicist will be ensuring image quality for the increasingly sophisticated imaging systems that will be available. Since these systems will include hybrid imaging components as well as increasingly complex RF systems for quantitative measurements of all types, it will be necessary for the medical physicist to develop routine quality assurance procedures and ensure that measurements are made and analyzed properly. Manual methods and handwritten log sheets are not likely to be enough to maintain the necessary records or allow facilities with several high-performance MR systems to properly monitor quality. Thus, new informatics tools will be needed with the use of computer software pipeline approaches to collect the data, automatically transmitting it to a quality assurance workstation where phantom data will be automatically analyzed possibly with deep learning technologies with the results populating a database for each system and qualiaty control (QC) test. A report generator will provide automatic notification of unsatisfactory results and automatic generation of reports, which will include long-term trend analyses. These databases can provide statistical prediction software with information that will enable assessment of the likelihood of a future QC failure before it happens. For all of this to function smoothly, the software systems must be in place and well-tested and the clinical medical physicist will need to be very comfortable not only with results reporting, but also with the general operation of the pipeline to be able to explain and educate interested physicians and technologists on the overall QC program. A comprehensive database for protocol maintenance will help ensure that there is uniformity of operation between identical machines at different working sites within a facility or between facilities. Protocols for each type of study, even advanced protocols, would be maintained in such a way so that changes can be readily downloaded to each client system by authorized personnel. Such informatics approaches mirror the use of informatics across the medical profession and will enable the medical physicists to do their jobs more efficiently and effectively in meeting the requirements of payer organizations and accreditation bodies. These capabilities will allow the consulting physicist to fully participate in each site's quality assurance program. Currently available software, both commercial and non-commercial, can provide an automatic analysis of the ACR phantom images, producing a full report. An example of this sort of automatic analysis is shown in Figure 21.6 for percent integral uniformity and percent signal ghosting. Such software can be setup for automated processing including receiving images, extracting analysis information, storage of the information in a database, and producing full reports. While useful, future requirements will dictate the need for much more sophisticated software systems than those currently available.

While automatic analysis of QC phantoms is available in limited form currently, advance automatic analysis of clinical images will be a capability that will become available over the next few

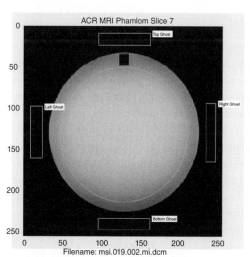

Table 1. Imaging Information

Institution	Vanderbilt Medical Center
Station	VUHMR1
Magnetic Field Strength	3
Protocol	T1-axial CLEAR
DICOM Slice Thickness(mm)	5
SOP Instance UID	1.3.46.670589.11.17047.5.05464.201306170649-0409127
Slice Location	60
Echo Time	20
Repetition Time	499.995

Table 2. Perecent Integral Uniformity

Perecent Integral Uniformity	82.25
Specification Minimum	82.00

Table 4. Perecent-Signal Ghosting

Perecent-Signal Ghosting	0.0020603
ACR Maximum	0.025
Pass-Fail	Pass

Figure 21.6 Percent uniformity calculated automatically from images of the ACR MR accreditation phantom using commercially available software. A complete report is automatically generated from the analysis of this slice and others from the phantom after.

years as advanced neural network techniques begin to be employed in imaging settings. This capability to evaluate the results of complex QC imaging sessions automatically will be important for ongoing quality assurance locally and will be especially important in inter-facility quality assurance, such as what would be needed in clinical trials involving MR imaging or in environments where there are several imagers of the same type. The goal is to generate reproducible and stable information so that a patient can be imaged at multiple sites with the expectation that the images will be quite comparable. This type of automated assessment should be independent of the MR system and software and will be important for quantitative analysis. Much work has been done and is available in the literature on mathematical observers and perceptual modeling of image quality. These techniques, modified for the environment of MR imaging, will move into automated assessment of clinical images.

There are some papers on automatic image quality determination that are in the current literature. In a clinical image there can be several specific problems that degrade image quality including various edge artifacts due to chemical shift, ringing, and ghosting. Also, there can be flow artifacts and aliasing from positioning problems. These types of artifacts propagate into the air background around the body and alter the noise distributions in the affected areas in 3D imaging. In Mortamet et al. two quality metrics are used that are extracted automatically from the background of head images [33]. These are artifactual voxel detection, quality index 1 (QI_1), and noise distribution analysis, quality index 2 (QI_2). The analysis methodology described in their paper demonstrates image quality in a multicenter trial environment with receiver operator characteristic curves (ROC) showing for these two metrics the performance of the authors' approach. The quality indices found automatically allow the authors to evaluate the attributes of accuracy and consistency as reflected in the ability to separate high quality verses low quality images.

21.4.4 Meaningful QC

The clinical medical physicist is and will be the resource for understanding new imaging technology and newly integrated technologies. Given that the state of MR imaging is evolving rapidly with new equipment and more sophisticated pulse sequences, the medical physicist will be the person with the responsibility to understand how to best apply this technology in the clinic in a manner that produces superior image quality with efficiency and safety. It is the bridging of the gap between clinical image quality and technical performance issues where the clinical medical physicist becomes a significant member of the clinical imaging team. Because of this important role in understanding equipment, imaging techniques, quality assurance, accreditation and compliance issues, and safety for all personnel and patients, the clinical medical physicist must keep in constant communication with all the facilities that they are responsible for, either in person or using electronic methods. This communication and providing expertise as a member of a team of professional individuals who perform MR imaging procedures is where the medical physicist will excel in the future.

Requirements for medical physicists' attention to the imaging environment will vary by the types of studies performed and equipment that is available at a site. What is necessary is that the medical physicist monitor quality assurance procedures, participate in the review of study types and protocols, evaluate the performance of the system in person on a regular basis for both imaging and therapeutic capabilities, review representative phantom and patient studies, and address safety concerns. How will this look in the coming years and how much time will it take? While it is hard to tell what future regulations might be imposed or relaxed, the fact remains that medical physicists will not be occasional participants in the ongoing work of each imaging site, Rather, they will need to be continuously engaged using the remote technologies mentioned earlier for those sites where the medical physicist is an outside consultant or meeting regularly for quality assurance and safety reviews as an in-house medical physicist, so that ongoing familiarity with each site is maintained. How often such meetings should occur will be a function of how closely integrated that medical physicist is within the clinical structure of each facility. However, the clinical physicist must be part of clinical processes at each site so that their expertise is part of the support team for providing the best care the facility can offer.

Much of the current requirements for testing and reporting for accreditation purposes will need to evolve to allow reasonable participation by the medical physicist while maintaining the high quality of the images and data obtained from each scan. Among the expected changes would be to the rules requiring testing of individual coil elements on systems with massively parallel transmit and receive components. These tests currently consume a large fraction of testing time for each system for each coil that is provided at the site and requires extending the amount of the time the system is unavailable for clinical work. Alternative methods are available to understand performance without individual testing of each element of a parallel receive array of 128 channels, for instance, as has been described earlier. Additionally, monitoring of clinical interventional studies in a systematic way by the medical physicist should be possible by remote access to images so that a representative sample can be evaluated for quality that can be reported back to the supervising radiologist, even during procedures, if appropriate. Routine testing will be implemented by technologists, but beyond routine testing, the evaluation of ongoing image quality on a study-by-study basis should be possible with some of the tools that are currently being evaluated in laboratory environments

21.5 Conclusion

The next few years will witness an expanding use of magnetic resonance systems with capabilities that are coming out of research environments and are being implemented in the clinic. New pulse sequences, new transmit and receive hardware, new integrated imaging systems as part of multi-imaging capabilities, improved extensive post-processing of images for quantitation of information, and the evolution of rules and regulations governing the use of this technology will require new approaches by each imaging site. With the introduction of 7.0 T systems and integrated systems using PET components for imaging or LINACs for treatment into the clinic, safety concerns will be at the forefront of medical physicists' responsibilities. It will no longer be sufficient to have a medical physicist evaluate a machine for basic low contrast detectability, spatial resolution, and image distortion once a year; it will be necessary for the medical physicist to be available as a direct participant in ongoing imaging issues to ensure that the technical and evolving regulatory issues are properly addressed along with patient and staff safety. Thus, the medical physicist will participate in the regular review of activities at each site using technologies for remote access, automated processing and review, and remote interactive communication. Making use of all the capabilities will permit the medical physicist to be an integral part of the imaging team, whether at a multi-unit university hospital or as a consultant servicing smaller facilities with single units. There is much for the medical physicist to learn and there are new requirements for the medical physicist, but the reward is full integration into the patient care stream as a fully invested participant in clinical practice.

References

1 (2015). *Magnetic Resonance Imaging: Quality Control Manual.* American College of Radiology.

2 Durand, D.J., Carrino, J.A., Fayad, L.M. et al. (2013). MRI psychophysics: an experimental framework relating image quality to diagnostic performance metrics. *J. Magn. Reson. Imaging* 37: 1402–1408.

3 Miao, J., Huang, F., Narayan, S. et al. (2013). A new perceptual difference model for diagnostically relevant quantitative image quality evaluation: a preliminary study. *Magn. Reson. Imaging* 31: 596–603.

4 Jiang, Y., Huo, D., and Wilson, D.L. (2007). Methods for quantitative image quality evaluation of MRI parallel reconstructions: detection and perceptual difference model. *Magn. Reson. Imaging* 25: 712–721.

5 Qian, D., El-Sharkawy, A.M., Bottomley, P.A. et al. (2013). An RF dosimeter for independent SAR measurement in MRI scanners. *Med. Phys.* 40 (12): 122303.

6 Umutlu, L., Ladd, M.E., Forsting, M., and Lauenstein, T. (2014). 7 Tesla MR imaging: opportunities and challenges. *RoFo* 186 (2): 121–129.

7 Webb, A.G. and Collins, C.M. (2010). Parallel transmit and receive technology in high-field magnetic resonance neuroimaging. *Int. J. Imaging Syst. Technol.* 20: 2–13.

8 Tang, L., Hue, Y.K., and Ibrahim, T.S. (2011). Studies of RF shimming techniques with minimization of RF power deposition and their associated temperature changes. *Concepts. Magn. Reson. Part B Magn. Reson Eng.* 39B: 11–25.

9 Burnner, D.O. (2011). Parallel transmit. ISMRM High Field Workshop, www.ismrm.org (accessed 11 October 2013).

10 Wald, L.L. and Adalsteinsson, E. (2009). Parallel transmit technology for high field MRI. *Magnetom Flash.* 1: 124–135.

11 Jackson, E. (2013). AAPM Annual Meeting Presentation July 30, 2012, handout downloaded from www.aapm.org on July 1.

12 Abramson, R.G., Arlinghaus, L.R., Weis, J.A. et al. (2012). Current and emerging quantitative magnetic resonance imaging methods for assessing and predicting the response of breast cancer to neoadjuvant therapy. *Breast Cancer (London).* 4: 139–154.

13 Raaymakers, B.W., Lagendijk, J.J., Overweg, J. et al. (2009). Integrating a 1.5T MRI scanner with a 6 MV accelerator: proof of concept. *Phys. Med. Biol.* 54: N229–N237.

14 Dietrich, O., Raya, J.G., Reeder, S.B. et al. (2007). Measurement of signal-to-noise ratios in MR images: influence of multichannel coils, parallel imaging, and reconstruction filters. *J. Magn. Reson. Imaging* 26: 375–385.

15 Hansen, M.S. and Kellman, P. (2014). Image reconstruction: an overview for clinicians. *J. Magn. Reson. Imaging* 41 (3): 573–585.

16 Gudbjartsson, H. and Patz, S. (1995). The Rician distribution of noisy MRI data. *Magn. Reson. Med.* 34 (4): 567–579.

17 Goerner, F.L. and Clarke, G.D. (2011). Measuring signal-to-noise ratio in partially parallel imaging MRI. *Med. Phys.* 38 (9): 5049–5047.

18 Goerner, F.L., Duong, T., Stafford, R.J. et al. (2013). A comparison of five standard methods for evaluating image intensity uniformity in partially parallel imaging MRI. *Med. Phys.* 40 (8): 082302.

19 Tsao, J. (2010). Ultrafast imaging: principles, pitfalls, solutions, and applications. *J. Magn. Reson. Imaging* 32: 252–266.

20 Oz, G. et al. (2014). Clinical proton MR spectroscopy in central nervous system disorders, appendix E1. *Radiology* 270 (3): 1–8. Supplementary Material.

21 Jackson, E.F. et al. (2010). AAPM Report 100: Acceptance testing and quality assurance procedures for magnetic resonance imaging facilities, report of MR subcommittee Task Group 1, AAPM.

22 Beyer, T., Freudenberg, L.S., Czernin, J. et al. (2011). The future of hybrid imaging – part 3: PET/MR, small-animal imaging and beyond. *Insights Imaging.* 2: 235–246.

23 Hamamura, M.J., Ha, S., Roeck, W.W. et al. (2010). Development of an MR-compatible SPECT system (MRSPECT) for simultaneous data acquisition. *Phys. Med. Biol.* 55: 1563–1575.

24 Brown, A.M., Elbuluk, O., Mertan, F. et al. (2015). Recent advances in image-guided targeted prostate biopsy. Abdominal Imaging. Published online 18 January 2015.

25 Partanen, A., Mougenot, C., and Vaara, T. (2009). Feasibility of agar silica phantoms in quality assurance of MRgHIFU. *AIP Conf. Proc.* 1113: 296. https://doi.org/10.1063/1.313143.

26 Ellis, S., Rieke, V., Kohi, M. et al. (2013). Clinical applications for magnetic resonance guided high intensity focused ultrasound (MRgHIFU): present and future. *J. Med. Imaging Radiat. Oncol.* 57: 291–399.

27 Waddell, K.W. and Checkmenov, E.Y. (2012). Chapter 22: Hyperpolarized MR of cancer. In: *Quantitative MRI in Cancer* (eds. T.E. Yankeelov, D.R. Pickens and R.R. Price). Boca Raton, FL: CRC Press, Taylor and Francis Group.

28 Couch, M.J., Blasiak, B., Tomanek, B. et al. (2015). Hyperpolarized and inert gas MRI: the future. *Mol. Imaging Biol.* 17 (2): 149–162. Published online April.

29 European Union Physical Agents Directive 2013/35/EU. 29.6.2013 Official Journal of the European Union L 179/1.

30 Criteria for significant risk investigations of magnetic resonance diagnostic devices: guidance for industry and Food and Drug Administration staff. U. S. Department of Health and Human Services, Food and Drug Administration. Issued June 20, 2014. https://www.fda.gov/regulatory-information/search-fda-guidance-documents/criteria-significant-risk-investigations-magnetic-resonance-diagnostic-devices-guidance-industry-and (accessed 29 November 2019).

31 Kanal, E. et al. (2013). ACR guidance document on MR safe practices. *J. Magn. Reson. Imaging* 37: 501–530.

32 Shellock, F.G. (2015). *Reference Manual for Magnetic Resonance Safety, Implants, and Devices: 2015 Edition*. Playa Del Rey, CA: Biomedical Research Publishing Group.

33 Mortamet, B., Bernstein, M.A., Jack, C.R. Jr. et al. (2009). Automatic quality assessment in structural brain magnetic resonance imaging. *Magn. Reson. Med.* 62: 365–372.

Part VIII

Imaging Informatics

22

Clinical Physics in IT: Perspective

Ehsan Samei

Departments of Radiology, Medical Physics, Physics, Biomedical Engineering, and Electrical and Computer Engineering, Duke University Medical Center, Durham, NC, USA

Information technology is not related to medical physics in the way the imaging modalities are. Physics is the foundation of medical imaging, but not of information technology. But IT is integrally related to the physics sphere of work which involves effective and safe use of imaging systems. Information technology is a subcomponent of imaging operation, an infrastructure that empowers the clinical operation and as such the clinical physicist needs to closely align and integrate their work with and through IT. Recent advances have further expanded the use of IT in imaging practice, offering new needs and opportunities for integration with clinical physics.

The exchange and integration of clinical physics and IT can be delineated into 12 systems, each of which can be represented in terms of three aspects: content, technology, and analytics (Table 22.1). Not all these prospective systems are at the same level of maturity. But the ones clinically deployed can operate in either isolation or ideally in integration within a comprehensive quality and safety IT system, further connected with the hospital information system. In this brief perspective we quickly go over these systems.

22.1 Imaging Informatics

Picture archiving and communication system (PACS) was the prelude of physics integration with IT. With the increased use of computers and digital technology in imaging departments, image archiving and communication systems have become commonplace in imaging clinics. This has necessitated the use of standard formats and communication protocols, which has been facilitated by the DICOM standard. As DICOM has become the essential standard and vocabulary of image exchange, communication, and archival, physicists need to be competent in understanding image handling issues to be able to address the needs of the imaging practice as they arise. For example, the current trend of using vendor neutral archives as separate units from PACS require physics input in terms of the needed features and ergonomics. This topic is well covered in Chapter 24.

Clinical Imaging Physics: Current and Emerging Practice, First Edition. Edited by Ehsan Samei and Douglas E. Pfeiffer.
© 2020 John Wiley & Sons, Inc. Published 2020 by John Wiley & Sons, Inc.

Table 22.1 IT systems and attributes with strong need for integration with clinical physics.

IT system	Attributes of each IT system
1) Imaging informatics	A) Content, involving the data themselves
2) Medical image displays	B) Technology involving formatting, transmitting, organizing, and communicating the data
3) Equipment status	C) Analytics, involving translating the data into actionable knowledge
4) Equipment performance	
5) Protocols	
6) Usage and workload	
7) Dosimetrics	
8) Qualimetrics	
9) Contrast and radioactive media	
10) Personnel dosimetry	
11) Clinical issues	
12) Decision support	

22.2   Medical Image Displays

Medical displays likewise have become a key component of current clinical practice. Effective use of medical images requires their high-quality display to interpreting physicians to ensure robust and confident decision-making. It is the responsibility of the clinical medical physicist to ensure the quality of the image display. This is an area where the discipline has taken full responsibility of its role, a topic that is well detailed in Chapter 23. New advances that require continuous investment and engagement of clinical physicists include the transition of imaging systems from monochromatic to color displays, static to dynamic displays, and stationary to portable displays. Further, the broad distribution of medical displays across the clinical enterprise requires semi-automatic remote monitoring systems that should be claimed and operated by clinical physicists who are responsible for the overall quality and safety of medical imaging operation.

22.3   Equipment Status

There is a tremendous value in tracking the configuration of an imaging system in terms of loaded features, loaded configuration and processing parameters, frequency of their use, software status and upgrades, repairs, and corrective actions. Often physicists face the dilemma of not being notified when a particular device has been upgraded. The upgrades can alter the system operation such that its high-quality and safe use cannot be assured without a physics inspection. An equipment status IT system can alert the physicist of such changes and ensure effective communication with service personnel and the users of the unit.

22.4   Equipment Performance

Equipment oversight is a core area of physics activity. The evaluations in terms of annual or intermittent testing are reflective of the performance of the imaging system. This data, however, can become more informative when they are put in the context of other similar imaging systems at any given point in time and across time. An informatics system that can keep track of the information and provide alerts (e.g. when the quality control (QC) data-point is below an acceptable limit) or system-wide reports on a frequent basis can be an effective tool to ensure maintenance of high-quality performance of the imaging systems.

22.5 Protocols

Protocols are an essential component of any medical imaging operation. They dictate not only the safety but also the quality of the resulting images. Thus, there is a need to ensure they are consistently defined and applied across the practice and over time. This necessitates an IT system to keep track of their definition, their changes, their distribution, and their improvement overtime. IT standards have been lacking in this area, but the need is so significant that some vendors have already started developing products. The physics insight is needed not only for the optimized definition of protocols, which has been highlighted in the earlier chapters, but in the way the IT system is set up and grouped and classified to ensure consistency across practice. Consistent definition and grouping of protocols is also paramount in the monitoring of dose and image quality noted below. Figure 22.1, as an example, shows how a single type of exam can be synthaxed in 100s of different ways, necessitating proper grouping of protocols for effective management and monitoring. This IT domain requires close integration with, and input from, imaging physics.

22.6 Usage and Workload

As image data and protocol data are sorted into their corresponding databases, pertinent data can be harvested and analyzed to indicate the usage of the equipment across different systems, protocols, and time. Figure 22.2, for example, shows such data. This data can be used to design better clinical workflow, ensure adequacy and consistency of resources across busy practices, and plan for future developments and upgrades. Clinical physics knowledge in handing complex numerical data can be used to help organize such multi-variant data and deduce insight from the data, thus help the institution for its planning purposes.

22.7 Dosimetrics

Dosimetrics is an area that has seen significant development through IT. Medical imaging systems can communicate dose related measures from the examinations to a server. Collecting and archiving such data enables monitoring of radiation dose across patients, to ensure their levels and their appropriateness in concordance with internal or external benchmarks. Mandated through accreditation and insurance systems, dose monitoring systems have become commonplace in most imaging practices. Physicists should actively engage with these systems to ensure their accuracy, the effectiveness of their claims, and proactive use of their output to optimize the imaging practice. New areas of advancement that physicists should promote and lead include upgrading the dose metrics to be more patient- and less modality-centered, ensuring integrity in data sorting and synthaxing, targeted analysis according to the needs of the practice, concordance with data registries, and expansion of the coverage beyond computed tomography (CT) and fluoroscopy which are the mainstay of the practice today [1].

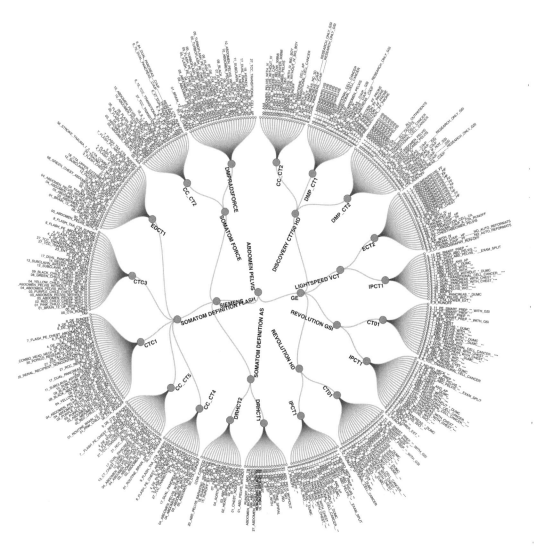

Figure 22.1 The 560 labels associated with a single type of CT examination at one busy institution.

StationName	1	2	3	4	5	6	7	8	9	10	11	12
CARYCT1	85	90	105	100	118	103	118	91	50	108	96	90
CCCT3REVO	188	220	243	217	271	222	193	256	114	213	234	224
CC_CT1	292	297	296	258	339	314	351	475	325	442	406	351
CC_CT2	306	316	358	341	353	368	477	550	425	547	494	452
CC_CT4	297	296	362	329	318	312	370	387	305	454	374	329
CC_CT5	285	317	351	327	341	320	334	391	291	382	340	312
CT01	451	453	506	547	503	538	553	545	409	577	492	429
CTC1	430	517	654	429	527	450	428	454	352	526	466	442
CTC3	459	472	525	461	510	432	424	493	358	510	479	364
CTJ1	135	122	132	120	129	103	118	120	90	112	108	101
CT_PETCT1	229	251	253	242	260	285	242	263	125	257	260	229
DMPRAD3FORCE	840	710	849	1024	961	871	905	917	794	892	890	523
DMP_CT1	439	418	371	369	409	416	365	481	365	395	413	418
DMP_CT2	806	794	772	818	926	817	798	790	716	826	799	795
DRAH_CT2	1200	1233	1398	1223	1258	1247	1201	1456	1312	1615	1365	1355
DRHCT1	851	842	975	896	879	915	873	937	909	1083	956	1011
DRHCT2	1020	892	1178	1158	1139	1038	1098	1127	960	1250	1120	1024
ECT2	1195	1158	1291	1295	1234	1313	1343	1373	1146	1291	1236	1221
EDCT1	1349	1276	1509	1490	1645	1423	1593	1594	1402	1662	1453	1574
HRCT	161	161	179	180	196	182	166	196	144	203	178	166
IPCT1	576	532	554	544	506	544	506	537	444	590	542	461
J3GECT750	197	199	197	155	195	193	201	182	146	178	181	126
MPCT1	126	111	120	95	104	89	82	100	114	136	123	115
P004	167	191	175	153	210	196	166	204	140	209	164	165

Month

Figure 22.2 The workload of multiple imaging systems (vertical) across 12 months of a year (horizontal).

22.8   Qualimetrics

While dose monitoring is an important area for integration of IT and physics, quality monitoring is perhaps a more impactful opportunity. Assuming radiation dose is managed and maintained below reasonable levels for each exam type and patient size, image quality takes prime importance to ensure the quality is adequate to provide the desired clinical benefit [2]. This calls for a monitoring system to assess image quality on an image by image basis. The data can then be collected and tracked, just like dose data, to analyze trends and ascertain adherence to predefined criteria. Prior work has shown how noise, resolution, and contrast can be measured *in vivo* (Figure 22.3) [3–6] toward improved consistency of image quality [7]. Medical physicists should be pioneers and instigators of such technologies to more directly fulfill the QC mandate of their charge not only in the context of phantoms but actual exam data.

22.9   Contrast and Radioactive Media

Similar to dose and image quality, other attributes of medical imaging can be monitored. Chief among them in the attributes of exams pertaining the administration of contrast media and radiopharmaceuticals. These administrations, taking place mostly in CT, magnetic resonance imaging (MRI), and nuclear imaging, should be tailored to the characteristics of the patient and the exam. This can be ascertained via an IT system that captures pertinent information from the media management system, integrates that with other patient information from the hospital information system, and provides analyses to ascertain trends and adherence pre-defined criteria; optimized prescriptions and the criteria should by themselves be optimized beforehand. Such a system will require active engagement of clinical physicist as the proper magnitude of contrast medium or radionuclides is dependent on the associated dose and image quality, matters that require physics input.

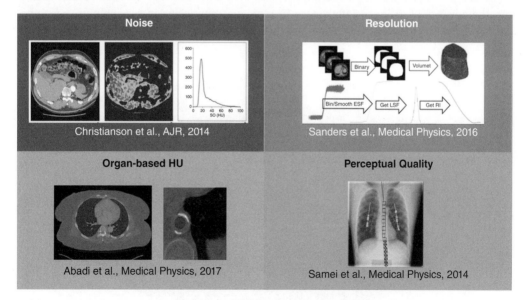

Figure 22.3   Four implementations of *in vivo* image quality assessment of individual clinical exams based on noise in uniform areas of the images, resolution from skin–air interface, Hounsfield unit (HU) values in organs, and perceptual quality.

22.10   Personnel Dosimetry

Personnel dosimetry is a regulatory requirement in interventional imaging. The IT system associated with that process can provide insight in the patterns of practice to which a physicist should provide input. Thus clinical physics should be closely involved in IT systems associated with personnel dosimetry. Further, the personnel dose should generally be relatable to the patient dose involved in the procedure; discrepancy between the two offers glimpses into the practice that can help optimize the patterns of practice. This is yet another opportunity for physicists to be involved.

22.11   Clinical Issues

Failures to communicate account for 80% of medical malpractice cases [8], and counter-intuitively, the digital era has made communication more difficult than ever. In spite of all attempts to optimize the clinical process, due to the complexities of clinical practice, issues often arise on a case by case basis. Examples include artifacts in certain clinical images, intermittent degradation of images from a particular shift or system, or changes in the imaging setup or applied protocol. It is ideal that an informatics system can be available to the interpreting physician to report such incidences to the physicist or the technologist in charge. An alert is generated and the issue is logged and tracked through the system till it is cleared. At one institution, such a system has been installed, a summary result of which can provide invaluable insight into issues that requires operational refinement (Figure 22.4). Clinical physicists should take an active role in promoting and using such systems.

22.12   Decision Support

Finally, decision support in image interpretation is a significant area of growth in medical imaging. With the advance of artificial intelligence in radiology, physicians increasingly use machine-learning algorithms to increase the efficiency, quantification, and analysis of their interpretations.

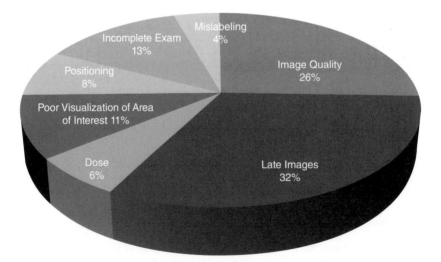

Figure 22.4   The percentage of types of issues reported through a clinical issues IT reporting system.

These systems are being actively integrated in the imaging IT infrastructure and the reading workstations. Medical physics knowledge is necessary to not only qualify the reliability and claims of the technologies, but also devise best integration models that can enhance the overall healthcare quality.

Any of the areas summarized above can and should be informed by active participation of seasoned medical physicists. Physicists should not only qualify the IT technologies involved, but use them toward their quality and safety mandate, and work alongside physicians, IT staff, and other healthcare providers to ensure their most effective use in the clinic.

References

1 Frush, D.P. and Samei, E. (2015). CT radiation dose monitoring: current state and new prospects *(invited article)*. *Medscape Radiol.* (March).

2 Samei, E., Jarvinen, H., Kortesniemi, M. et al. (2018). Medical imaging dose optimization from ground up: expert opinion of an international summit. *J. Radiol. Prot.* 38 (3): 967–989.

3 Abadi, E., Sanders, J., and Samei, E. (2017). Patient-specific quantification of image quality: an automated technique for measuring the distribution of organ Hounsfield units in clinical chest CT images. *Med. Phys.* 44 (9): 4736–4746.

4 Christianson, O., Winslow, J., Frush, D.P., and Samei, E. (2015). Automated technique to measure noise in clinical CT examinations. *AJR Am. J. Roentgenol.* 205: W93–W99.

5 Samei, E., Lin, Y., Choudhury, K.R., and McAdams, H.P. (2014). Automated characterization of perceptual quality of clinical chest radiographs: validation and calibration to observer preference. *Med. Phys.* 41: 111918.

6 Sanders, J., Hurwitz, L., and Samei, E. (2016). Patient-specific quantification of image quality: an automated method for measuring spatial resolution in clinical CT images. *Med. Phys.* 43 (10): 5330–5338.

7 Ria, F., Davis, J.T., Solomon, J.B. et al. (2019). Expanding the concept of diagnostic reference levels to noise and dose reference levels in CT. *AJR Am. J. Roentgenol.* 213 (4): 889–894.

8 Berlin, L. (2010). Failure of radiologic communication: and increasing cause of malpractice litigation and harm to patients. *Appl. Radiol.* 39: 17–23.

23

Clinical Physics in Informatics Display: Current and Emerging Practice
Michael Flynn

Diagnostic Radiology, Henry Ford Health System, Henry Ford Hospital, Detroit, MI, USA

23.1   Current Practice (Medical Physics 1.0)

23.1.1   Introduction

About 20 years ago (~1995), the technology for picture archive and communication systems (PACS) had matured and early adopters began converting enterprise radiological imaging operations to eliminate the use of film as a display. Ten years ago (~2005) such conversions were widespread. At the time of this writing (2019), film is rarely used even in small clinics. This operational change eliminated previous clinical physics responsibilities involving film selection, processing, and quality assurance and introduced new roles for electronic display performance specification, testing, and quality assurance.

In the early portion of the electronic imaging transition period, cathode ray tube (CRT) devices were the only available technology for image presentation. Specialized monochrome CRT devices were developed for medical applications; however, these had significant performance limitations. CRT specific problems included blur from electron beam spot size, glare from the glass faceplate, noise from phosphor granularity, geometric distortion, and amplifier drift that affected brightness and contrast.

Significant change in electronic display technology began with the introduction of liquid crystal display (LCD) devices and, most recently, the introduction of organic light emitting diode (OLED) devices [1]. By about 2005, CRT production had become limited and most medical centers had upgraded their workstations with LCD devices. Early LCD devices had limited brightness and significant contrast changes for oblique viewing angles. Brightness was improved for medical monochrome LCD monitors by removing the color filter layer. Viewing angle performance was improved by the use of dual domain pixel structures with advanced pixel structures using vertical alignment (VA) or in plane switching (IPS) [2]. More efficient backlights using light emitting diode (LED) lamps have recently improved the brightness of color LCD monitors. Specialized monochrome LCD monitors are thus disappearing from the medical market. OLED handheld devices are now widely available with excellent display performance and have recently been introduced for television devices. In general, OLED devices have high brightness and minimal change in luminance response with viewing angle. In the near future, low cost professional OLED monitors may provide important advantages for medical applications.

Clinical Imaging Physics: Current and Emerging Practice, First Edition. Edited by Ehsan Samei and Douglas E. Pfeiffer.
© 2020 John Wiley & Sons, Inc. Published 2020 by John Wiley & Sons, Inc.

Methods to measure the display performance of medical display devices along with recommendations for acceptance testing and quality control were considered by Task Group 18 (TG18) of the American Association of Physicists in Medicine (AAPM) between 1998 and 2003. The TG18 committee included extensive participation from the medical display industry as well as medical physicists with special expertise in display performance measurement. The final report described visual, quantitative, and advanced methods for the assessment of display performance in nine categories along with expected response (Section 4 of AAPM On-Line report no. 03 April 2005). A comprehensive set of display test patterns was developed as shown in Figure 23.1. The design rule for each

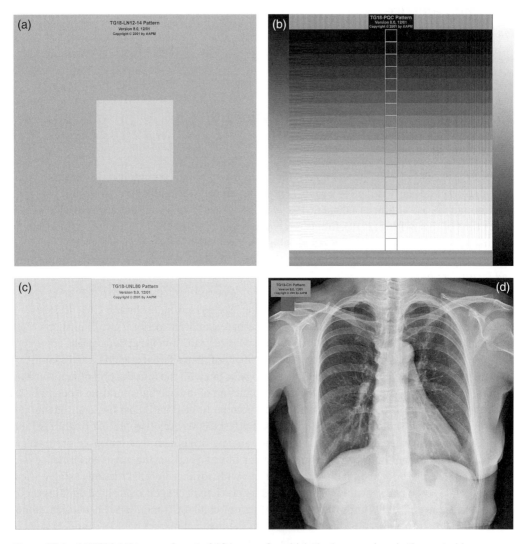

Figure 23.1 (a) TG18-LN is one of a set of 18 images for which the image values in the central box vary from black to white in uniform steps. The set is used for manual measures of the luminance response. (b) TG18-PQC presents an 18-step pattern with low contrast modulation at two spatial frequencies. The pattern is used to visually verify proper DICOM GSDF calibration. (c) TG18-UNL-1 k-02 presents constant image values for the evaluation of luminance uniformity. Defining lines are added to establish measurement regions. (d) TG18-CH presents a normative chest image that can be used to establish subjective appearance among displays and over time.

image is documented in the report and electronic image sets are available[1] in both TIFF and Digital Imaging and Communications in Medicine (DICOM)[2] formats. Important aspects of the full report were published in Medical Physics [3]. During the period when the report was developed, CRT devices were in common use. Some of the performance tests described are no longer relevant to modern LCD devices as summarized in Table 23.1. In 2009, the TG18 evaluation methods and terms for luminance and chromaticity were adopted as an international standard (IEC 62563-1, edition 1.0 2009-12) [4] along with revised versions of the test patterns. These TG18/IEC test methods have been referenced in various guidelines including

- JESRA X-0093: "Quality Assurance (QA) Guideline for Medical Imaging Display Systems" formulated by Japan Industries Association of Radiological Systems (JIRA).
- European Commission/EUREF: EC "European guidelines for quality assurance in breast cancer screening and diagnosis" and EUREF "Monitor QC Test Patterns."
- DIN V 6868-57, PAS 1054: "Requirements and Testing of Digital Mammographic X-ray Equipment."

While the TG18 test methods are now well established, the expected values suggested in the TG18 report were based on the performance of CRT devices and are consequently outdated.

23.1.2 System Performance

23.1.2.1 Workstation Characteristics

The display device used to present the medical imaging studies from various modalities, along with the associated workstation, is a critical element in the communication of image information to

Table 23.1 The AAPM task group 18 report [3] (AAPM On line report 03) detailed the assessment of display performance in 10 categories with most directed at display characteristics relevant to CRT systems.

	Performance (AAPM, On line report 03)	CRT	LCD	IEC
4.1	Geometric Distortion	✓		
4.2	Display Reflection	✓	✓	
4.3	Luminance Response	✓	✓	✓
4.4	Luminance spatial/angular dependency	✓	✓	✓
4.5	Display Resolution	✓		
4.6	Display Noise	✓	✓	
4.7	Veiling Glare	✓		
4.8	Display Chromaticity	✓	✓	✓
4.9a	Misc. tests – CRT	✓		
4.9b	Misc. tests – LCD		✓	✓
4.10	Overall evaluations	✓	✓	✓

The LCD specific tests are addressed in an IEC standard [4].

---

1 http://deckard.mc.duke.edu/~samei/tg18.

2 DICOM is an international standard for medical images and related information (ISO 12052) developed and maintained by the member organizations and companies of the DICOM standards committee. The current standard is available at http://medical.nema.org/standard.html.

technologists, radiologists, and clinical practitioners. The medical physicist needs to consider this with the same professional approach as used to address the image quality of acquisition devices.

23.1.2.1.1 *Monitor Classification*

In TG18, monitors were classified as either primary or secondary devices. Primary devices were those used for the interpretation of medical images by either radiologists or medical specialists. Secondary systems were those used for viewing medical images for purposes other than for providing a medical interpretation. The ACR-AAPM-SIIM guidelines discussed below are primarily directed at Radiologist's workstations with a few comments regarding appropriate differences for secondary devices. A more granular classification is now being considered by AAPM TG270.

1) *Diagnostic*: image presentation monitors used for radiology interpretations
2) *Modality*: monitors integrated on acquisition devices (DX/CR, CT, MR, US, …)
3) *Clinical*: clinical specialist workstations (ED, orthopedics, dermatology, etc.), and
4) *EHR*: workstations used to access patient electronic health records (EHR).

Modality monitors are now recognized as devices that need to be specified and maintained for consistent image presentation. The image viewed by a modality operator, who may make processing or window/level adjustments before releasing the image, should be consistent with that viewed by the interpreting radiologist. Modality monitor performance is now commonly included as a part of accreditation requirements.

The requirements for clinical image presentation vary significantly for different specialists. In orthopedic surgery and in the emergency department, physicians are often making medical management decisions based on a radiology examination prior to interpretation by a radiologist. Performance similar to the diagnostic category is thus needed. In dermatology, color accuracy becomes an important factor. In ophthalmology, images with large array sizes containing fine detail are presented.

For handheld devices, a separate classification is not considered. Rather, the image presentation requirements are considered to be the same. Modern handheld devices have particularly good performance characteristics with respect to pixel pitch, maximum luminance, and viewing angle. However, the ergonomic and workflow characteristics of the handheld device are likely to be significantly different than for workstations. In particular, the size of the presented image is necessarily small and comparison to prior studies is more difficult. Additionally, they are used at close viewing distance which leads to eye strain.

23.1.2.1.2 *Purchase Specification*

Information technology (IT) specialists are essential for support computer hardware, managing operating systems, deploying health business applications, and insuring privacy. However, IT staff typically do not have training or expertise in those aspects of computer image presentation that are important for the consistent presentation of high-fidelity images. While IT staff may have operational responsibilities for medical display devices, radiology administrators and leaders need to ensure that appropriate advice and management for image presentation is being provided by medical physicists.

---

cMP#1: A clinical medical physicist should be able to make expert recommendations regarding the purchase of medical monitors and the display related configurations of workstations used for image presentation.

Presently, medical physicists are primarily focused on providing device specifications for radiologist's displays and modality monitors. In some organizations, recommendations may also be made for enterprise systems. For clinical specialists, image presentation may involve specifications for color accuracy and consistency as discussed later in this chapter.

The current monitor market has extensive variation in display size, pixel pitch, pixel structure, and integrated features. With numerous manufacturers in the market, the number of monitor devices to be considered is extremely large. In most cases a monitor product is listed under the manufacturer's model name even though the LCD internal panel is made by one of a few companies that specialize in panel fabrication. In general, a monitor manufacturer does not identify the LCD panel used. In some cases the pixel structure may be identified only as a generic type (i.e. IPS rather that S-IPS, H-IPS, e-IPS, p-IPS, etc.). Independent reviews are an important source of detailed information that should be considered as a part of the purchase specification process.[3]

Cost is always a factor in purchase specification and the clinical medical physicist will generally be challenged to defend the need for higher cost devices. The available devices to be considered can be group into four categories: *consumer*, *enterprise*, *professional*, and *medical* in order of increasing price. *Consumer* devices are used typically in the home are the least expensive. They often have glossy faceplates for viewing movies in dimly lit rooms. Still modestly priced, *enterprise* devices offer improved viewing angle and brightness. They often have energy saving features including ambient light sensors which are features that may interfere with consistent presentation of images. DICOM calibration of *enterprise* devices can usually only be done with graphic card look up tables (LUT), although a few products now provide internal firmware DICOM settings. The *professional* monitors have high performance LCD panels and good color rendering with internal OSD settings that may include DICOM grayscale standard display function (GSDF[4]) luminance response. They typically have high bit depth for the internal panel drivers that allow for precise calibration of the grayscale and color. The *medical* monitors have several value added features to maintain calibration and remotely monitor performance status, but come with a significant premium in price. These feature differences are summarized in Table 23.2.

23.1.2.2 Visual Quality Assurance

A visual check of image quality can be easily done by inspecting an appropriate quality assurance test pattern (see Figure 23.2). In the film era, the Society of Motion Picture and Television Engineers (SMPTE) test pattern [5] was used to check the performance of video monitors in fluoroscopy, angiography, and for cross sectional imaging devices. Multi-format film printers were also checked using this test pattern. In addition to a series of gray level regions, the patterns include tests of resolution, distortion, and video artifacts which were relevant to CRT devices. The AAPM TG18 final report included a somewhat improved version of the SMPTE test pattern that includes a CX pattern designed to evaluate blur associated with CRT beam focus. Three regions at the bottom were added to verify contrast in dark, medium, and bright regions using faint block characters with the words "QUALITY" and "CONTROL" each of which has different contrast. In 2009, the IEC 62563 standard removed the no longer relevant CX pattern and renamed the TG18-QC as TG18-OIQ. These test patterns are all commonly used today despite design characteristics that are no longer relevant to modern LCD and OLED monitors.

---

3 Presently, www.tftcentral.co.uk provides current reviews on new products, maintains a database of LCD panel structures, and has useful articles on LCD technology including pixel structures and backlights.
4 Part 3.14 of the DICOM standard defines a GSDF used for the luminance response of medical display devices.

Table 23.2 The current monitor market can be considered in four categories.

Category	Monitor Characteristics	Cost
Medical	• Internal firmware GSDF calibration (12+ bits). • Integrated photometer to measure luminance. • Software for remote calibration and monitoring • Anti-reflective coatings on faceplate. • 450+ cd/m^2 brightness. • Good viewing angle performance (LCD: VA, IPS).	\$\$\$\$\$
Professional	• Internal color calibration (12+ bits, GSDF options). • Software for workstation color calibration. • Diffuse faceplate with minimal specular reflection. • ~350 cd m^{-2} brightness. • Good viewing angle performance (LCD: VA, IPS).	\$\$\$
Enterprise	• Graphic LUT needed for GSDF calibration (8 bits). • Diffuse faceplate with minimal specular reflection. • ~350 cd m^{-2} brightness. • Good viewing angle performance (LCD: VA, IPS).	\$\$
Consumer	• Graphic LUT needed for GSDF calibration (8 bits). • Smooth faceplate with specular reflection. • ~200 cd m^{-2} brightness. • Limited angular response (low cost LCD panel).	\$

Consumer devices used typically in the home are the least expensive. Still modestly priced, *enterprise* devices offer improved viewing angle and brightness. The *professional* monitors have high performance LCD panels and good color rendering with internal OSD settings that may include DICOM GSDF luminance response. The *medical* monitors have several value added features to maintain calibration and remotely monitor performance status, but come with a significant premium in price.

The most common use of these three test patterns (SMPTE, TG18-QC, and TG18-OIQ) involves verification of the luminance response and LR using low contrast features in a dark and bright region. This is better done using a test pattern designed to check that the grayscale is properly calibrated to the GSDF and that the LR is appropriate. The TG18-QC test pattern is useful for this purpose. A version of this pattern that has been modified for used with LCD panels in included in the pacsDisplay[5] open source software package (see Figure 23.2d). The test pattern has 18 rows with uniform steps of luminance that have low contrast modulation patterns with two different contrast levels and four spatial frequencies that are similar to the contrast threshold psycho-visual basis of the DICOM GSDF. With proper GSDF calibration and LR, the contrast of the modulation patterns is similar for most of the 18 Gy levels with the exception of reduced contrast in the very dark regions associated with visual adaptation.

cMP #2: Clinical medical physicists should ensure that workstations provide easy access to a quality assurance test pattern. The physicist should also provide instruction on how to interpret the test pattern and encourage routine use.

---

5 www.pacsdisplay.org.

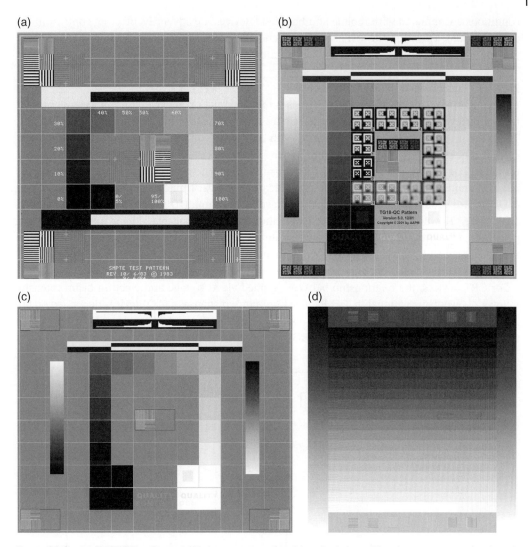

Figure 23.2 (a) SMPTE Test Pattern [5]: A test pattern for video displays and hard-copy cameras developed by a subcommittee of the Society of Motion Picture and Television Engineers (SMPTE). (b) AAPM TG18-QC test pattern [3]: A multi-purpose test pattern developed by AAPM task group 18. The black and white bars at the top test for CRT video ringing. The CX patterns in the center test for resolution degradation due to CRT beam spread. The horizontal and vertical matrix organization allows the assessment of distortion in CRT system. (c) IEC 62563-1 TG18-OIQ [4]: A revised version of the TG18-QC pattern with some of the CRT specific features removed. (d) pd iQC: A visual QC test pattern included displayed by the iQC application in the pacsDisplay open source software package. The test pattern demonstrates uniform contrast for modulated regions when monitors are calibrated to the DICOM GSDF.

Quick visual inspection of a quality assurance test pattern can be very helpful in identifying display performance characteristics that are significantly different than expected. For example, a good luminance response and LR test pattern should be able to easily establish that the appropriate calibration LUTs and monitor firmware settings are in place. Software updates, IT service, or monitor replacements can often leave a system with incorrect configurations which these tests can easily identify. This type of test is also good for establishing when the ambient light viewing conditions encountered with mobile and handheld devices are adversely affecting contrast in the darker regions. However, the visual tests are generally not sensitive enough to evaluate whether the luminance response is within acceptable limits as determined with a photometer.

23.1.2.3 Luminance Response Assessment

The luminance response of a display device is simply the relation between luminance and the digital driving level (DDL) which is often referred to as the grayscale or the tone scale for color devices. Target features in the displayed image array with DDL values different than the surrounding background region are presented with a luminance difference that is determined by the luminance response. For relatively bright scenes, the human visual system perceives contrast based on the relative luminance change, $\Delta L/L$, of the target feature. A logarithmic luminance response (log (L) $\propto$ DDL) thus produces similar perceived contrast for the same DDL change for any background DDL value.[6] However, for darker scenes where the cone cells of the eye become unresponsive, the perception of contrast is reduced. To compensate for this, the logarithmic slope of the luminance response is generally increased in the low luminance region. Figure 23.3 illustrates three common luminance response relationships plotted at log-luminance versus DDL.

For CRT devices, the relationship between applied video voltage and electron beam intensity follows a power law relationship, $I_e \propto V^\gamma$. The luminance response of CRT devices depended on the power law exponent, γ, which could be varied. It was thus common to describe a luminance response by a "gamma" value. In the sRGB color space definition [6], luminance response is

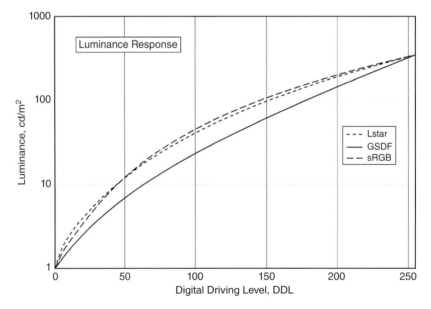

Figure 23.3 The luminance response of a display device refers to the relationship between luminance and the digital driving level or gray level. When plotted using a log luminance scale, the slope of the curve is associated with the image contrast presented to the viewer. At low luminance, contrast is increased to account for decreased visual contrast sensitivity. The DICOM GSDF is compared to the CIE L* and the sRGB luminance response.

---

6 In psychophysics, Weber's law indicates that the just noticeable difference between two stimuli (visual, auditory, etc.) is proportional to the magnitude of the stimuli (i.e. a relative stimulus change). Fechner's law indicates that subjective sensation is proportional to the logarithm of the stimuli.

specified by an equation that is equivalent to a gamma of 2.2. As an international standard, this is still used for digital monitors (see Figure 23.3, sRGB).

The International Commission on Illumination[7] (CIE) has defined color spaces that represent color and brightness in perceptual coordinates. The 1976 L*a*b* or CIELAB color space represents perceived brightness, L*, as proportional to luminance to the 1/3 power. This relationship is based on data for the visual perceptions of relatively large regions of a scene with varied brightness and was defined primarily for plastic, textile, and paint industries. Some professional monitors used for graphic design can be configured with a luminous response base on this color space (see Figure 23.3, Lstar). Historically, it was used in Europe for medical monitors prior to the now more common DICOM GSDF luminance response. CIE technical committee 1-93 is now considering neutral (gray-scale) response for self-luminous surfaces which might compliment L* for reflective surfaces. The Whittle model being considered has been shown to be consistent with the DICOM GSDF [7].

About 20 years ago, DICOM working group 11 evaluated human visual models for the just-noticeable detection of small target regions with sinusoidal modulation [8]. Using the Barten model [9], just-noticeable luminance differences (displayed one at a time) were considered for a specified standard target (a grating pattern with sinusoidal modulation of 4 cycles/°, a 2°×2° area, and a uniform background with a luminance equal to the mean target luminance). The peak to peak luminance modulation relative to the background luminance that is just detectable (i.e. the contrast threshold) is about 0.007 at high brightness but increased markedly below $10\,\mathrm{cd\,m^{-1}}$ [2] (see Figure 23.4). The standard uses this to build a table of luminance values from 0.050 to $3993\,\mathrm{cd\,m^{-1}}$ [2] where the relative luminance between successive values is equal to this contrast

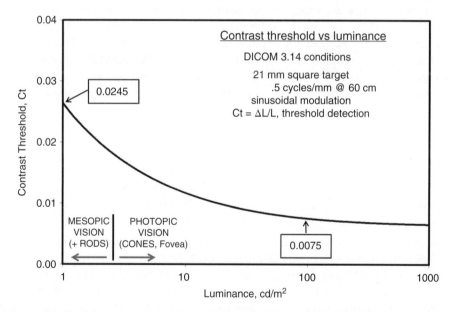

Figure 23.4 Contrast threshold is the just noticeable contrast for a small modulated target in a uniform background field. The contrast shown here is the peak to peak modulation of a sinusoidal pattern of the type used to define the DICOM GSDF. The contrast threshold increases at low luminance as the visual system shifts from cone cell to rod cell response.

---

7 www.cie.co.at.

threshold. This is used as the basis for establishing the luminance response of a monitor (see Figure 23.3, GSDF). The GSDF luminance response distributes contrast for subtle, detailed structures uniformly over the full range of gray values which has proven useful for the types of diagnostic features found in medical images and has become universally adopted. In comparison, sRGB and Lstar luminance response has increased contrast in darker regions and less contrast in bright regions.

> cMP #3: The clinical medical physicists should assume overall responsibility for establishing luminance response conditions that provide consistent image presentation on monitors of all classes (siagnostic, modality, clinical, and EHR).

When introduced, the GSDF was said to provide a perceptually linear grayscale that would provide consistent presentation on different monitors. However, the perception of real structures with supra-threshold contrast and/or primarily low spatial frequency content varies from the standard target conditions of the GSDF. Additionally, due to visual adaptation the contrast of very dark features is somewhat diminished. The term "perceptually linear" is thus not appropriate. Rather the GSDF is simply a recommended standard luminance response for consistent presentation. Consistent presentation also requires that the ratio of the maximum luminance to the minimum luminance be the same on all devices which is discussed below.

The GSDF is defined in DICOM part 3.14 for which Annex B has a list of 1023 sequentially increasing luminance values. A second column with index numbers from 1 to 1023 is labeled JND since the difference between successive luminance values is just noticeable according to the Barten model. The GSDF itself is defined by two mathematical functions from which the JND index, as a fractional number, can be computed as a function of luminance and from which luminance can be computed for any fractional JND index value within the valid range. For a display having a specific minimum luminance at DDL = 0 and maximum luminance at DDL = 255 for 8 bit graphics, the desired luminance values at all other DDLs are determined using these functions:

- Step 1: compute the JND index values for the luminance at DDL 0 and 255.
$$JND_0 \text{ and } JND_{255}.$$
- Step 2: identify the set of intermediate JND index values with uniform spacing.
$$JND_0, JND_1, JND_3 \ldots JND_{255} \text{ with uniform } \Delta JND.$$
- Step 3: compute the luminance for each of the 256 JND values.
$$L_0, L_1, L_3 \ldots L_{255} \text{ with varying } \Delta L/L.$$

To calibrate a monitor to follow the GSDF luminance response, internal or graphic controller LUTs are used to closely match these 256 luminance values.

In Annex C of DICOM part 3.14, a method is described to assess how closely the luminance response of a display is to the GSDF. For the calibrated display, luminance is measured using a photometer at uniformly spaced gray level intervals. For an 8 bit graphic system this could be all 256 Gy values, or could be 18 measures with a gray level interval of 15 as described in the TG18 report. For each of the measured luminance values, the JND index fractional value is determined using the defined equation along with the JND difference. Typically, this is plotted as ΔJND per gray level as a function of gray level and should closely follow a constant value for a well calibrated system (see Figure 23.5a).

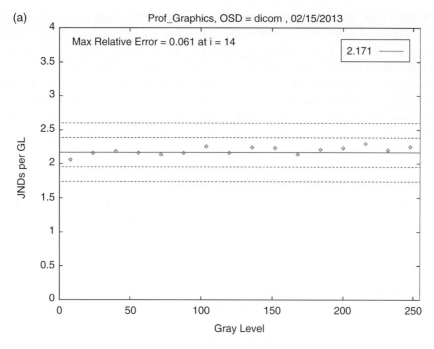

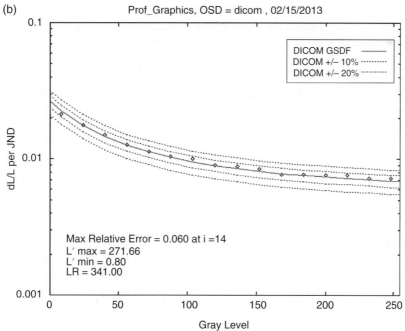

Figure 23.5 (a) Part 3.14 of the DICOM standard suggests that the luminance response of a display be evaluated by measuring the luminance at uniformly spaced gray level intervals. For each, the JND index from the GSDF is determined and the JNDs per gray level deduced. A properly calibrated display will have constant JNDs per gray level. For 8 bit graphic systems, the average value is typically a little more than two. The graph below was obtained as a part of a quality control assessment for which relative luminance contrast was measured at 16 Gy levels. (b) The AAPM task group 18 report recommends that GSDF calibration be evaluated by plotting the contrast, dl/l, per JND versus gray level and comparing that to the GSDF expected contrast. This plot uses the same measurement data at (a). Both JNDs per gray level and dl/l per JND are appropriate for evaluating luminance response. The dl/l per JND additionally shows the increased contrast at low luminance.

The TG-18 report describes an alternative method where the relative contrast, $\Delta L/L$, from luminance measures at uniformly spaced gray level intervals is compared to that expected from the Barten contrast threshold model [9] (see Figure 23.5b). The relative luminance change over each interval is normalized by the mean number of JND indices over the gray level interval used. The result is somewhat more intuitive in that the relative contrast, i.e. the slope of the luminance response in a log luminance versus gray level plot, is shown. However, both methods are equivalent and appropriate for assessing the luminance response of a monitor purported to be calibrated to the GSDF.

23.1.3   Testing Paradigm and Clinical Implementation

The modern era of electronic imaging has introduced new and important needs to maintain consistent display quality for all persons who view medical imaging studies. When film recording was prevalent, the display characteristics were cast when the study was acquired. While film processing quality control was important, once the images were recorded all persons would subsequently view the same presentation. With electronic imaging, the technologist (radiographer), interpreting physician, and clinical management staff are viewing imaging studies on different workstations and monitors. Yet all persons should be viewing scenes with consistent characteristics.

For the technologist, parameters affecting image presentation may be adjusted to obtain the correct appearance for each view. In ultrasound, amplifier gain and depth compensation are adjusted to obtain echo signal with appropriate amplitude. For MRI, window and level default settings are adjusted to provide appropriate initial views during interpretation. For digital radiography, adjustments sometimes need to be made to correct issues with image processing. It is therefore important that the presentation on the modality display be consistent with that of the interpreting radiologist.

During interpretation, several radiologists may participate in the interpretation. In academic centers, radiology residents will first review the study and render a preliminary interpretation. This can be reviewed by a staff radiologist at a different workstation. In the evenings and weekends, on call staff may review a study at a home workstation or using a handheld device. In emergency medicine services and for certain clinical specialists, clinical management decisions may be made immediately after the study is performed and prior to interpretation by a radiologist. It is therefore important that image presentation to all physicians reviewing a study for interpretation or clinical management be consistent.

Typically, imaging studies will be viewed several times during patient visits subsequent to the acquisition and interpretation of the study. This may be at clinical stations located in consultation areas or within patient rooms. Often key images are noted within the study interpretation. To effectively communicate the interpretation, the image presentation on EHR monitors should be consistent.

> cMP #4: The clinical medical physicists should be competent to test display performance at acceptance and for periodic quality control for monitors of all classes (diagnostic, modality, clinical, and EHR).

Acceptance testing and quality control processes are required to insure consistent image presentation. Section II.C.6 of the AAPM TG-18 report executive summary [3] states:

The acceptance and quality control (QC) testing of a display system must be performed by an individual(s) having appropriate technical and clinical competencies. Even though the vendor is expected to perform some testing before turning a display system over to the user, the user must independently test the system(s). For acceptance testing and annual QC evaluation, the tests should be performed by a medical physicist trained in display performance assessments.

Table IV then summarizes eight performance tests for acceptance test along with acceptance criteria. Table V summarizes six performance tests for quality control. While the need for testing by or under the supervision of a medical physicist is well accepted, the test schedule from TG-18 in now outdated. Many tests were important for CRT devices but are no longer relevant to digital LCD panels. For example, geometric distortion is not present, resolution does not change over time, and veiling glare is relatively insignificant. In the next section, recent professional guidelines for electronic imaging display that pertain specifically to LCD devices are reviewed in detail.

23.2 Medical Physics 1.5

Recently, a joint effort of the American College of Radiology (ACR), the AAPM, and the Society for Imaging Informatics in Medicine (SIIM) developed guidelines for the electronic practice of medical imaging that include recommended display device specifications [10]. The section on workstation characteristics makes specific recommendations pertaining to the graphic adapter, the graphic interface, and LCD viewing angle. The section on display characteristics makes recommendations on the luminance response as well as pixel pitch and display size. The ACR-AAPM-SIIM Technical Standard provides useful criteria for specifying *diagnostic* displays used by radiologists as well as displays used for other purposes.

23.2.1 L_{amb}, L_{min}, L_{max}, and LR

Recommendations on display characteristic pertaining to the luminance response are considered in Section 23.1.2.1. Ambient luminance (L_{amb}), maximum and minimum luminance (L_{max} and L_{min}), and the luminance ratio (LR) are considered at the beginning of Section 23.1.2.1.

- 2-a1: L_{amb}: *"When the power to the display device is off, the display surface will still show some brightness due to diffusely reflected room lighting. This is called the ambient luminance. The ambient luminance should be less than one fourth of the luminance of the darkest gray level."*

  When a monitor is unpowered and emitting no light, the surface will reflect incident light from environmental lighting in the room. The incident light can be measured with an ambient light meter in units of lux. Historically, CRT devices had high diffuse reflectance because of the granular phosphor layers used to produce the image. In this era, incident light was kept very low for diagnostic workstations (i.e. 20–50 lx). Modern digital monitors have pixel structures that can absorb incident light which significantly reduces diffuse reflection. Thus, typical diagnostic reading rooms now use somewhat higher environmental light (i.e. 50–80 lx). These low reflectance devices perform better than CRT devices in bright rooms where modality and clinical displays are placed and handheld devices are used.

  When evaluating the ambient reflections on a monitor surface, the medical physicist should first sit in the normal viewing position and verify that the light sources in the room do not appear on the screen as specular reflections. If present, either the workstation or the light source needs to be moved. The diffuse ambient luminance, L_{amb}, then needs to be measured using a spot photometer held at the approximate position of the observer's eye and pointed toward the center of the display surface. It is important to understand that L_{amb} is highly variable and may change by simply the number of persons at a workstation and the clothing that they wear. With experience, a nominal value for L_{amb} can be established for a particular monitor model.

The ambient luminance of the display is added to the emissive luminance of the display device. In the dark regions of the display, the added ambient luminance can significantly reduce image contrast. The guideline recommendation that L_{amb} be less than 1/4 of the luminance of the darkest gray level is consistent with the TG18 recommendations, although TG18 also indicates that less than 2/3 is acceptable if it is accounted for in the calibration. Most GSDF calibration software will specifically account for L_{amb} and one should always be sure that appropriate values are being used, particularly when the room lighting may cause elevated L_{amb} values.

- *2-a2: L'_{min}:* "*Since the contrast response of the adapted human visual system is poor in very dark regions, the luminance of the lowest gray value, L_{min}, should not be extremely low. The minimum luminance including a component from ambient lighting, $L'_{min} = L_{min} + L_{amb}$, should be at least 1.0 cd/m² for diagnostic interpretation and 0.8 cd/m² for other uses.*"

The guideline begins with the important recommendation that L_{min} needs to be sufficiently high for the human visual system to adequately respond to the contrast of structures with image value near the lower level of the presentation. The cones in the fovea of the human eye become less effective below about $5\,cd\,m^{-2}$ and at $1\,cd\,m^{-2}$ the contrast threshold is over three times larger than at $100\,cd\,m^{-2}$ (see Figure 23.4). The guideline recommendation on L_{amb} is an often overlooked display specification. Typically, more attention is paid to L_{max}.

In the CRT era, medical CRT devices adjusted the contrast and brightness controls (i.e. amplifier gain and offset) to obtain appropriate contrast in the dark region of the grayscale. For LCD devices, the only control is that for the backlight brightness. Most LCD panels are designed with a much darker minimum luminance which provides the dark black that is often desired in graphic applications. As a consequence, the display calibration needs to elevate L_{min} using either graphic card or internal monitor LUTs.

- *2-a3: L_{max}:* "*The perceived contrast characteristics of an image depend on the ratio of the luminance for the maximum gray value (L_{max}) to L_{min}. This is the luminance ratio (LR), which is not the same as the contrast ratio often reported by monitor manufacturers. Ideally, all display devices in a facility should have the same LR so that the presentation is consistent for all viewers of a study.*"

Consistent image presentation on all devices requires the both the tone scale, the DICOM GSDF for medical images, and the LR be the same. When calibrating or setting up a monitor, an appropriate LR should be used. DICOM part 14 defines only the GSDF. The guidelines define L_{max} simply as the result of a recommended L_{min} and LR value.

- *2-a4: LR:* *The LR must be large for good image contrast; however, an excessively large LR will exceed the range of the adapted human visual system. A LR of 350, which is equivalent to a film OD range from 0.20 to 2.75, is effective. For acceptable contrast, LR should always be greater than 250.*

The contrast sensitivity of the human visual system, when adapted to a single image with bright and dark regions, covers a relatively narrow range of luminance. Figure 23.6 shows the approximate contrast threshold as a function of luminance for an observer adapted to a single image. This curve is based on the biologic contrast response reported by Flynn in 1999 which was derived from experimental photoreceptor data [11]. The precise nature of adapted contrast response is complex and depends on the type of scene observed, the position within the scene that the observer is looking at, and the background luminance surrounding the image. Using test

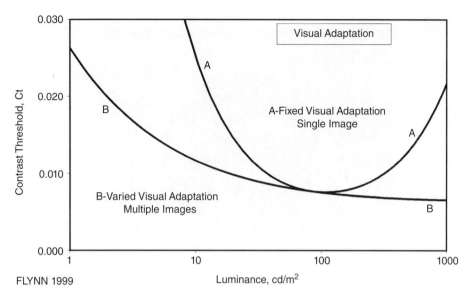

Figure 23.6 A representative curve for contrast threshold versus luminance is shown for an observer viewing various regions of a single image that has regions with varying brightness (curve A). The curve is based on the biological contrast response reported by Flynn [11] that is based on measured photoreceptor neural activity. For comparison, the contrast threshold from Figure 23.4 is shown (curve B). This represents measures from many images with uniform luminance and a central grating pattern (sinusoidal modulation).

patterns displayed on a medical LCD monitor, Tchou measured the contrast threshold under conditions designed to change the state of adaption by changing the brightness of the region surrounding a test pattern (Figure 23.7) [12]. The results are consistent with those in Figure 23.6 with the contrast threshold being adversely affected when the test pattern region is surrounded by very bright regions.

Flynn suggested in the 1999 report that LR should be 240. General experience indicates that 350 produces better contrast with a deeper black and an acceptable LR. The guideline points out that this corresponds to a film with densities ranging from 0.20 to 2.75. In the era when radiographic films were interpreted on an illuminator, regions with a film density above about 2.75 could not be inspected. Common practice was to use a small light source with higher luminance (hot light) to inspect these regions. Today, when an image in encountered that has particularly low signals, window width and level adjustments are made to inspect those regions. This technique is, in effect, an electronic answer to the hot light practice.

For a monitor calibrated over a luminance range of 350 to the DICOM GSDF, the grayscale appearance can be visually evaluated using a step function test pattern such as the AAPM pQC test pattern (Figure 23.1b) which has added low contrast modulation at each step. In general, the perceived contrast at each step will be similar in the middle gray and bright regions. However, some loss of contrast is perceived for the darkest steps. This is because the DICOM GSDF does not account for the effects of adaptation for single images with varying luminance.[8]

---

8 The past literature has referred to calibration with the DICOM GSDF as producing a "perceptually linear" condition for contrast detection at different brightness. This is a misconception since the Barten contrast threshold model [9] used to derive the GSDF is based on experiments with many images of different uniform brightness and does not represent human visual performance adapted to a single image with varying brightness.

(a)

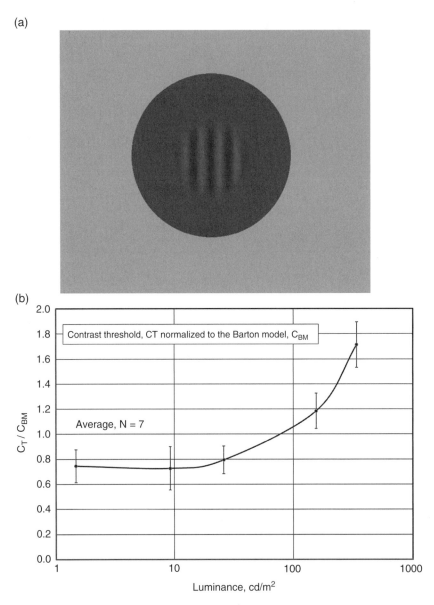

Figure 23.7 (a) Using a 2AFC experiment, Tchou measured the contrast threshold for seven observers using a calibrated medical LCD monitor under conditions having different states of visual adaptation [12]. The detection target was a 10 mm circular grating pattern with sinusoidal 0.5 cycles/mm modulation of varying contrast. The target was surrounded by a 20 mm circular region with luminance equal to the mean luminance of the grating pattern which was fixed at 9.3 cd mm^{-2}. Beyond this 20 mm diameter, the luminance was uniform and set to five different values: 1.5, 9.3, 26.0, 155.4, and 339.1 cd mm^{-2}. Contrast threshold was measure for each of these five surrounding brightness levels. (b) The measure contrast threshold, CT, was normalized to the contrast threshold predicted by the Barten model [9] for patterns with the same frequency, size, and mean target luminance. For the reference condition when the surrounding luminance was equal to the mean target luminance, i.e. 9.3 cd mm^{-2}, the result is less than predicted by a factor of 0.73 ±0.17. This is because the 2AFC experimental method is more sensitive than the variable threshold method used as the basis for the Barten model. When the surround brightness is a factor of six less than the reference conditions, the contrast threshold is not significantly different. When the surround value is brighter the contrast threshold is larger indicating poor visual performance. For a surround value that is a factor of 36 larger than the reference value, the contrast threshold is elevated by a factor of 2.4.

- *2-a5: L_{max} and L'_{min}:* The L_{max} of diagnostic monitors used for interpretation should be at least 350 cd m^{-2} with an L'_{min} of 1.0 cd m^{-2}. For the interpretation of mammograms, L_{max} should be at least 420 cd m^{-2} with an L'_{min} of 1.2 cd m^{-2}. The monitors used for other purposes should have an L_{max} of at least 250 cd m^{-2} with an L'_{min} of 0.8 cd m^{-2}. For brighter monitors, L'_{min} should be proportionately larger to maintain the same LR.

The recommend maximum luminance for diagnostic monitors comes from the recommend L'_{min} of 1.0 cd m^{-2} and suggested LR of 350. These recommended values are based on psychovisual data along with the consensus opinion of the three participating professional societies. It is otherwise difficult to experimentally establish the significance of these recommendations given the variety of modalities and anatomic scenes along with variations in subtle image patterns that indicate the possible presence of an abnormal condition. Walz-Flannigan [13] recently reported a trend for improved performance with increasing L_{max} from 100 to 400; however, the only statistically significant difference was between $L_{max} = 100$ cd m^{-2} and $L_{max} = 400$ cd m^{-2}. The study used contrast-detail observer experiments using spherical nodules projected on a uniform background. This study also demonstrated improved performance when high L_{amb} values were accounted for in the GSDF calibration. In an ROC experiment using chest radiographs with subtle nodules, Krupinski [14] showed statistically significant differences when using a medical class monitor ($L_{max} = 500$) and an enterprise class monitor ($L_{max} = 342$), however this could be due to performance factors other than the maximum luminance.

A slightly higher L_{max} of 420 cd m^{-2} is recommended for mammography based on the practice history of brighter illuminators for film mammography and for consistency with other practice guidelines. A significant difference in performance is otherwise unlikely between L_{max} values of 350 versus 420 cd m^{-2}. For other monitor types (i.e. modality and EHR class monitors), an L_{max} of 250 is recommended. For L'_{min} of 0.8 cd m^{-2}, this results in a LR of 312. Ideally, a somewhat higher value of 280 cd m^{-2} with an LR of 350 should be used.

Until recently, monitor products that meet these L_{max} recommendations have been limited and expensive. Most medical monitors easily meet the recommendations. Using active L_{max} tracking systems, the backlight power is slowly increased to keep L_{max} constant as the backlight lamp ages. The brightness of professional class monitors currently on the market meets the requirement for initial use, but may have limited lifetime due to backlight aging. With the introduction of LED backlights with continually improving luminance efficiency and the expected availability of OLED devices, professional and enterprise monitors that can meet the requirements with good lifetime is anticipated.

23.2.2 Luminance Response, Calibration, Quality Control, White Point

Section 23.1.2.1 on luminance response display characteristics then continues with recommendation pertaining to the grayscale, calibration, quality control, and white point.

- *2-a6: Luminance versus gray level:* In addition to having similar LR, the luminance of intermediate gray values between L'_{min} and L_{max} should follow the same response function for all monitors in a facility. It is recommended that the DICOM GSDF be used to set the intermediate gray values.

Most consumer and enterprise class monitors are designed to meet sRGB specifications which have a gamma 2.2 luminance response [6]. Some professional monitors also support the Adobe RGB (aRGB) specifications[9] which have a larger color gamut and also use a gamma 2.2

---

9 https://www.adobe.com/digitalimag/adobergb.html.

luminance response. Optionally, most professional monitors allow the user to change the luminance response using on screen controls (OSD) to follow the CIELAB L, and some allow the GSDF to be used along with specific settings for L_{max} and L_{min}. It is the medical class monitors that use by default the DICOM GSDF which has been widely adopted for radiology, cardiology, and dental systems. Its use in other specialties is still evolving (digital pathology, dermatology, etc.).

- *2-a7: Calibration: The luminance response, LR and GSDF, of some medical and professional graphics monitors can be selected using the monitor on screen display controls. Other medical/ professional devices require software from the monitor manufacturer to load LUTs to the monitor that set the luminance of each gray level. For business class monitors used by technologists and clinical care staff, the calibration can be achieved by loading a LUT to the driver of the graphic control card.*

  Professional and medical class monitors use display panels that set the luminance with digital signals have 12 bits of precision or more. As such, the desired luminance for each of 256 Gy levels can be set with good accuracy the relative luminance change between successive DDL will closely follow the desired DICOM GSDF. These systems generally have internal monitor LUTs that transform each 8 bit DDL to the desired high bit depth value. These LUTs are also used to calibrate the color response of professional class monitors. Enterprise class monitors may use only 8 bit display panel drivers and thus would not have internal LUTs. For these, the calibration must be done using LUTs in the graphic controller that are supported using standard driver calls. To achieve improved accuracy in setting the desired luminance, a larger palette of gray values may be used that contain gray values for which the R, G, and B components are allowed to vary by 1 DDL [15]. This results in slight luminance changes but not a discernable color tone shift. Some low-priced consumer class monitors use only 6 bit drivers on the display panel and, as such, are not appropriate for medical display.

- *2-a8: Quality control: All display devices should be periodically checked to verify that the luminance response is correct. Basic verification can be done using a visual test pattern designed for evaluating contrast response. Advanced tests, done on an annual or quarterly basis, measure the luminance in relation to gray value and evaluate the contrast. The contrast response of monitors used for diagnostic interpretation should be within 10% of the GSDF over the full LR. For other uses, the contrast response should be within 20% of the GSDF over the full LR.*

  DICOM part 3.14 and the AAPM TG18 report both describe methods to evaluate the luminance response by assessing contrast as a function of DDL (see Medical Physics 1.0 Section 23.1.3 above). This approach is widely accepted and photometer software is broadly available. The TG18 report recommends that diagnostic devices should have a contrast response within 10% of the GSDF and 20% for other display devices. These criteria have been found acceptable by both manufacturers and health users. The ACR-AAPM-SIIM guidelines simply adopt the TG18 GSDF criteria. Not mentioned in the ACR-AAPM-SIIM guideline is the need to assess other performance characteristics such as pixel defects.

- *2-a9: White point: The color characteristics of a display with respect to the presented color space are not considered in this technical standard. However, the white point associated with presentation of grayscale images is important for medical imaging systems. It is recommended that monitors be set to a white point corresponding to the CIE daylight standard D65 white point. This corresponds to a color temperature of about 6500 K.*

  In the film era, the neutral tone of film basis was clear for some products and blue toned for others. Prior CRT devices varied in the neutral tone depending on the phosphors and glass faceplate used in manufacturing. For current LCD devices, the backlight neutral tone varies as well as the color of red, green, and blue filters. Current OLED products have distinctly different color emission properties than LCD devices. Thus, the presentation of monochrome images can vary significantly among products. Furthermore, the neutral tone can change with aging of a device.

The TG18 report only considered the need to match the neutral tone of multiple displays on a workstation. Using the CIE 1976 u', v' color coordinate, the report recommended that the vector difference between monitors be no more than 0.010 which is about twice the noticeable difference in neutral tone for two monitors [16].

Neutral tones are commonly described by the tone produced by an ideal black body radiator with a specified temperature. A color temperature of 2700 K corresponds to a warm tone seen with incandescent lamps. A color temperature of 6500 K corresponds to average daylight illumination. Larger color temperatures correspond to increasingly blue toned colors. No definitive data exists to indicate that visual detection for monochrome images is influenced by the absolute value of the color temperature. However, it can be argued that effective visual performance will be achieve when the red, green, and blue cones in the fovea are all stimulated. The recommendation of the CIE D65 illuminant with a color temperature of about 6500 K nicely matches the response of the cone cells. Most modern display devices can be set to this tone without significant loss of brightness.

23.2.3   Display Size and Pixel Pitch

Section 23.1.2.2 makes recommendations on display characteristics pertaining to display size and pixel pitch.

- *2-b2: Display size*: "*When interpreting images, the attention of the viewer is not limited to the center of the display but extends to the edges as well* via *peripheral vision. Good visualization of the full scene is achieved when the diagonal display distance is about 80% of the viewing distance.*"

  When interpreting or reviewing a medical image, a person directs attention to a particular position in the scene where high detail can be perceived by the closely spaced photo-receptors in the fovea of the eye. As attention is drawn to other regions, the scene is scanned by the fovea response region which covers about 1° (i.e. about 1–2 cm for workstation viewing). The peripheral vision from rod receptors in other regions of the eye's retina draws attention to features in the scene that the observer may want to look at more closely. These receptors are highly interconnected and respond to moving object as the eye is panning the scene. The rod density remains high in a region that is 22° from the fovea [17] for which the peripheral vision is good (i.e. a cone of about 44°).

  If the size of the display is larger than the peripheral vision cone, portions of the scene may never be viewed. The guideline recommendation is based on a 44° cone (80% of the viewing distance) which is consistent with home entertainment recommendations (THX1[10]). Table 23.3 lists the maximum diagonal size recommended for four different types of display devices at their typical viewing distance. For workstations, the 22 in. portrait monitors that have been commonly used by radiologists are just below this limit. Notably, the display industry is moving to wide format monitors. For these devices, images are typically presented with the presentation split into two side by side frames. Thus a 32 in. wide format (16:9 aspect) monitor will have two frames that meet the guideline recommendation.
- *2-b1: Pixel pitch*: "*For monitors used in diagnostic interpretation, it is recommended that the pixel pitch be about 0.200 mm and not larger than 0.210 mm. For this pixel pitch, individual*

---

10 https://www.thx.com/.

Table 23.3 The ACR-AAPM-SIIM guidelines recommend that the diagonal size of a monitor be no larger than 80% of the viewing distance.

Display Type	Viewing Distance Inches (cm)	Diagonal Size Inches (cm)
Small Handheld	10 (25)	8 (20)
Large Handheld	14 (36)	11 (28)
Laptop	20 (51)	16 (40)
Workstation	30 (76)	24 (61)

Typical viewing distances for four types of display devices are listed with the corresponding diagonal size.

pixels and their substructure are not visible and images have continuous tone appearance. No advantage is derived from using a smaller pixel pitch since higher spatial frequencies are not perceived."

A variety of test patterns have been used to assess visual acuity. Clinical measures are done typically with a Snellen eye chart having rows of letters that vary in size. Psycho-visual research has been done using scenes with a small target region with sinusoidal luminance modulation surrounded by a uniform field equal to the mean target luminance (Figure 23.8). In much of the literature, the contrast of the target pattern that is just visible (i.e. the contrast threshold, C_{TM}) is based

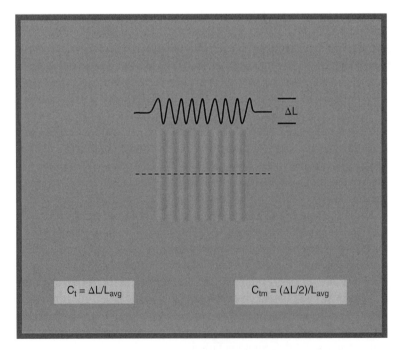

$$C_t = \Delta L/L_{avg}$$

$$C_{tm} = (\Delta L/2)/L_{avg}$$

Figure 23.8 Contrast threshold is measured in psycho-visual experiments using square test target regions with sinusoidal modulation having a uniform background equal to the average of the modulation region. Contrast is defined at the relative luminance modulation, dl/l. The modulation can be either the peak to peak relative modulation which is used in DICOM part 3.14 or the amplitude of the modulating sine function which is used in the psycho-visual literature and is known as the Michelson contrast.

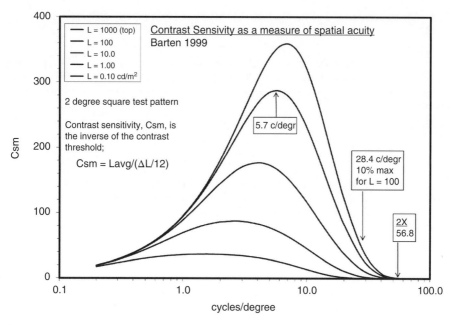

Figure 23.9 The contrast sensitivity of the human eye is illustrated as a function of spatial frequency (cycles per degree) based on the Barten model [9]. Contrast sensitivity is the inverse of the relative contrast, $(\Delta L/2)/L_{avg}$, for a grating pattern (sinusoidal modulation) that is just visible. Above a frequency of 28.4 cycles/degree, the human visual system is unresponsive.

on the Michelson definition of contrast which is the amplitude of the modulating sine function. However, DICOM uses the peak to peak contrast, C_T, in part 3.14 of the standard. Frequently the inverse of the contrast threshold is used which is known at the contrast sensitivity (i.e. either $C_{SM} = 1/C_{TM}$ or $C_S = 1/C_T$). The visual acuity is thus good when contrast sensitivity is high.

Contrast sensitivity depends on several factors. Most important are the spatial frequency of the modulation which is described in units of cycles per degree[11] and the uniform field luminance. The size of the modulated test target and the orientation of the modulation also influence the result. Figure 23.9 illustrates contrast sensitivity, C_{SM}, as a function of frequency and luminance for the test target size and orientation that was used in DICOM 3.14 to derive the GSDF. We see first that visual acuity is sharply peaked in relation to spatial frequency. At 100 cd m^{-2} the maximum occurs at a frequency of 5.7 cycles per mm. At higher frequencies the contrast sensitivity drops rapidly due to the finite size and spacing of the cones in the retinal fovea. For 100 cd m^{-2}, the sensitivity drops to 10% of the maximum at a frequency of 28.4 cycles per degree.

The pixel pitch of a display device determines the maximum spatial frequency that can be presented to the human eye. The Nyquist sampling theorem indicates that the maximum frequency will be at one cycle every for every two sample in distance. Using this, the maximum spatial frequency in cycles per degree for a pixel pitch of P_P mm will be $1/(2P_P)$. Since there is no value in presenting spatial frequencies that are greater than the eye can perceive, this can be converted to cycles per degree (see footnote 4) and set equal to a limit of 28.4 cycles per degree

---

11 Data on visual performance can easily be converted from cycles/° to cycles/mm at a specified viewing distance using the relation cycles/mm equals cycles/° times 57.3 divided by the viewing distance in mm.

Table 23.4 The acuity of the human visual system limits its ability to perceive very high spatial frequencies.

	View distance Inches (cm)	Diagonal size Inches (cm)	Pixel pitch μm	Pixels per inch PPI
Small Handheld	10 (25)	8 (20)	78	325
Large Handheld	14 (36)	11 (28)	109	232
Laptop	20 (51)	16 (40)	156	163
Workstation	30 (76)	24 (61)	234	108

Image signals above 28.4 cycles/degree are not perceived. The pixel pitch desired to present all spatial frequencies up to this limit is tabulated as a function of the distance of the viewer from the display. The corresponding diagonal size from Table 23.3 is repeated for convenience. The pixels per inch, which is often specified for display devices, is shown in the right column.

(i.e. the 10% limit noted above). The desired pixel pitch which delivers all frequencies up to the limits of the eye is then found to be equal to $D_V/3255$ where D_V is the viewing distance.[12] For a viewing distance of 650 mm, the desired pixel pitch is 0.200 mm which is what the ACR-AAPM-SIIM guideline recommends.

Table 23.4 lists the desired pixel pitch for four different types of display devices along with the corresponding pixels per inch. The values for the small handheld and tablet handheld are nearly identical to the specifications of devices made by Apple under the brand name of "Retina Display." According to Apple, these devices have a high enough pixel density that the human eye is unable to notice pixelation at a typical viewing distance.[13] In principle, some improvement would be achieved with a pitch that is a factor of two smaller corresponding to a limiting spatial frequency of 56.8 cycles per degree as shown in Figure 23.9. In practice, the added value is negligible.

The ACR-AAPM-SIIM guidelines are based on a conservative viewing distance of 65 cm for radiologists interpreting images at a workstation. For 22 staff radiologists at Henry Ford Health System, viewing distance was measured as each person was interpreting a case (see Figure 23.10). The mean viewing distance was 76 cm which is used in Table 23.4 for workstation devices with a desired pitch of 234 μm (microns). However, a significant number of individuals read with a lower viewing distance. Using the ACR-AAPM-SIIM guideline helps ensure good quality presentations for all individuals. In this sample, 19 of 22 individuals were above the viewing distance of 65 cm corresponding to a 200 μm pitch.

When specifying the needed pixel pitch for monitors, the intended application should always be considered along with the expected viewing distance. The ACR-AAPM-SIIM guideline notes that "*Monitors used by technologists and clinical care staff are often not viewed at a desk, and the viewing distance is larger than for diagnostic interpretation. For these monitors, a pixel pitch of 0.250 mm (not larger than 0.300 mm) is appropriate.*" The same approach can be used to specify monitors for conference and consultation applications where the expected viewing distance is large.

---

12 The constant of 3255 is computed as $2 \times 57.3 \times 28.4$. The length unit for P_p is the same as D_v.

13 http://en.wikipedia.org/wiki/Retina_Display.

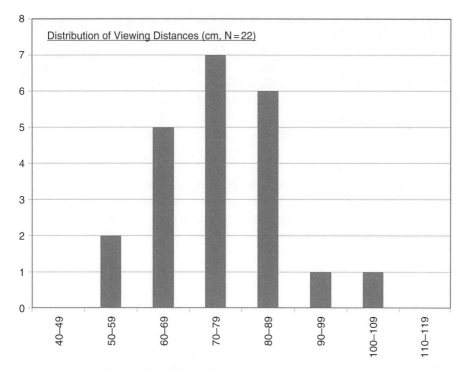

Figure 23.10 Distribution of viewing distance for 22 staff radiologists at Henry Ford Health System (Detroit, MI). All individuals were reading alone at workstations with two medical grade monitors for image presentation and two enterprise monitors for navigation and report authoring. The workstation was on a split deck computer desk with adjustable height. Individuals were sitting on ergonomic office chairs. Measurements were made with a 1 m long ruler by carefully interrupting each radiologist being careful to keep their position. The minimum is 54 cm, the maximum is 104 cm, and the distribution mean is 76 cm.

23.2.4 Technology, Graphic Interface, Presentation Size

The ACR-AAPM-SIIM guidelines also include recommendations for workstation characteristics that impact display quality that should be consider when configuring workstations. These are covered in display Section 23.1.1.

- *1-b: LCD technology: "TN devices should not be used. Several advanced pixel structures are now available to provide improved viewing angle performance (vertical alignment, in-plane switching, and dual domain structures). The viewing angle characteristics of any LCD device should be evaluated using contrast transfer test patterns prior to purchase."*

The first monochrome medical LCD monitor made by IBM used an IPS pixel structure. Today most IPS panels are made by LG Display. However, different variations have been produced which vary with respect to performance (viewing angle, response time, etc.) and production cost. S-IPS, AS-IPS, S-IPS II, H-IPS, UH-IPS and e-IPS are all terms that LG Display or other monitor manufacturers have used to denote the type of panel. Recently, Samsung has used a plane to line structure (PLS) which is similar to IPS and has been used in Samsung and Apple products. VA pixel structures were originally developed by Fujitsu and rapidly move to multi-domain vertical alignment designs (MVA). Today, Samsung makes numerous VA panels using patterned structures (PVA). These similarly have numerous variations including S-PVA, cPVA, A-PVA, and SVA. All of the different IPS and VA pixel structure variations can be recognized by inspecting individual pixels with a 5X to 10X loupe or with a macro photograph. While the guideline suggestion to use advanced structures is sound, when purchasing monitors one should look closely at the performance characteristics and understand what specific pixel structure is used in the monitor's panel.

- *1-c: Graphic interface: "The interface between the graphic controller and the LCD device should transfer the image data using a digital format such as DVI-D (either single-link or dual-link) or DisplayPort. For optimal resolution, the graphic controller device driver should always be set to the native rows and columns of the LCD device."*

All modern monitors, LCD and OLED, set the brightness of each pixel based on a value stored in the monitors digital memory. The graphic interface rapidly updates this memory by transferring the image frame digital content to the monitors. Thus, the graphic card should always be set to the row and column size corresponding to the panel in the monitor. The two digital communication channels now in use are the DVI and the more recently introduced DisplayPort which has performance advantages. The legacy analogue graphic controller channels that send a raster scanned voltage signal to CRT devices are inappropriate for digital monitors.

- *1-d: Presentation size: "For optimal image resolution, the interpolation of each displayed pixel, whether up- or down-sampling, should consider more than the closest four acquired pixel values. Cubic spline and cubic polynomial interpolation algorithms are commonly used for high quality interpolation with the graphic controller providing acceleration so that images are presented with negligible delay."*

The image obtained from a modality device is rarely the same size at the monitor pixel array used to present the image. Radiographs are typically presented in a smaller array (i.e. down-sampled) while CT, MRI, US, and NM are typically presented in larger arrays (i.e. up-sampled). When re-sampling the acquired image, a best estimate of each presented image can be done using interpolation algorithms that consider a four by four set of values in the acquired image. The cubic spline and cubic polynomial interpolation noted in the guideline are two common implementations.

For images that are modestly minified, the cubic interpolation algorithms control the presentation noise, and retain a best estimate of edge features. For images that are significantly minified, advanced algorithms that extract only the low spatial frequencies in the image are more effective in controlling presentation noise.

The re-sampling operations are done by the application software used to select and present images in conjunction with standardized procedure calls implemented by the graphic card. Many applications provide configuration options to set the type of interpolation used. When deploying monitors on workstations or configuration web services for image presentation, these settings should be examined.

The guideline also has useful information on graphic bit depth (1-a), image presentation support features (1-e), and ergonomic factors (1-f).

23.2.5 Significance

> cMP #5: Medical physicists should be familiar with the display recommendations of the ACR-AAPM-SIIM electronic imaging guideline and be able to explain the rationale for each as discussed in this section.

As a recent professional guideline on electronic imaging the display related recommendations provide a useful basis for current medical physics practice. The active participation of three professional societies enhances the significance. For the medical physics society, AAPM, the full membership had opportunity to comment in additional to the participation of members in writing the draft. The final document was approved by the ACR Medical Physics Commission prior to final approval by the ACR Council.

23.3 Emerging Practice (Medical Physics 3.0)

23.3.1 Philosophy and Significance

Clinical medical physicists need to understand their responsibilities for the quality of images presented to technologists, radiologists, clinical specialists, as well as persons viewing EHR. For areas of delineated responsibility, the physicist will provide professional support in three areas:

- Display technology purchase recommendations
- Display device acceptance testing
- Quality assurance program management

Presently, specification and testing of diagnostic monitors is done primarily at some larger centers that have full time staff physicists who assume the needed responsibility. In the future, consulting service groups are likely to provide such support on a routine basis to smaller centers in a manner similar to the support provided for modality purchasing and testing.

Most medical physicists, whether consulting or directly employed, have responsibilities for modality devices and should routinely be specifying and testing the display performance of monitors used by the modality operators. Unfortunately, the expectation of consistent presentation has not been fully understood by manufacturers. Inclusion of specific display performance requirements in purchasing documents will help convey this expectation to suppliers. To support routine testing, all modality devices should be able to easily present a contemporary visual QC test pattern and should have graphic application to facilitate verification of the luminance response with an external photometer (i.e. L_{min}, L_{max}, and a GSDF luminance response).

Workstations used by radiologists typically have two to four monitors with some used for image presentation and some for study navigation and report authoring. Because of the strategic role that radiology reports have on patient management, performance specifications and display quality control are of particular importance. While the ACR-AAPM-SIIM guidelines provide useful professional recommendations, these workstations are not presently accredited by ACR as are modality imaging services. It is likely that diagnostic display performance in the context of electronic imaging will become a part of hospital accreditation requirements.

At present, display testing is appearing in ACR modality accreditation requirements, US state regulations, hospital accreditation requirements, and various national regulations (i.e. EU, DIN, JESRA...). The specific testing requirements and frequency are not always consistent. As an example, the state of New York (USA) expects health providers to have a QA program in place for primary diagnostic monitors as a part of the Radiation Safety/Quality Assurance program of a facility.[14] A published guide suggests the following:

- Biweekly – clean and visual check
- Quarterly – L_{max} and GSDF verification

---

14 https://www.health.ny.gov/environmental/radiological/radiation_safety_guides/diagnostic_monitors.htm.

- Annual:
  - Licensed medical physicist (with photometer)
  - Luminance (L_{max}) and LR
  - Viewing conditions
  - Review QC documentation
  - Document findings and recommendations

While the inclusion of frequent cleaning is laudable, the guide omits consideration of non-uniformities or small-scale artifacts. In the coming decade, medical physics professional guidelines should be published which will lead to harmonization of these requirements.

The presentation of images to clinical specialists also requires consistent presentation. Specifically, physicians in orthopedic surgery, neurology, and emergency medicine have skills for evaluating imaging studies in the context of the patient's immediate clinical condition and will make immediate patient management decisions based on their review of imaging studies. For these situations, a subsequent interpretation by a radiologist provides confirmation but may also identify unexpected findings not related to the patient's immediate clinical condition. An active role by a medical physicist in providing specifications and testing of these workstations is warranted; however, these operations are outside of radiology where medical physicists have traditionally worked. Facility management should understand this need and seek support from a clinical medical physicist.

The workstations used for accessing patient information as a part of enterprise health records usually have application support to view medical imaging studies but rarely have monitors that can provide consistent presentation. In the past, this would require a significant increase in cost. Presently, low cost monitors with good performance can be economically configured for consistent configuration. IT staff responsible for these systems need to be taught the importance of consistent presentation. Periodic audits of L_{max} and GSDF graphic configurations can help identify when particularly systems need to be replaced or when the enterprise graphic configurations need to be reviewed.

In general, workstations used by radiologists and clinical specialist should have a display performance acceptance test. This is only now starting to become a part of typical clinical medical physics responsibilities. For monitors on modality devices, these should be routinely tested as a part of the device acceptance. For monitors used in the general health enterprise, the large volume precludes testing of all workstations. Rather, by working with purchasing and IT departments, several representative monitors should be test. Ideally this can be done prior to order placement.

As for modality devices, the acceptance test affirms performance specified in a purchase contract. Some performance characteristics reflect design elements of the monitor display panel. Specifically, diffuse reflection, viewing angle characteristics, and fixed panel pixel noise. Ideally, these should be evaluated prior to purchase. When many devices are purchased, these can be confirmed by checking the performance of a few selected monitors. The luminance response, pixel defects, luminance uniformity, and color can vary among monitors of the same model and should be evaluated for each monitor. The recorded baseline values can then be used as reference for subsequent quality assurance tests.

Quality assurance test frequency is driven by the probability that performance will change. Most agree that quick visual tests should be done by the workstations' users more frequently. These tests can quickly detect problems with operating system or monitor configurations that result in significant luminance response changes. Some application software products, particularly for handheld devices, present a visual test image when the user logs on and requires affirmation that the appearance is correct. Users should also be trained to report any suspected non-uniformity present on a monitor. These can occur suddenly due to a defective fluorescent or led backlight lamp element. Testing by a medical physicist can then establish whether the non-uniformity is out of acceptable limits.

The luminance response (i.e. grayscale) and color of LCD and OLED monitors tends to change gradually as a part of device aging. For current technology, an annual performance test by a medical physicist is appropriate. Some workstations used as a part of emergency medicine or intensive care services are used every day on all shifts. Present aging characteristics result in a lifetime of only a few years for these monitors. Workstations in other services will have monitor lifetimes on the order of five years. Annual testing of these workstations can help predict when replacement is going to be required and facilitate budget planning.

23.3.2 Metrics and Analytics

23.3.2.1 Workstation Configuration Management

When purchasing recommendations for image display are being considered for any monitor class, it is important for IT staff (radiology or enterprise) to appreciate their limitations regarding display performance specifications as well as important operating system display configurations that impact image quality. The medical physicist needs training and experience in this area and relevant managers and purchasing agents need to understand the importance of this professional input. A technology "enthusiast" is often encountered among the user groups to whom the detailed rationale for professional recommendations needs to be explained. As a part of the purchasing process, the medical physicist should establish appropriate inventory management processes that can be used to record performance at acceptance and subsequent test intervals.

When testing display performance on installed workstation, it is important to document the make, model, and serial number of all monitors on the workstation along with all display related graphic configuration settings. This can be quickly done using an application that reads graphic configurations from the OS registry (Windows OS) and obtains monitor data from the data structure[15] stored in all monitors. The EDID profile application distributed with the pacsDisplay open source software identifies all active monitors from information in the Windows registry and parses the EDID of each. The application creates a table in a text file having monitor identification information (monitor descriptor, serial number, week and year of manufacture) that can be used to associate performance test results with an inventory database (see Table 23.5). The native vertical and horizontal array size is reported along with the sizes configured in the graphic driver so that one can easily confirm that the workstation is correctly configured to use the native display size. Quickly obtaining identification and configuration data is an essential first step for all medical physicists, either consulting or facility staff.

> cMP #6: Inventory tracking: When assessing workstation display performance, monitor make and model along with display configuration settings should be recorded and results associated with a display tracking and QA database.

---

15 The VESA Extended Display Identification Data (EDID) data structure is currently stored in digital monitors and can be read by operating system drivers. The VESA DisplayID standard was recently released and is designed to eventually replace the EDID standard.

Table 23.5 When evaluating the display performance of a set of monitors on a workstation, graphic information related to each monitor should be documented.

Adapter display ID	DISPLAY2	DISPLAY3	DISPLAY1	DISPLAY4
Adapter string	RealVisionVR/MD	RealVisionVR/MD	NVIDIAFX4600	NVIDIAFX4600
Monitor Descriptor	MD21GS-3MP	MD21GS-3MP	DELL 2007FP	DELL 2007FP
Extended S/N (L/R)	79E00741YW	79E00741YW	G324H95I2HDL	G324H06I2NVL
Week of manufacture	38	38	21	25
Year of manufacture	2007	2007	2009	2010
Max. horizontal image size (mm)	432	432	367	367
Max. vertical image size (mm)	324	324	275	275
Native vertical resolution	1536	1536	1200	1200
Current vertical resolution	1536	1536	1200	1200
Native horizontal resolution	2048	2048	1600	1600
Current horizontal resolution	2048	2048	1600	1600
Est. hor. pixel size (microns)	210.9	210.9	229.4	229.4
Est. ver. pixel size (microns)	210.9	210.9	229.2	229.2

The pacsDisplay open source software provides a utility called EDIDprofile to make a table using information stored in the windows OS registry include data extracted from the EDID data structure stored within each monitor.

Several companies with medical display products provide network inventory management software tools that can be very helpful for tracking displays within an organization. Once the client software is installed on all display workstations, a central server application managed by a medical physicist can track identification information, configuration settings, and available performance information. Typically, more detailed performance information will be available for monitors manufactured by the company providing the client and server software applications. In 2014, the DICOM standard incorporated methods for the communication of display parameters[16] including a display system information object and an SOP class allowing retrieval of standardized display system characteristics and performance information including image quality factors. This will permit implementation of client and server applications that provide complete information for all types of monitors.

23.3.2.2 Visual Performance Evaluation

Visual test patterns that are routinely used by workstations users will continue to be important to identify malfunctions or improper configurations that are easily recognized. Most frequently, these problems manifest themselves as alterations of the luminance response. Currently available test patterns often have excessive complexity in an attempt to detect all possible display quality problems. However, these can often be confusing to the workstation user. Simplified test patterns that focus on the most likely problem with the luminance response are now being considered with the expectation that they will be used more frequently. However, more detailed test patterns (see Figure 23.2d) are more appropriate for the medical physicist doing monthly or quarterly quick evaluations that do not involve photometric measurements.

---

16 DICOM Supplement 124: Communication of Display Parameters, Final Text April 22, 2014.

Whenever a medical physicist is evaluating display performance, each monitor should be examined for possible pixel defect, line defects, or small scale non-uniformities that can result from panel deterioration. For evaluating pixel or line defects, both a near black and a near white image should be used with gray values of about 5 and 250 for 8 bit graphic systems. For evaluating small scale panel deterioration, an image with uniform mid gray values of about 135 is best. This can be done by storing three images with uniform values of 5, 135, and 250 and using a simple image viewer to pan a small window over the full display field. Pixel or line defects can be one of the following: always black, always white, or sometimes flickering. Modern monitors should have no defects. For small scale non-uniformities, professional judgment must be used to decide whether a monitor should be taken out of service. Documentation the problem should be done with using a camera. Any non-uniformity that is clearly seen and could interfere with the presentation of subtle clinical detail in a medical image should be reason to replace the monitor (see Figure 23.11).

It should be obvious to all that the surface of a monitor needs to be optically clear; however, the responsibility to periodically clean the surface is frequently not delegated. Over time dust and lint will accumulate and stains may appear from spills or coughing. Oil stains often appear from persons pointing to detail in an image. These can usually be quickly cleaned with an optical cleaning solution and lint free cloth. As a part of any workstation performance test, a subjective statement regarding the display surface cleanliness should be made and included in the test report. This is generally best done with the monitor off or with a full black presentation. For performance tests involving photometric measurement discussed in the next section, it may be necessary to clean the surface before proceeding.

23.3.2.3 Luminance Response Assessment (i.e. Grayscale)

The first step is evaluating the luminance response is to measure or determine L_{amb}. A spot photometer is used to measure the luminance with the display device turned off. The meter needs to be sufficiently far from the display surface so as not to shield the device from room lighting. Sitting in the position of a viewer, the meter should be pointed toward the center of the device in a direction perpendicular to the surface. The spot photometer will typically be about 50 cm from the surface. Alternatively, L_{amb} can be inferred from the known diffuse reflection coefficient for a particular display model and the ambient illumination on the display surface. When sitting in the position of

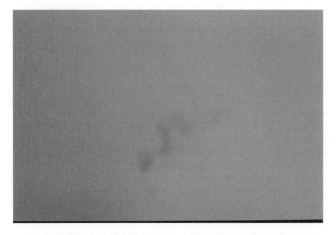

Figure 23.11 A small scale non-uniformity detected using a visual test evaluation with a uniform mid gray pattern. Each of the diffuse oval dark regions is 1–2 cm is size. Artifacts of this type can result from LCD panel material deterioration or delamination.

a viewer, an illuminance meter is placed at the center of the device to record the amount of light incident on the surface. The diffuse reflection coefficient is the ratio of luminance to illuminance with units of cd m^{-2} per lux. For a facility with many monitors of the same model and with room lighting designed to establish a nominal average ambient illuminance, a nominal L_{amb} may be used and the illuminance simply verified to be within a specified range.

The device luminance, L_{nn}, is then measure as a function of gray level (i.e. *nn*) using a contact photometer placed on the surface of the monitor so as to record only light emitted from the surface. For each measurement, the value of L_{amb} is added to deduce the luminance in the presence of ambient light, L'_{nn}.[17] This is then compared to the luminance response of the DICOM GSDF between L'_{min} and L'_{max} as was described earlier in this chapter (see Figure 23.5a and b). To date, 18 measurements are typically made with intervals of 15 between gray level 0 and 255 which was recommended in the TG-18 report. While this can be done quickly, it can fail to detect anomalies in the luminance response that can be seen with smaller gray level intervals. Figures 23.12 and 23.13 illustrate two examples of anomalies detected by measuring luminance at each of 256 Gy levels. Both anomalies were present for monitors of a particular manufacturer's model used with a

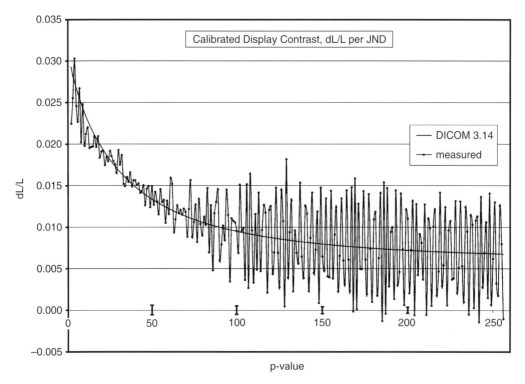

Figure 23.12 The luminance measured for gray values from 0 to 255 (DICOM p values) with an interval of 1 is evaluated for the contrast of the luminance response, dl/l, and compared to the GSDF in DICOM part 3.14. This diagnostic medical grade monitor demonstrates an oscillation of the slope for bright gray values corresponding to a luminance response with a staircase pattern. The artifact is not detected with QC measures of 18 Gy levels.

---

17 IEC 62563–1 standardized the terminology and symbols for luminance response with unprimed symbols referring to device luminance only (i.e. L_{min}, L_{max}) and primed symbols referring to device plus ambient luminance (i.e. L'_{max}, L'_{min}). The ACR-AAPM-SIIM guidelines use the same terminology and we do so in this chapter.

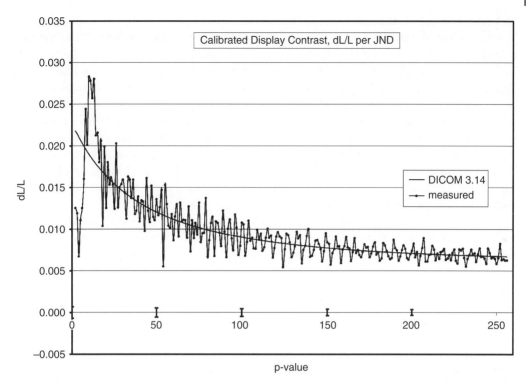

Figure 23.13 The luminance measured for gray values from 0 to 255 (DICOM p values) with an interval of 1 is evaluated for the contrast of the luminance response, dl/l, and compared to the GSDF in DICOM part 3.14. This diagnostic medical grade monitor demonstrates an initially low contrast followed by abnormally high contrast that corresponds to an S shaped deviation of the luminance response in the region of the first 15 Gy levels. The artifact is not detected with QC measures of 18 Gy levels.

particular version of that manufacturer's software. When performing acceptance tests on a set of new monitors, a detailed measurement of this type should be performed on a few systems to establish that the performance is acceptable. While 18 measurements with increments of 15 are likely to remain common for routine testing, low noise photometers with fast response time may permit routine use of tests with 51 measures in increments of 5.

Luminance response assessment can be done by manually stepping through a series of images or panning a test image position, recording the luminance of each DDL (i.e. gray value) in a spread sheet, and using a spread sheet to evaluate the response relative to the DICOM GSDF. However, this can be tedious and time consuming. Software to automatically change the gray value, record luminance, and perform the evaluation is now readily available[18] and allows the luminance response to be assessed in a few minutes. Using the pacsDisplay open source software referred to above, the results are reported as a document suitable to storing in a test database or sending to a client which includes a table of results compared to recommended performance along with plots (see Figure 23.16).

---

18 Many monitor manufactures supplying products to health systems provide software applications for luminance response assessment including Barco, NEC, and Eizo. Qubyx specializes in monitor calibration software compatible with numerous photometers including a product for medical displays. pacsDisplay (www.pacsdisplay.org) is open source software compatible with several photometers.

23.3.2.4 Uniformity Evaluation

The human visual system is insensitive to very low spatial frequencies (see Figure 23.9) and thus gradual differences in luminance over the full field of display are not problematic. Most monitor backlights are now designed with a set of LED lamps mounted on the sides of a panel and optical light transport components that produce a relatively uniform luminance distribution. However, individual lamps can become defective and the luminance reduces in corners or along sides of a display.

The TG18 report recommended measuring luminance in the center of rectangles formed by dividing the display surface into a 3×3 array. The report recommends that five measurements should not have a deviation of more than 30% with respect to the maximum to minimum luminance difference relative to the average of the measurements. The report further recommends making measures with a uniform field set at two different gray levels which was deemed necessary because of CRT performance characteristics.

Measuring nine regions in a 3×3 array of positions using a single uniform test pattern with a mid to high gray is recommended for the type of backlight defects now encountered with LCD panels and can be done quickly with a software controlled photometer. Comparison of individual values to the median of the nine measurements is recommended since the median is less influenced by a single low measurement. In general, one expects a defect to involve one of the nine measures being different than the median. A value less by 30% should be considered defective and a value less than 15% should be carefully reviewed (i.e. for a median of $350\,cd\,m^{-2}$, a value less than 245 would be defective and 298 would be suspect). When performing this test, the display should be visually examined along the edges for short range uniformity changes that may not be detected with a photometer centered in the 3×3 array of test positions.

For OLED panels now becoming available, uniformity testing may become unnecessary. As emissive devices with no backlight component, the devices are not susceptible to the type of sudden change that occurs with LCD backlights. However, aging of the emissive materials has been a materials problem in the development of this technology and may manifest itself in a non-uniform manner. There is simply not enough experience at this time to make recommendations for OLED devices.

23.3.2.5 Fixed Pattern Pixel Noise

The majority of LCD and OLED panels now being manufactured have six sub-pixels for each pixel (i.e. dual domain RGB devices) and the physical dimensions of each subpixel is very small. As such, it is reasonable to expect that some variation is the light emitted by each sub-pixel will be present. While a small pixel pitch makes this sub-pixel structure not visible at a normal viewing distance, the perceived luminance may still vary from pixel to pixel with a fixed pattern.[19] This is typically uncorrelated white noise similar to the quantum mottle in a digital radiograph and as such can limit the visual detection of small low contrast image features.

Evaluation of LCD fixed pattern noise done with scientific CCD camera recordings can document the noise power spectrum (NPS) of the fixed pattern noise [18–20] and has been considered for quantitative testing of noise [3]. However, the measurement is difficult to perform since the subpixel structure creates high frequency peaks in the NPS that can distort the low frequency spectrum unless the recording camera pixels are carefully aligned with the display pixels [21]. This can be done with scientific CCD cameras having monochrome rectangular detector elements but is particularly difficult with a graphic camera having an RGB color filter in a Bayer array pattern. As a consequence, quantitative assessment of noise is not currently done as a part of medical physics testing.

---

19 For static image presentation, once the voltage signal has been set in the pixel structure of an LCD or OLED panel, the temporal noise of the pixel is negligible.

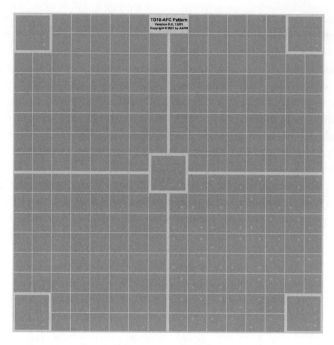

Figure 23.14 Fixed pattern pixel noise is difficult to quantitatively measure. Show here is the TG18-AFC visual test pattern with the image contrast increased by a factor of 4 to make the small low contrast targets more clearly seen. Each square has a small low contrast target in one of four positions making it possible to evaluate the pattern using 4 alternative forced choice methods. In practice, a subjective decision is made as to whether the position of the small targets can be seen in each of the four quadrants. The 58 target objects in the four quadrants have sizes of 2, 3, 4, and 6 pixels and contrast of 2, 3, 4, and 6 DDL units for 8 bit images. For radiologist's workstations, all but the smallest targets should be visible.

A visual test was suggested in the TG-18 report using a contrast detail test pattern (TG18-AFC, see Figure 23.14). In each quadrant of the pattern, about 60 small boxes have a uniform mid-gray background and a small square target object positioned randomly in one of four positions. The target objects in the four quadrants have sizes of 2, 3, 4, and 6 pixels and contrast of 2, 3, 4, and 6 DDL units for 8 bit images. For radiologist's workstations, all but the smallest targets should be visible. The pattern is similar to contrast detail mammographic test objects and in principle can be evaluated using 4 alternative force choice (4AFC) scoring. In practice, a subjective determination is typically made. In lieu of a practical NPS evaluation method, a visual evaluation is needed which will generally be done as a part of the purchasing process when comparing alternative products. The fixed pattern noise of modern LCD panels is low and the NPS of OLED devices has been reported as better than LCD devices [22]. A revised version of the TG18-AFC test pattern designed for current viewing distance recommendations and the noise characteristics of modern LCD and OLED monitors should be anticipated.

23.3.2.6 Color

Imaging studies from radiology, cardiology, and dental studies are usually reviewed using a gray-scale presentation. This follows the traditional presentation when studies were reviewed on film recordings. For both film and electronic imaging, there is a long history of discussions regarding the preferred color tone of gray. Some have preferred a slightly blueish daylight tone and some preferring a warmer tone with a lower color temperature. No definitive studies have established a difference in visual performance and the gray tone remains largely a matter of preference.

The ACR-AAPM-SIIM guidelines recommend a gray tone (i.e. white point) corresponding to the CIE D65 illuminant with a color temperature of about 6504 K, which nicely matches the response of the cone cells as noted above. For consistent presentation of images, this daylight white tone represents a consensus recommendation and is easily achieved by present display products.

For workstations with multiple monitors, differences in white point can be distracting. The TG18 report recommends that the white point of all monitors be within a vector difference of 0.010 in the CIE 1976 u',v' color coordinates. While Groth reported that 0.004 is a detectable difference to radiologists [16], differences up to 0.010 will usually be acceptable.

For LCD display panels, the changing orientation of liquid crystals with gray level can result in a shift in gray tone with luminance. When assessing the luminance response of a monitor, the u'v' color coordinate can be simultaneously measured at each gray level. Figure 23.15a and b illustrate

(a)

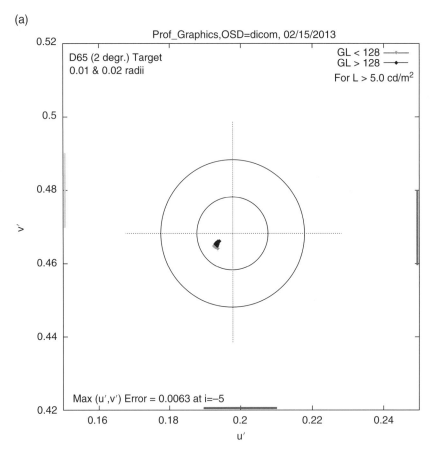

Figure 23.15 (a) The (u', v') color coordinates measured for gray values differing by 15 are plotted to evaluate gray tracking. The D65 target white point is shown by the dotted lines. The circles represent deviations of 0.01 and 0.02. The colored bars at the left, right, and bottom represent the directions of the red, green, and blue primaries in the color space. This professional graphics LCD monitors with internal DICOM GSDF calibration and a luminance ratio of 350 has excellent gray tracking characteristics with a maximum deviation from the D65 coordinate of 0.006 in the blue-green direction. Only gray levels with a luminance in the photopic vision region above 5 cd m^{-2} are considered.

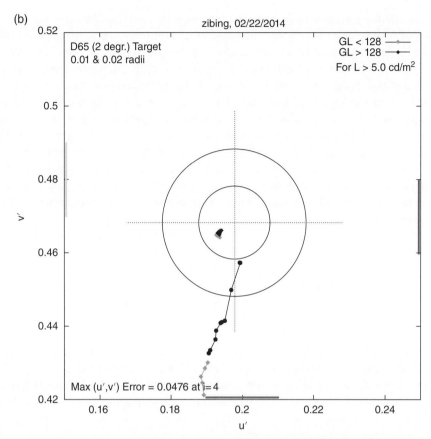

Figure 23.15 (Continued) (b) The (u',v') color coordinates measured for gray values differing by 15 are plotted to evaluate gray tracking. The D65 target white point is shown by the dotted lines. The circles represent deviations of 0.01 and 0.02. The colored bars at the left, right, and bottom represent the directions of the red, green, and blue primaries in the color space. This full HD wide viewing angle laptop monitor has poor gray tracking characteristics with a maximum deviation from the D65 coordinate of 0.048 in the blue direction. The monitor was calibrated for a GSDF luminance response with a luminance ratio of 350 by using graphic controller LUTs. Only gray levels with a luminance in the photopic vision region above 5 cd m^{-2} are considered.

the gray tracking characteristics of two different monitors. The color coordinate is plotted with the desired D65 white point shown as a target point and circles representing 0.010 and 0.020 vector deviations. Ideally, the color coordinate would be within 0.004, but within 0.010 would be considered acceptable. Only gray levels above 5 cd m^{-2} should be considered since the RGB cone cells of the eye become less responsive below that level.[20]

> cMP #8: The gray tracking characteristics of all monitors should be evaluated as an integral part of the luminance response assessment. For some specialties, the RGB color space should also be evaluated.

---

20 At high luminance, the human eye uses the color sensitive cone cells to process light (i.e. the photopic vision). A low luminance, the eye uses the monochrome rod cells (i.e. scotopic vision). For luminance between about 0.005 and 5.0 cd m^{-2} a combination of rods and cones is used (i.e. mesopic vision).

For some radiology images, images may be presented by replacing the grayscale with a color scale such as with color coded nuclear medicine images. In other cases, selected information is included as a color overlay such as with ultrasound Doppler images. While consistent color is desirable, the specific color coordinates used as represented by the RGB color space is not likely to affect interpretation. However, for other specialties that acquire, store, and view color images accurate color space rendering can be important. For example, in dermatology and wound management images need to be rendered so as to appear similar to direct viewing of the patient's lesion under specific illumination conditions. In digital pathology, a broad color space with highly saturated colors can help distinguish color differences between stains or fluorescent emissions. The International Color Consortium (ICC) is now actively considering recommendations for color presentation in these specialties.[21] A need is rapidly developing for experts in color image presentation to manage the display characteristics of the workstations used in these specialties. This need could be effectively met by medical physicists.

To manage workstations with color monitors, including radiologist workstations, one must understand the basic concepts of color vision and colorimetry for which the book by Daniel Malacara is an excellent resource [23]. Secondly, it is becoming important to understand how operating systems and applications manage color presentation using ICC profiles as described in the specifications and resources of the ICC (www.color.org). Modern operating systems (Linux, Microsoft Windows, and Apple OS X) provide color management services that involve use of the display device color profile used by the graphic pipeline to render images with desired color characteristics. Many applications, including recent versions of various web browsers, can render color images by considering the ICC acquisition profile stored in an image tag and the ICC profile of the display registered in the operating system. Understanding these configurations is essential for managing the configurations of workstations used for medical imaging. In some cases, the operating system color management configurations can interfere with the DICOM calibration of a display causing improper display characteristics.

23.3.3 New Display Technologies

The last decade has been a disruptive era in display technology. LCD displays have seen dramatic improvement in performance and significant decreases in price. We are now in a period where LCD devices with impressive performance are common for handheld devices, desktop monitors, large format television and conference displays, and for signage. Medical displays have benefitted significantly from this technology change. A decade ago, the desired medical display performance was available only with specialized monitors sold in the health care market at high price. Today, prices have decreased significantly for medical market products and some professional grade monitors are meeting the performance requirements of the ACR-AAPM-SIIM electronic imaging guideline that has been reviewed in this chapter.

Notably, this high rate of technology change is likely to continue in the coming decade. In 2012, standards for ultra-high definition television (UHD TV) were approved by the International Telecommunication Union (ITU) in ITU-R Recommendation BT.2020. These include both 4 K (3840×2160) and 8 K (7680×4320) formats, 12 bits/color (RGB), and an extended color space with highly saturated red and green primaries. Using IGZO technology[22] for thin film transistor circuits,

---

21 ICC Medical Imaging Workgroup, http://www.color.org/groups/medical/medical_imaging_wg.xalter.
22 Developed by Sharp and the Semiconductor Energy laboratory Co., Ltd., IGZO TFT circuits made with Indium (In), Gallium (Ga), Tin (Zn), and oxygen (O) are an alternative to amorphous Silicon TFT circuits. Improved mobility facilitates the design of high-resolution low-power circuits.

Sharp is now producing UHD 4 K panels with a 31.5 in. diagonal size that has 0.180 mm pixel pitch and L_{max} of 350 cd mm^{-2}. This is used by three manufactures that include configuration settings for DICOM GSDF luminance response. For these devices, the specification of concern is only the limited lifetime due to backlight aging. Further developments in LCD pixel structures, backlight efficiency, and OLED materials are likely.

Technology change will continue to challenge the medical physicist who is asked to specify and maintain display equipment. In the coming decade, professional and business class monitors are likely to routinely meet and exceed the performance needed. For professional class monitors internal photometers for calibrating and monitoring luminance response are likely to be more widely available. Uncertain is whether new devices will be less prone to artifacts such as pixel defects or more stable with respect to loss of brightness with age.

23.3.4 Medical Physics Implementation

The clinical medical physics competencies described in this chapter are summarized in the outline below.

- Purchase specifications:
  - Evaluate design specific performance of display devices being considered
    - Pixel pitch
    - Luminance response versus viewing angle
    - Fixed pattern pixel noise
    - Ambient light reflection
    - Color gray tracking
    - Color space (for clinical specialties)
  - Establish performance specifications for purchasing orders
  - Recommend monitor models
- Acceptance testing measurements:
  - Verify the pre-purchase performance measurements (see above)
  - Luminance response
    - L_{amb}
    - L_{min}
    - L_{max}
    - GSDF max deviation
  - Uniformity
  - Pixel defects and small-scale non-uniformities
  - For each display, enter the workstation, monitor SN, and acceptance test results in a display tracking database
- User QC:
  - Recommend user visual QC test patterns
  - Ensure that visual QC test patterns are available
  - Provide training for the use and importance of visual QC
  - Establish processes to ensure monitor surfaces are kept clean
  - Implement processes for rapid reported of suspected monitor problems
- Physics QC
  - Establish physics QC test frequency consistent with professional guidelines
  - Provide a QC report with
    - Luminance response (L_{amb}, L_{min}, L_{max}, GSDF deviation)
    - Gray tracking

      ○ Color space (clinical specialties)
      ○ Pixel defects and small-scale non-uniformities
   – Enter test results keyed to monitor SN and workstation in a display tracking dB

To perform display measurements, Medical physicist require a colorimeter capable of measuring luminance, illuminance, and u'v' color coordinates along with a software application to automatically record and evaluate luminance response and gray tracking. Most modestly priced colorimeters use an array of about four silicon photodiodes with filters to separate the photometric response and the color primary response. They are generally very good for making photometric measures of luminance but may have small errors with respect to the accuracy of the measured u'v' color coordinates due to variations in the display emission light spectrum relative to the filters in the colorimeter. Argyll CMS is an open source software package for colorimetric measurements and ICC

Display ID	Prof_Graphics,OSD=dicom
Date	02/15/2013
Time	12:00:03
LumResponse version	1.9

Monitor Evaluation Summary

	Measured Values	Criteria
L'_{max} (cd/m^2)	271.66	Mammo: ≥ 420 Diagnostic: ≥ 350 Other: ≥ 250
L'_{min} (cd/m^2)	0.80	Diagnostic: ≥ 1.0 Other: ≥ 0.8
L_{amb} (cd/m^2)	0.06	[See AR below]
LR, L'_{max}/L'_{min}	341	350 +/- 50
AR, L_{amb}/L_{min}	0.08	Acceptable: ≤ 2/3 Desired: ≤ 1/4
dL/L per JND Max Error	6.00%	Diagnostic: ≤ 10% Other: ≤ 20%
Mean JND/GL	2.171	2.25 +/- 0.25
JND/GL Max Error	6.07%	Diagnostic: ≤ 10% Other: ≤ 20%
Max (u',v') error (D65 gray, L>5)	0.0063	≤ 0.01

Figure 23.16 The pacsDisplay (pd) open source software produces a table in html format having nines measures of the luminance response reported along with the performance criteria for each. A link to this html file can be place in a display tracking database as a way to document the findings of a QC evaluation. Four graphic plots are included below the table but are not shown in this illustration.

profile generation that includes colorimetric drivers for numerous devices (www.argyllcms.com). The Argyll colorimeter driver is used in the pacsDisplay open source software package referred to previously in this chapter. The X-Rite i1 Display Pro colorimeter is currently recommended for use with pacsDisplay. The device provides photometric measures of luminance with good precision at a relatively rapid rate. The integration time varies with luminance in order to maintain good precision at low luminance values. The device uses a lens collimator that enables it to be used on contact with the display surface, or at 50 cm for measures of L_{amb}. The devices also provides u',v' color coordinates suitable for gray tracking assessments. Using this colorimeter, the pacsDisplay software produces a QC report in html format (see Figure 23.16) along with four image files having plots of the luminance response, luminance response deviation and gray tracking results. The html report with embedded plots can be included as a link in a display tracking database.

References

1 Badano, A., Flynn, M.J., and Kanicki, J. (2004). *High-Fidelity Medical Imaging Displays*. SPIE Press.
2 Lu, R., Zhu, X., Wu, S.-T. et al. (2005). Ultrawide-view liquid crystal displays. *J. Disp. Technol.* 1 (1): 3–14.
3 Samei, E. et al. (2005). Assessment of display performance for medical imaging systems: executive summary of AAPM TG18 report. *Med. Phys.* 32 (4): 1205–1225.
4 IEC 62563-1 (2009). *Medical electrical equipment - Medical image display systems - Part 1: Evaluation methods.*
5 Gray, J.E., Lisk, K.G., Haddick, D.H. et al. (1985). Test pattern for video displays and hard-copy cameras. *Radiology* 154 (2): 519–527.
6 I.E. Commission and others (1999). IEC 61966-2-1: Multimedia systems and equipment-Colour measurement and management-Part 2-1: Colour management-Default RGB colour space-sRGB, Geneva Switz. Int. Electrotech. Comm.
7 Carter, R.C. and Brill, M.H. (2014). Calculation of self-luminous neutral scale: how many neutral steps can you see on that display? *J. Soc. Inf. Disp.* 22 (4): 177–186.
8 Blume, H.R. (1996). ACR/NEMA proposal for a gray-scale display function standard. pp. 344–360.
9 Barten, P.G.J. (1999). *Contrast Sensitivity of the Human Eye and Its Effects on Image Quality*. SPIE Press.
10 Norweck, J.T. et al. (2012). ACR–AAPM–SIIM technical standard for electronic practice of medical imaging. *J. Digit. Imaging* 26 (1): 38–52.
11 Flynn, M.J., Kanicki, J., Badano, A., and Eyler, W.R. (1999). High-fidelity electronic display of digital radiographs. *RadioGraphics* 19 (6): 1653–1669.
12 Tchou, P.M. (2007). *Visual Performance in Medical Imaging Using Liquid Crystal Displays*. The University of Michigan.
13 Walz-Flannigan, A., Babcock, B., Kagadis, G.C. et al. (2012). Human contrast-detail performance with declining contrast. *Med. Phys.* 39 (9): 5446–5456.
14 Krupinski, E.A. (2009). Medical grade vs off-the-shelf color displays: influence on observer performance and visual search. *J. Digit. Imaging* 22 (4): 363–368.
15 Flynn, M.J. and Tchou, P. (2003). Accurate measurement of monochrome luminance palettes for the calibration of medical LCD monitors, in Proceedings Volume 5029, Medical Imaging 2003: Visualization, Image-Guided Procedures, and Display, pp. 438–448.
16 Groth, D.S., Bernatz, S.N., Fetterly, K.A., and Hangiandreou, N.J. (2001). Cathode ray tube quality control and acceptance testing program: initial results for clinical PACS displays. *RadioGraphics* 21 (3): 719–732.

17 Osterberg, G. (1935). Topography of the layer of rods and cones in the human retina. *Acta Ophthalmol.* 13 (S6): 1–103.

18 Saunders, R. and Samei, E. (2006). Resolution and noise measurements of five CRT and LCD medical displays. *Med. Phys.* 33 (2): 308–319.

19 Roehrig, H., Krupinski, E.A., Chawla, A.S. et al. (2003). Spatial noise and threshold contrasts in LCD displays. In: *Proceedings Volume 5034, Medical Imaging 2003: Image Perception, Observer Performance, and Technology Assessment*, 174–186.

20 Fan, J., Roehrig, H., Sundareshan, M.K. et al. (2005). Evaluation of and compensation for spatial noise of LCDs in medical applications. *Med. Phys.* 32 (2): 578–587.

21 Badano, A., Gagne, R.M., Jennings, R.J. et al. (2004). Noise in flat-panel displays with subpixel structure. *Med. Phys.* 31 (4): 715–723.

22 Yamazaki, A., Wu, C.-L., Cheng, W.-C., and Badano, A. (2013). Spatial resolution and noise in organic light-emitting diode displays for medical imaging applications. *Opt. Express* 21 (23): 28111.

23 Malacara, D. (2002). *Color Vision and Colorimetry: Theory and Applications*. Society of Photo Optical.

24

Clinical Physics in Imaging Informatics: Current and Emerging Practice

Donald Peck

Department of Radiology, Michigan Technological University, Henry Ford Health System, Houghton, MI, USA

24.1 Philosophy and Significance

The use of digital medical information has become a requirement to function in today's health environment. This data identifies the patient; specifies the procedures performed, or those that are ordered to be performed; and includes quantitative and qualitative results. How this data is moved and stored throughout a health system (and between heath systems), a process termed *medical informatics,* is important to understand. Information stored with an image or that is associated with an acquisition provide the direct link between the patient and the system that acquired the data. This information is used to direct the study to the correct location, for continued care of the patient, and to enhance the interpretation of the study by providing technical information about the acquisition. This information can also be used for optimizing operations and improving healthcare by analyzing all data associated with the patient population or equipment utilization. This is often done through internal health system analytic programs and external registries (e.g. dose, disease, etc.). When using and combining this type of information, it is important to understand how the data is input into an image or file. In imaging this data defines the acquisition and technical parameters that were used in the acquisition. The medical physicist should be considered the primary person to assist the informatics technology (IT) team on all imaging equipment integration, use, and maintenance. This is because the medical physicist understands the acquisition systems and should know how this data is stored within the image or file. Therefore, the medical physicist needs to have knowledge of how the systems interact and where data is stored.

All data communication and storage have defined structures and formats. The development of these formats is done through standards developing organizations (SDO). The two largest SDO for imaging systems in the world are the International Electrotechnical Commission (IEC) and the International Organization for Standardization (ISO). In medicine, the Health Level 7 International (HL7) standard develops requirements for the exchange, integration, sharing, and retrieval of electronic health information in all areas of healthcare. All systems should be compliant with all three of these primary SDOs, but the more fundamental SDO for all imaging systems is the digital imaging and communication in medicine (DICOM) standard [1–3]. DICOM is an ISO reference standard. The medical physicist needs to be an expert in the use and interpretation of the DICOM

Clinical Imaging Physics: Current and Emerging Practice, First Edition. Edited by Ehsan Samei and Douglas E. Pfeiffer.

standard. With knowledge of the DICOM standard and the physics of the acquisition device, the imaging data can be correctly used in the healthcare environment.

Therefore, the medical physicist must have a complete understanding of how information moves into and out of systems. This chapter will focus on the fundamental DICOM concepts a physicist should be knowledgeable about.

24.2   Metrics and Analytics

At any point in time, the official DICOM standard consists of the most recent edition published on the DICOM website (http://medical.nema.org) with additional content being considered part of the standard if it was approved since the last publication date. At the time of this writing, the DICOM standard was being published on at least a semi-annual basis, so the content on the website can be considered at most only six months out of date. Since it can take months to years for any part of the DICOM standard to be implemented by a manufacturer, this delay should never be an issue.

The DICOM standard is divided into 18 parts (parts 9 and 13 have been eliminated), and the names of each part are shown in Figure 24.1. The standard is published in multiple formats

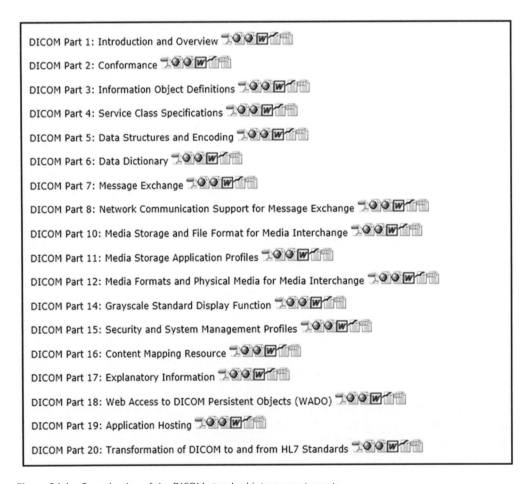

Figure 24.1   Organization of the DICOM standard into separate parts.

(e.g. HTML, PDF), with the PDF version being the official documentation of the standard. The parts are all related but are considered independent documents. The title of each part explains the content and, depending on what information is needed, the review of a single part may be sufficient to accomplish many tasks. When these different parts are referenced in the DICOM standard, they will be listed as PS3.XX, where the "XX" is the part number. The "PS3" portion of this reference is based on the history of the DICOM standard development through the ACR-NEMA terminology to DICOM, where the current version of the standard is version 3, i.e. PS3. The parts that may be used most frequently will be discussed next.

PS3.1 Introduction and Overview is a summary of the standard and provides a brief description of each of the other parts. Although it is not very verbose, a review of PS3.1 can provide a general understanding of the standard organization. PS3.2 Conformance provides the information required for claiming conformance with the standard. This section defines the content of a conformance statement that a manufacturer would publish for a system. PS3.3 Information Object Definitions (IOD) is one of the primary sections used by physicists to understand the content of DICOM images and files. The IOD attributes in PS3.3 describe how data is represented and the rules that define the requirements for including the information in a data file. An attribute is the name given to each item of information stored in a DICOM object. Attributes are designated by a numerical tag number that defines each element within the IOD. The tag numbers are organized into two parts; a four digit group number followed by a four digit element number (see Figure 24.2). In this manner, similar information will all have the same group tag number, but each item will have its own element number. All DICOM applications

C.8.15.3.8 CT Exposure Macro

Table C.8-124 specifies the attributes of the CT Exposure Functional Group Macro.

Table C.8-124. CT Exposure Macro Attributes

Attribute Name	Tag	Type	Attribute Description
CT Exposure Sequence	(0018,9321)	1	Contains the attributes defining exposure information. Only a single Item shall be included in this sequence.
⋮	⋮	⋮	⋮
>CTDIvol	(0018,9345)	2C	Computed Tomography Dose Index (CTDI$_{vol}$), in mGy according to IEC 60601-2-44, Ed.2.1 (Clause 29.1.103.4), The Volume CTDI$_{vol}$. It describes the average dose for this frame for the selected CT conditions of operation Required if Frame Type (0008,9007) Value 1 of this frame is ORIGINAL. May be present otherwise.
>CTDI Phantom Type Code Sequence	(0018,9346)	3	The type of phantom used for CTDI measurement according to IEC 60601-2-44. Only a single Item is permitted in this Sequence.

Figure 24.2 DICOM Information Object Definition attributes requirements.

use the tag number to differentiate elements and do not use the attribute name or description. It is therefore important to use this convention when discussing DICOM elements to clarify what is being referred to. Also, all even number groups are reserved for DICOM use while odd group tag numbers are called "private" groups and can be used without any DICOM requirements imposed. This is done to allow manufacturers to include proprietary information or information that DICOM has not yet defined to be included if necessary. It is important to know that the tag numbers are hexadecimal, so care must be taken when determining if a group number is odd or even. The information in private tags does not have to follow any convention, and what is stored can change without any justification. Consequently, this information is inherently unreliable unless it is known how a manufacturer encodes and presents the information. In addition, the format of the information is not defined in the DICOM standard as are DICOM attributes, which have value representative (VR) constraints. Therefore, private tags, without VR constraints, can be of any length and have any units desired by the manufacturer. A complete registry of data elements is given in PS3.6 Data Dictionary and in this section the required VR is given.

Every DICOM attribute will have a Data Element Type defined. The Type determines if the attribute is always included in a DICOM compliant object (see Figure 24.2). Data Element Type requirements are defined as follows:

- Type 1 = mandatory attribute that must always be included
- Type 2 = mandatory attribute that must be included if known
- Type 3 = optional attribute

In addition, an attribute may be conditional based on specified criteria; if this occurs the Type is followed by a "C," (i.e. Type 1C, 2C, or 3C). The rules for inclusion are always given in the Attribute Description. The reason all attributes are not Type 1, i.e. mandatory, is because at the time the attribute is included in the standard this information may not be available on all systems or may not be an option for every system to populate this information. Once the Type is defined for an attribute as anything other than Type 1, by convention that attribute can never be changed to Type 1. For example, when the standard is initially published if an attribute is Type 3 it can never be changed to Type 1 in future published versions of the standard for this IOD. The reason for this convention is that once a manufacturer has developed a system that is compliant with the DICOM standard, a change in the next version of the standard cannot make that system now non-complaint by changing the Type to mandatory. This makes it very important to either make as many attributes as possible Type 1 upon initial development of the standard, or to try to make the attributes Type 2 or conditional such that the condition can make the attribute required as systems change. Another option to include more Type 1 attributes for an existing DICOM object is to create a new object, often termed an "enhanced" object. This has been done for CT, MR, and US objects, and the new enhanced objects have substantially more Type 1 attributes than the original IOD for these objects.

For many DICOM objects there are some attributes that are the same in all objects, e.g. patient identification and pixel size. To reduce the redundancy in the DICOM standard, attributes are combined into Functional Group Macros. By using Group Macros, the IOD in PS3.3 can just list the link to the macro without repeating the content. In Figure 24.3, a partial list of the Functional Groups for the Enhanced CT Image object is shown. Note that the CT Exposure attributes shown in Figure 24.2, are referenced here. The requirement for whether a Functional Group Macro is included in an IOD is defined by the Usage Type. This is similar to the attribute Type and uses the following codes:

A.38.1.4 Enhanced CT Image Functional Group Macros

Table A.38-2 specifies the use of the Functional Group Macros used in the Multi-frame Functional Group Module for the Enhanced CT Image IOD.

Table A.38-2. Enhanced CT Image Functional Group macros

Functional Group Macro	Section	Usage
Pixel Measures	C.7.6.16.2.1	M
• • •	• • •	• • • -
Frame VOI LUT	C.7.6.16.2.10	U
• • •	• • •	• • • -
CT Exposure	C.8.15.3.8	C - Required if Image Type (0008,0008) Value 1 is ORIGINAL or MIXED, may be present otherwise.

Figure 24.3 DICOM Functional Group Macro attributes requirements.

- M = module support is mandatory
- C = module support is conditional
- U = module support is optional

If a Functional Group Macro is mandatory, then it must always be included for the system to be complaint with the DICOM standard. But if it is conditional or optional, then the entire Functional Group Macro, and all attributes defined in the IOD, may not be included. If the Functional Group Macro is included, then the attribute Type requirements for each attribute must be used for a system to be considered complaint with the standard.

To determine which IOD a manufacturer's system is using, e.g. CT Image or Enhanced CT Image, it is important to understand where to find this information in the DICOM standard. All manufacturers of imaging equipment will have a DICOM compliance statement for each of their products, as defined by PS3.2. In this statement they will list the Service-Object Pairs (SOP) that the equipment will allow an association to occur. The associations are grouped into what are termed Classes. The SOP Classes that the equipment uses are given a Unique Identification Number (UID). An example of the DICOM SOP Class UID from PS3.4 Service Class Specifications is shown in Figure 24.4. The registry of each UID is also given in PS3.6. Also shown in Figure 24.4 is the attribute for the modality, tag (0008, 0060). Note that the modality tag can be the same for several different IOD and is not the information to use to determine the IOD requirements that the equipment will use. It is the SOP Class UID that should be used to find the attribute requirements.

In Figure 24.5, the location of the SOP Class UID is shown in the metadata from a DX object under tag (0002, 0002) Media Storage SOP Class UID. The listings of Media Storage SOP Class UID are in PS3.10 Media Storage and File Format for Media Interchange. When viewing a

SOP Class Name	SOP Class UID	Modality Data Element (0008, 0060)
Computed Radiography	1.2.840.10008.5.1.4.1.1.1	CR
Digital X-Ray - For Presentation	1.2.840.10008.5.1.4.1.1.1.1	DX
Digital X-Ray - For Processing	1.2.840.10008.5.1.4.1.1.1.1.1	DX
Digital Mammography - For Presentation	1.2.840.10008.5.1.4.1.1.1.2	MG
Digital Mammography - For Processing	1.2.840.10008.5.1.4.1.1.1.2.1	MG
Breast Tomosynthesis	1.2.840.10008.5.1.4.1.1.13.1.3	MG
CT	1.2.840.10008.5.1.4.1.1.2	CT
Enhanced CT	1.2.840.10008.5.1.4.1.1.2.1	CT
MR	1.2.840.10008.5.1.4.1.1.4	MR
Enhanced MR	1.2.840.10008.5.1.4.1.1.4.1	MR
MR Spectroscopy	1.2.840.10008.5.1.4.1.1.4.2	MR
Enhanced MR Color	1.2.840.10008.5.1.4.1.1.4.3	MR

Figure 24.4 DICOM SOP Class versus modality designation.

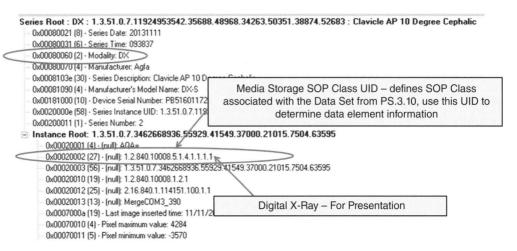

Figure 24.5 DICOM Meta data.

stored image, it is the storage SOP Class that should be used to determine what IOD to review for compliance.

In addition to image objects, there are many non-image IOD's in the DICOM standard. One form of non-image IOD that is important for medical physicists to understand is the DICOM Structured Report (see Figure 24.6). Structured Reports are organized by templates of information. Templates are designated by UIDs, the template ID (TID), and each TID is used similarly to a Functional Group Macro in an image IOD. The contents of each TID have a different configuration as compared to the attributes of an image IOD, and this information is located in PS3.16 Content Mapping Resource.

Figure 24.7 shows how the data presented in a TID. The definition for the content listed in each column is given below:

- NL = nesting level
  - Represented by ">" symbols, one per level of nesting. This is similar to the nesting in Module tables in PS3.3. If the nesting level is blank, this is considered to be the "source" Content Item

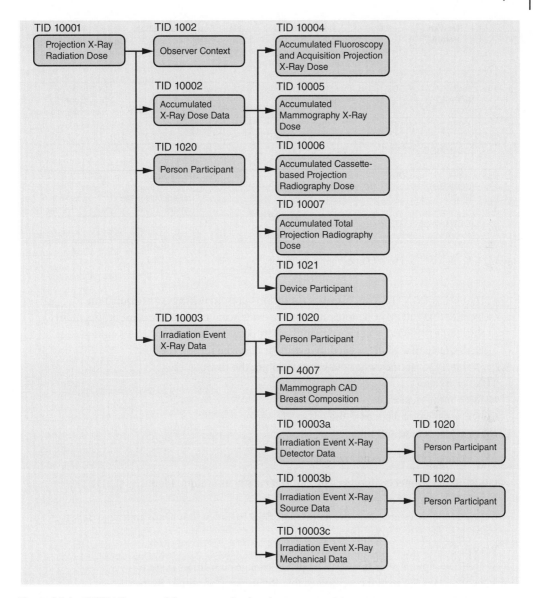

Figure 24.6 DICOM Structured Report organizational arrangement.

in the TID and the nested levels underneath this level are all considered to be the information specific to this Content Item.

- Relation with Parent,
  - The type of relationship between the above nested source content and the information given in this row, i.e. the target content.
    - CONTAINS = information relative to the source is enclosed in the target, this is a very generic designation
    - HAS PROPERTIES = description of properties
    - HAS OBS CONTEXT = description of observations

	NL	Rel with Parent	VT	Concept Name	VM	Req Type	Condition	Value Set Constraint
1			CONTAINER	EV (113706, DCM, "Irradiation Event X-Ray Data")	1	M		
2	>	HAS CONCEPT MOD	CODE	EV (113764, DCM, "Acquisition Plane")	1	M		DCID 10003 "Equipment Plane Identification"
3	>	CONTAINS	UIDREF	EV (113769, DCM, "Irradiation Event UID")	1	M		
4	>	CONTAINS	TEXT	EV (113605, DCM, "Irradiation Event Label")	1	U		
5	>>	HAS CONCEPT MOD	CODE	EV (113606, DCM, "Label Type")	1	MC	IF the value of Row 4 is the value of an Attribute in the images.	DCID 10022 "Label Types"
6	>	CONTAINS	DATETIME	DT (111526, DCM, "Date Time Started")	1	M		

Figure 24.7 DICOM Structured Report content layout.

    ○ HAS ACQ CONTEXT = describes conditions present during data acquisition
    ○ INFERRED FROM = denotes supporting evidence for a measurement or judgment
    ○ SELECTED FROM = conveys spatial or temporal coordinates
    ○ HAS CONCEPT MOD = used to qualify or describe the source item
- VT = Value Type, defines what the information in the row is.
  - TEXT = free text
  - NUM = numerical value
  - CODE = categorical coded value
  - DATETIME = date and time
  - DATE = date
  - TIME = time
  - UISREF = reference to another DICOM IOD using its Unique Identifier (UID)
  - PNAME = name of a person
  - COMPOSITE = reference to one composite SOP instance that is not an image or waveform
  - IMAGE = reference to an image
  - WAVEFORM = reference to waveform
  - SCOORD = spatial coordinates in a DICOM image coordinate system
  - SCOORD3D = 3D spatial coordinates in a Reference Coordinate System
  - TCOORD = temporal coordinates
  - CONTAINER = groups content items and defines the heading or category of observations
  - INCLUDE = another TID is to be included or linked to this Content Item
- Concept Name = coded entry defining the content. The code information will have at a minimum the first three entries listed below, but may contain more.
  - Code Value = a code value
  - Coding Scheme Designator = identifies the coding scheme in which the code is defined
  - Code Meaning = text that defines the code
  - Coding Scheme Version
  - Long Code Value = present and the Code Value is not a URN or URL
  - URN Code Value = present and the Code Value is a URN or URL

In Figure 24.7, the abbreviation in front of the coded information (e.g. EV or DT) designates the terminology for the code. These abbreviations are described in the definitions section of the standard. Also, when VT = INCLUDE, the Concept Name field specifies the template to be included.

- VM = Value Multiplier, indicates the number of times a separate entry may be included for this content.
  - 1, 1-n, ...
- Requirement Type, similar to the attribute and Module requirements for inclusion.
  - M = Mandatory
  - MC = Mandatory conditional
  - U = User optional
  - UC = User option conditional.
- Condition = specifies any conditions upon which presence or absence of the content or its values depends.
  - XOR = Exclusive OR
  - IF = Shall be present if the condition is TRUE; may be present otherwise
  - IFF = If and only if. Shall be present if the condition is TRUE; shall not be present otherwise
- Value Set Constraint specifies a default value for the content if no information is present.

The most important difference in a structured report IOD from an image IOD is that in a structured report, all information is linked to coded information (i.e. Concept Name). Although the Value Type can be other than a code (e.g. date, number, text), the Concept Name uses a code so the data can be searched, parsed, etc. more efficiently. There are many organizations that define codes, such as the International Classification of Diseases (ICD), Current Procedural Terminology (CPT), and Systematized Nomenclature of Medicine-Clinical Terms (SNOMED-CT). If the content does not have a well-established classification, then the code can be defined within the DICOM standard. In these cases, the Coding Scheme Designator will be DCM.

The information in a TID is not differentiated by single tag numbers for individual structured reports as in a single image IOD. The tag numbers are used to define the content information, but the relationship of this content to the structured report TID must be understood to use the data correctly. The tags are used multiple times in a single structured report. Figure 24.8 shows the metadata from a Radiation Dose Structured Report (RDSR). As can be seen in this Figure, the tag numbers for coded information are given: (0008, 0100) = Code Value, (0008, 0102) = Coding Scheme and (0008, 0104) = Code Meaning. In the example shown in Figure 24.8, these tag numbers include the code for "Dose Area Product," Code Value = 113 722, Code Scheme = DICOM (DCM), and Code = Meaning Dose Area Product. But these same tag numbers also designate the units of measure for the Dose Area Product later in the metadata to be $Gy*m^2$. The value for this irradiation event is given in tag (0040, a30a) as 0.00318572. This tag designation is then repeated for the next values in the report for "Dose." Therefore, the use of the data needs to be based on the TID structure, not just reading tag number data without using the relation to the entire structured report.

24.3 Testing Implication of New Technologies

The actual testing of informatics systems is not a primary role of a medical physicist in most clinics. Instead, current testing in informatics may consist of simply following the workflow to validate that the end results are accurate or acceptable. This would include monitoring functions such as:

- Modality Worklist configuration and function
- Validate that correct orders go to correct devices
- Verify that patient identifiers are accurately transmitted and populated

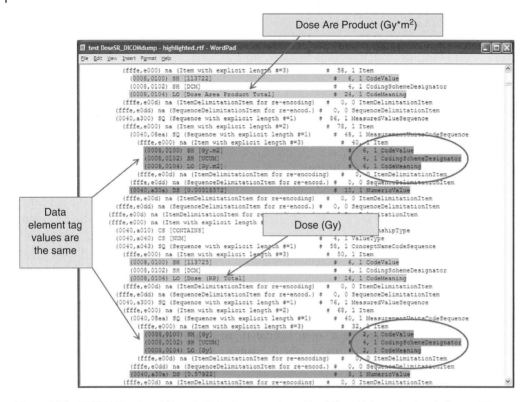

Figure 24.8 DICOM Structured Report attributes are not used to differentiate content as in image IOD.

- Assist in the setup of procedure code mapping to acquisition parameter function
- Following data from acquisition to storage and display to authenticate continuity
- Fault Tolerance
- What happens when a component of the system goes down
- Follow vendor-suggested strategy for component failure
- Correction Workflow
- How to correct manual entry errors or mismatched studies/patients
- Network Performance
- Verifying required bandwidth is available

Instead of doing direct testing of IT equipment, the majority of medical physics interactions are assisting the IT department, picture archiving and communication system (PACS) Administrator, or equipment service personnel through problem analysis and determination of a resolution by combining their knowledge of the acquisition system and the IT component functionality. The medical physicist may be considered the expert on the use and interpretation of the information received, stored, or exported by a system.

24.4 Clinical Integration and Implementation

Informatics is an integral part of the clinical operation. Most systems rely on the digital information from images to be communicated automatically between systems. Therefore, when new equipment is installed, the validation that this communication is working correctly must be done.

Even prior to this, the informatics features of a system should be reviewed so this integration can be assumed to be available prior to purchase. The medical physicist should be considered part of the team in making this evaluation. The informatics evaluation should include a review of the DICOM conformance statement to understand what SOP Classes are supported. It also should include review of what interfaces are needed with the system, e.g. HL7, and if there are any additional fees associated with the integration.

Gaining knowledge of the how different components within a health system or department communicate and exchange data can be a daunting task. Integrating the Health Enterprise (IHE) is both a process and a forum for encouraging integration efforts between manufacturers of healthcare equipment and healthcare institutions. IHE does not make standards, but instead utilizes existing standards to develop profiles to help improve integration. IHE Profiles describe specific solutions to integration problems. A Profile documents how standards will be used by each system. In IHE terms, each system is called an "Actor." Actors includes systems such as the Electronic Health Record (EHR), Radiology Information System (RIS), the acquisition system (i.e. modalities. A medical physicist can use an IHE Profile to understand how the Actors should be interacting. When a failure occurs, the IHE Profile may assist in determining where to look for the solution.

As an example, the IHE Radiology Scheduled Workflow (SWF) Profile will be used. Figure 24.9 shows the basic components in the workflow. The details for this workflow can be shown in a

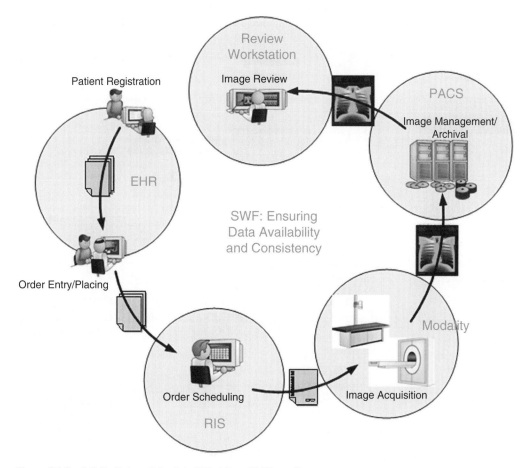

Figure 24.9   IHE Radiology Scheduled Workflow (SWF) profile.

Process Flow diagram. Figures 24.10–24.12 show some of the actors involved and the processes that are included in the workflow. In the diagrams, the green boxes represent processes that are performed by a user, the orange boxes designate processes that are performed by the informatics system (usually automatically) and yellow boxes are systems that may require user input and may be new to some health systems. Also, the solid lines between the processes are associations that will occur, while the dotted lines may or may not occur.

At the beginning of the IHE SWF, an operator must register the patient in the system and input some history providing the reason for the procedure that is to be performed. The ICD version 10 (ICD-10) codes include very detailed diagnosis information and, if used, can help automate the ordering processes. But this only works if the operator inputs the correct history/ICD-10 information at the time of the order. With the history defined, an order can be made. The order can be generated automatically directly from the system that is used to input the history. For billing purposes, the orders must be associated with the applicable CPT codes. This is done within the RIS through pre-defined look-up tables, although complex procedures may require an operator to add additional CPT codes or modify the standard assigned codes. In addition, the procedure can be scheduled directly from the ordering system within the EHR or the RIS system.

Decision Support systems assist in directing the referring physicians to the correct procedure or exam based on the patient history. These systems use evidence-based guidelines to assist referring physicians and other providers in making the most appropriate decision on the procedure to order for a specific clinical condition. The appropriateness criteria are developed by organizations that have an established knowledge base from their members for the type of orders being generated.

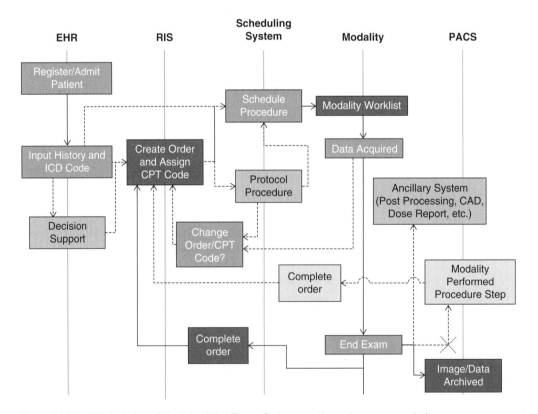

Figure 24.10 IHE Radiology Scheduled Workflow – Order entry through exam completion.

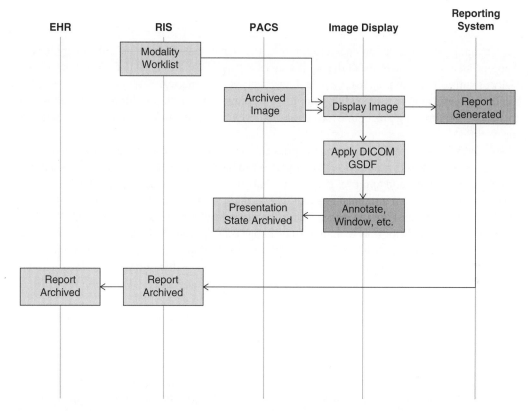

Figure 24.11 IHE Radiology Scheduled Workflow – Image display and report generation following the traditional methodology.

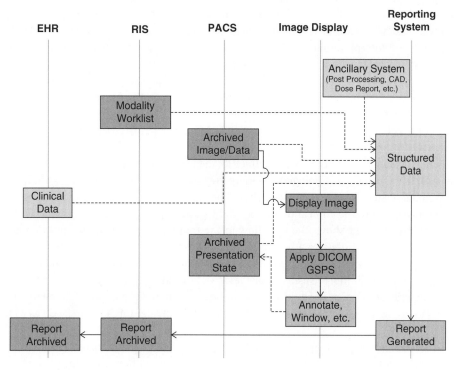

Figure 24.12 IHE Radiology Scheduled Workflow – Optimized image display and report generation using structured data from the EHR, PACS, and any additional system that has relevant data for the report.

For imaging and image guided procedures, the American College of Radiology (ACR) Appropriateness Criteria is one of the main sources of this information, but there are other subspecialty organizations that are creating guidelines, such as the American College of Cardiology. The use of Decision Support systems for complicated exams or invasive procedures will continue to expand beyond imaging procedures, which should assist in automating the ordering and scheduling workflow.

Following the creation of the orders, the protocol to use must be defined for complicated exams or procedures, such as computed tomography. This can be automated, but it often requires a physician to at least review and approve. This is especially true for larger advanced care health systems where complex patient conditions may require special protocols. Based on the protocol decision, the order or the device that was schedule for the procedure may need to be changed. The SWF Profile includes details for how to manage the change order processes. It also defines how to handle exceptions for data that is sent to the PACS or RIS that does not meet all requirements for accurate association with a patient. In Figure 24.10, the RIS and Scheduling systems are separated even though the processes listed under each may be combined in the RIS, may be in the HER, or may be a separate system.

The orders and protocols are automatically sent to the modality through the DICOM Modality Worklist. Depending on what actually occurs during the procedure, the order and CPT code may again need to be changed to accurately reflect what was done. The ending of the exam on the modality usually initiates the archiving of the images and data in the PACS. This archiving would include all images and other data (e.g. structured reports) that the modality is set up to archive or that the technologist selects. The completion of the order in the RIS starts the next processes for reviewing and interpreting the images and data. The ending of the exam can be set to automatically complete the order in the RIS through the DICOM Modality Performed Procedure Step. Although this process has been included in the SWF from its creation, the use of the DICOM Modality Performed Procedure Step has not been utilized widely. The reason for this is to allow time for technologists to complete other functions relative to the images and data prior to its release for reviewing and interpretation, e.g. quality control, annotation, or correction of any exceptions. In addition, it may be appropriate to require a technologist to verify in the PACS that all images and data that is supposed to be archived is in the PACS and associated with the correct patient prior to completion of the exam in the RIS. This is why this association in the figure has a red "X" on it and the boxes are blurred. In addition to being sent to the PACS for archiving, the images and data can also be sent to other systems for post-processing or storage, e.g. 3D processing, Computer-Aided Detection (CAD), or dose reporting.

Following the completion of the order in the RIS, the images are ready for review and interpretation by a clinician, usually a radiologist. In emergency situations, this process can be initiated prior to the completion step in the RIS, but care should be taken to ensure errors in the images and data are not propagated into the clinical treatment of the patient, or lead to the treatment of an incorrect patient. Figure 24.11 shows the workflow in the traditional paradigm where the images are viewed and a radiologist dictates a report, through transcription service or a speech recognition system. For proper viewing, the DICOM Gray Scale Display Function (GSDF) should be applied to all display systems, including the technologist review workstations and any clinical review displays in physician offices or clinics. In addition, any annotations or image manipulation that the radiologist wants to use with their interpretation of the images should be stored in the PACS as a DICOM Presentation State.

Although the workflow in Figure 24.11 is used in many clinics, an optimized image display and interpretation workflow is shown in Figure 24.12. In this workflow, data from many sources relevant to the interpretation of the images and data are automatically sent to the reporting system. This information must be sent in a structured manner to be input into the correct location of the report. Many systems that utilize structured data in a reporting system often include required dictation fields to be completed by the radiologist or interpreting physician. These required fields make sure that important clinical information needed in the patient's care are not overlooked, or the information for correct billing is included. The required information can be driven by the ICD and CPT codes or by the protocol.

Obtaining knowledge in the application and use of DICOM Standards will allow a medical physicist to be an integral part of all areas within a health system. This does not fall into the traditional role of testing a system. To be an integral part of the imaging team, the medical physicist should use this knowledge to assist in making the correct purchase of a system, tracking down problems with data communication and storage, and, perhaps more importantly, in the use of all of the informatics data available to analyze the entire imaging architecture and ultimately the entire health record.

References

1 DICOM. website http://medical.nema.org.
2 Pianykh, O. (2008). *Digital Imaging Communications in Medicine (DICOM): A Practical Introduction and Survival Guide*. Berlin-Heidelberg: Springer-Verlag.
3 Clunie, D. (2000). *Digital Imaging Communications in Medicine (DICOM): A Practical Introduction and Survival Guide*, Structured Reports. Bangor, Pennsylvania: PixelMed Publishing.

Abbreviations

AAPM	American Association of Physicists in Medicine
ACR	American College of Radiology
ACRIN	American College of Radiology Imaging Network
AEC	automatic exposure control
AERC	automatic exposure rate control
AGD	average glandular dose
ALARA	as low as reasonably achievable
AP	anterior–posterior
CAD	computer aided detection
CC	craniocaudal
CMS	Centers for Medicare and Medicaid Service
CNR	contrast to (relative) noise ratio
CR	computed radiography
CRCPD	Council of Radiation Control Program Directors
CRT	cathode ray tube
CsI	cesium iodide
CT	computed tomography
CTDI	computed tomography dose index
DAP	dose area product
DBT	digital breast tomosynthesis
DICOM	digital imaging and communications in medicine
DLP	dose length product
DQE	detective quantum efficiency
DR	digital radiography
EDAK	entrance detector air KERMA
eDQE	effective detective quantum efficiency
EI	exposure index
EPA	Environmental Protection Agency
ESAK	entrance skin air KERMA
ESE	entrance skin exposure
FBP	filtered back projection
FDA	Food and Drug Administration
FFDM	full-field digital mammography

Clinical Imaging Physics: Current and Emerging Practice, First Edition. Edited by Ehsan Samei and Douglas E. Pfeiffer.
© 2020 John Wiley & Sons, Inc. Published 2020 by John Wiley & Sons, Inc.

FOV	Field of View
FPD	flat-panel display or flat-panel detector
HL7	health level 7
HU	Hounsfield unit
HVL	half value layer
ICRU	International Commission on Radiation Units & Measurements
IEC	International Electrotechnical Commission
IHE	Integrated Health Enterprise
IR	iterative reconstruction
KAP	KERMA area product
KERMA	kinetic energy released per unit mass
kV	kilo volt
kVp	kilo volt peak
MEE	mammography equipment evaluation
MLO	mediolateral oblique
MP	medical physicist
MQSA	Mammography Quality Standards Act
MRI	magnetic resonance imaging
MTF	modulation transfer function
NEMA	National Electrical Manufacturers Association
NEQ	noise equivalent quanta
NIH	National Institutes of Health
NPS	noise power spectrum
PA	Posterior–Anterior
PACS	picture archiving and communication system
PBL	positive beam limitation
PET	positron emission tomography
QA	quality assurance
QC	quality control
RIS	radiology informatics system
ROI	region of interest
RSNA	Radiological Society of North America
SNR	signal to noise ratio
SPECT	single photon emission computed tomography
SSDE	size-specific dose estimate
TCM	tube current modulation
TGC	time gain compensation
TJC	The Joint Commission
US	ultrasound
VCR	video cassette recorder

Index

Page locators in **bold** indicate tables. Page locators in *italics* indicate figures. This index uses letter-by-letter alphabetization.

Clinical Imaging Physics: Current and Emerging Practice, First Edition. Edited by Ehsan Samei and Douglas E. Pfeiffer.
© 2020 John Wiley & Sons, Inc. Published 2020 by John Wiley & Sons, Inc.